Current Research in Rheumatology

Current Research in Rheumatology

Edited by Ross Hill

STATES
ACADEMIC PRESS
www.statesacademicpress.com

States Academic Press,
109 South 5th Street,
Brooklyn, NY 11249, USA

Visit us on the World Wide Web at:
www.statesacademicpress.com

ISBN: 978-1-63989-140-5

Cataloging-in-Publication Data

Current research in rheumatology / edited by Ross Hill.
p. cm.
Includes bibliographical references and index.
ISBN 978-1-63989-140-5
1. Rheumatology--Research. 2. Connective tissues--Diseases. 3. Joints--Diseases. I. Hill, Ross.
RC927 .C87 2022
616.723--dc23

Table of Contents

Preface

The world is advancing at a fast pace like never before. Therefore, the need is to keep up with the latest developments. This book was an idea that came to fruition when the specialists in the area realized the need to coordinate together and document essential themes in the subject. That's when I was requested to be the editor. Editing this book has been an honour as it brings together diverse authors researching on different streams of the field. The book collates essential materials contributed by veterans in the area which can be utilized by students and researchers alike.

Rheumatology is the branch of medicine that is concerned with the diagnosis and therapy of rheumatic diseases. These encompass immune-mediated disorders of musculoskeletal system and soft tissues, vasculitides, autoimmune diseases and inherited connective tissue disorders. Diagnosis of these diseases can be done by physical examination or specialized examination. Some examples of the methods used for physical examination are multiple joint inspections, Schober's test, and musculoskeletal examination such as screening musculoskeletal exam, general musculoskeletal exam and regional musculoskeletal exam. Specialized examinations include laboratory tests, X-rays, ultrasounds, and cytopathology and chemical pathology of fluid aspirated from affected joints. Rheumatic diseases are treated with monoclonal antibodies such as adalimumab and infliximab, analgesics, TNF inhibitor etanercept, etc. This book contains some path-breaking studies in the field of rheumatology. It provides significant information of this discipline to help develop a good understanding. A number of latest researches have been included in this book to keep the readers up-to-date with the global concepts in this area of study.

Each chapter is a sole-standing publication that reflects each author's interpretation. Thus, the book displays a multi-facetted picture of our current understanding of application, resources and aspects of the field. I would like to thank the contributors of this book and my family for their endless support.

Editor

1

Synoviolin is a Novel Pathogenic Factor of Arthropathy and Chronic Inflammation

Naoko Yagishita, Satoko Aratani, Hidetoshi Fujita, Yoshihisa Yamano, Kusuki Nishioka and Toshihiro Nakajima

Abstract

Inflammation is classical pathogenic concept, but still very crucial for understanding many disorders even in twenty-first century. The purpose of inflammation is to eliminate the damaged tissues and to initiate tissue repair. By contrast, chronic inflammation leads to intractable diseases, including rheumatoid arthritis (RA), atherosclerosis, cancer, diabetes mellitus, and obesity. We recently cloned synoviolin, an E3 ubiquitin ligase, as an overexpressing molecule in rheumatoid synovium and has been verifying its critical roles in RA, inflammatory cytokine signaling, and fibrosis. Moreover, *synoviolin*-deficient mice exhibited severe anemia caused by defective nursing activity of erythrocytes in the fetal liver. This phenomenon resembles of RA that accelerates nursing activity. Our data indicate a close relationship between embryogenesis and RA. We successfully discovered synoviolin inhibitors, LS-101 and LS-102. These drugs have inhibitory effects to synoviolin in vitro and in vivo. We are now proceeding with the optimization of small compounds, and we hope our research will lead to the development of a new therapy for RA and fibrosis and other synoviolin-related diseases.

Keywords: synoviolin, synoviocyte, ubiquitin ligase, ERAD

1. Introduction

Rheumatoid arthritis (RA) has a tremendous negative impact on quality of life and affects nearly 1% of the adult population worldwide [1, 2].

Clinically, RA is characterized by multiple joint pain, stiffness, and swelling due to synovial inflammation and effusion [3–6]. The pathological features of RA result from multiple processes including chronic inflammation, overgrowth of synovial cells, bone and joint destruction, and as terminal phase tissue fibrosis.

2. Synoviolin is a causative factor for arthropathy

We cloned "synoviolin" by immunoscreening using anti-rheumatoid synovial cell antibody [7]. Synoviolin is a RING-type E3 ubiquitin ligase and is highly expressed in rheumatoid synovial cells [7]. Synoviolin is a mammalian homolog of Hrd1p/Der3p [8–10] and is involved in endoplasmic reticulum(ER)-associated degradation (ERAD) [7].

In eukaryotic cells, the balance of protein synthesis and degradation is strictly regulated, and the selective degradation of protein is carried out *via* the ubiquitin-proteasome system (UPS) [11, 12]. The proteins targeted for proteasomal degradation are ubiquitinated by three enzymes: ubiquitin-activating enzyme E1, ubiquitin-conjugated enzyme E2, and E3 ubiquitin ligases [11, 12]. Newly synthesized proteins are correctly folded in the ER and transported to the secretory pathway. When the amount of misfolded protein exceeds the protein folded capacity, result from ER stresses, it is eliminated by UPS-dependent degradation process of ERAD [13]. Synoviolin plays an important role in ERAD as an E3 ubiquitin ligase and involved in quality control of proteins.

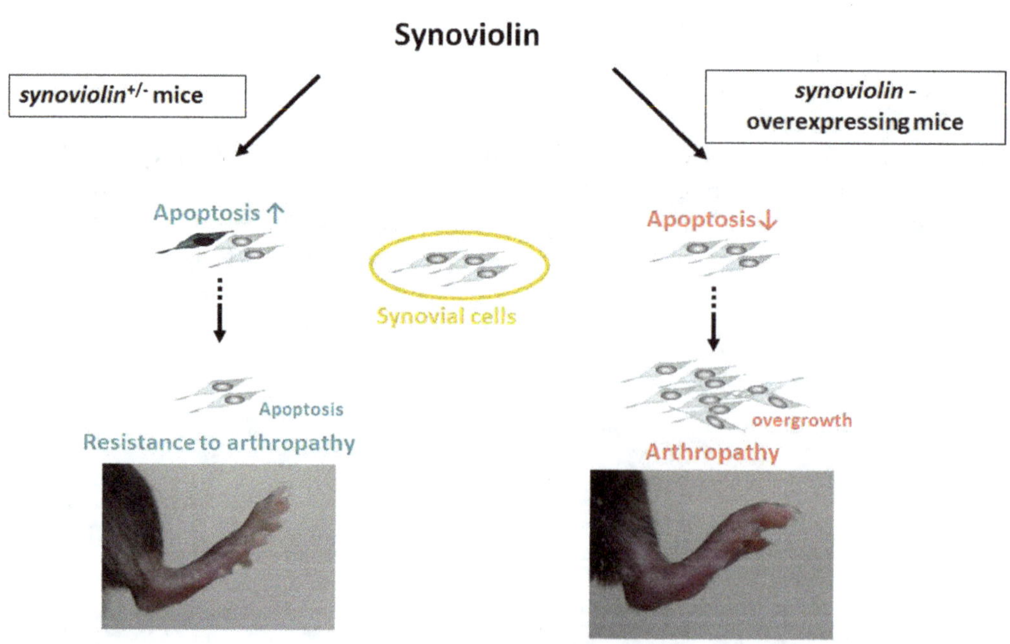

Figure 1. Synoviolin is a causative factor for arthropathy. "Gain-of-function" of synoviolin results in the development of spontaneous arthropathy through the anti-apoptotic effects of synoviolin. On the other hand, *syno*$^{+/-}$ mice are resistant to CIA model. Therefore, synoviolin is a novel causative factor for RA.

Synoviolin is ubiquitously expressed in whole body, especially highly expressed in synoviocytes of patients with RA. Approximately 30% of overexpression of synoviolin in transgenic mice leads to advanced arthropathy caused by reduced apoptosis of synoviocytes (**Figure 1**) [7]. On the other hand, synoviolin-heterozygous mice demonstrate resistance to the development of collagen-induced arthritis (CIA) because of enhanced apoptosis of synovial cells (**Figure 1**) [7]. We postulate that the overexpression of synoviolin leads to hyperactivation of the ERAD and results in synovial hyperplasia. In addition, synoviolin negatively regulates the tumor suppressor p53 in the cytoplasm by ubiquitinating p53 [14]. Therefore, synoviolin regulates both apoptosis in response to ER stress and a p53-dependent apoptotic pathway. These studies indicate that synoviolin is a novel pathogenic factor of arthropathy through its anti-apoptotic effects [15].

3. The reason for death of *syno*$^{-/-}$ mice in utero

To gain insight into the function of synoviolin in vivo, we generated *synoviolin*-deficient (*syno*$^{-/-}$) mice by gene-targeted disruption. Strikingly, all fetuses lacking *synoviolin* died in utero by embryonic day 13.5 (E13.5) [16]. It is surprising that loss of synoviolin only can cause embryonic lethality, since Hrd1p/Del3p, a yeast homolog of synoviolin, is nonessential for survival [8]. Then, why is synoviolin deficiency associated with embryonic death? Morphologically, there was no remarkable difference between E13.5 wild-type and *syno*$^{-/-}$ embryos; however, the *syno*$^{-/-}$ fetal liver looked pale, suggesting an abnormal hematological status in *syno*$^{-/-}$ embryos, since the liver becomes the main hematopoietic organ by E12.5 [17–20]. Indeed, the number of peripheral blood cells was decreased in *syno*$^{-/-}$ embryos, and the level of β-major globin, which first appears in the fetal liver during definitive erythropoiesis, was markedly reduced in *syno*$^{-/-}$ embryos [16]. Subsequently, we examined erythropoiesis in *syno*$^{-/-}$ in vitro by colony-forming assay. Unexpectedly, we found that erythrocyte progenitors of *syno*$^{-/-}$ could differentiate in vitro to produce hemoglobin. Definitive erythropoiesis in embryos is controlled by cell autonomous and non-cell autonomous mechanisms. Therefore, it is expected that the abnormal cell morphology in *syno*$^{-/-}$ erythroid is secondary to changes in the local environment, that is, liver. Consequently, we analyzed the *syno*$^{-/-}$ fetal liver and found reduced number of hepatocytes and their augmented apoptotic cell death in *syno*$^{-/-}$ embryos compared to wild-type embryos [16]. Considered together, the above results indicate that the death in utero of *syno*$^{-/-}$ around E13.5 is caused by abnormal erythropoiesis in a non-cell autonomous manner, which depends on aberrant apoptosis in the liver.

4. Symmetric features of synoviolin in RA and embryogenesis

At a glance, embryogenesis and RA are non-related events. However, when considered through synoviolin, commonness becomes apparent. What is the common feature between these two processes? One answer could be the nurse-like cells. Nurse cells were first recognized in a cell suspension from the thymus [21, 22]. Wekere and Ketelsen concluded that thymic nurse cells played an important role in the differentiation of thymocytes [23–25]. They referred to this phenomenon as pseudoemperipolesis. Pseudoemperipolesis has been observed also in the interaction between murine lymphocytes and murine bone marrow (BM) stromal cells [23–25]. Iwagami et al. [26] and Shimaoka et al. [27] reported cloning of nurse cells from synovial tissue of patients with RA. Moreover, BM stromal cells migrated from the BM into the affected joint cavity and contribute to synovial proliferation [28]. Clinically, BM stromal cells derived from donors show very little pseudoemperipoletic activity, and thus, nurse cell activity is considered a unique feature of BM stromal cells derived from RA [29]. That is, RA is a disease with accelerated nurse cell activity of BM stromal cells. In other words, increased nursing cell activity would enhance the cooperation between surrounding cells, BM stromal cells, and synovial cells.

When one compares RA with *syno*$^{-/-}$, these processes are symmetrical. In *syno*$^{-/-}$ fetal liver, there is a complete loss of nurse activity to erythrocytes. The excessive amount of synoviolin in RA and the lack of synoviolin in *syno*$^{-/-}$ are quite a symmetrical feature. These observations suggest the possible involvement of synoviolin in promoting the nursing activity in RA, a topic for future research. A more thorough analysis of *syno*$^{-/-}$ indicates that RA and embryogenesis are closely related processes (**Figure 2**).

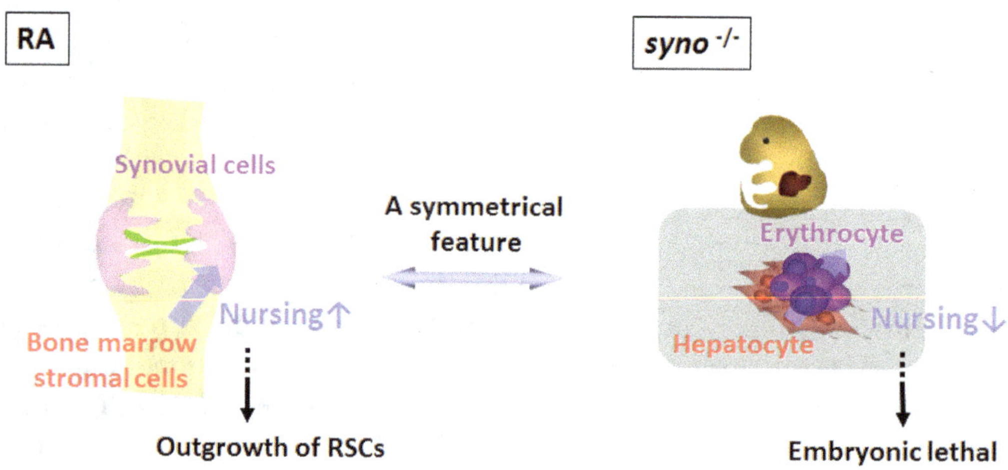

Figure 2. RA and embryogenesis have shared features. RA is a disease with accelerated nursing activity of bone marrow stromal cells. On the other hand, *syno*$^{-/-}$ fetal liver shows loss of nursing cell activity of erythrocytes. In this regard, RA and *syno*$^{-/-}$ demonstrate a symmetrical feature. The study of *syno*$^{-/-}$ has allowed the elucidation of new etiological factors of RA.

5. Impact of synoviolin on RA and embryogenesis

Embryogenesis, in which a single fertilized egg forms an individual consisting of millions of cells, is the most complicated process in higher eukaryote. That synoviolin shoulders this process highlights the importance of this protein. On the other hand, RA is a complex disease, in which all the details of its pathology are not yet understood. That this fundamental molecule is involved in the crisis of RA makes it conceivable that synoviolin is implicated in the intricacy of this disease. Furthermore, the joint cavity, representing the nidus of RA, is a complex space; it is formed of several types of cells, such as synovial cells, chondrocytes, osteoblasts, osteoclasts, and bone marrow cells. Just as there are many contacts with all sorts of cells in embryogenesis, the same is true for contacts between these numerous types of cells in the RA joint cavity. Except for the joint and eye, there is no space in our body formed by so many types of cells. In this regard, RA is a disorder of this complex space which needs to connect with the periphery, and the crisis of RA requires making sense of synoviolin function. Therefore, analysis of *syno*$^{-/-}$ has indicated that synoviolin is a molecule that connects embryogenesis and RA, and studies involving both processes would be the cutting edge in elucidating the pathogenesis of RA.

6. Synoviolin is participated in multiple processes of RA

RA consists of multiple processes including chronic inflammation, overgrowth of synovial cells, bone and joint destruction, and tissue fibrosis. Synoviolin plays an important role in over growth of synovial cells through hyperactivation of ERAD.

Inflammation is the most important process of RA. The synovial cells, macrophages, T cells, and B cells produce many kinds of cytokines, such as interleukin (IL)-1, IL-6, IL-10, tumor necrosis factor (TNF), and transforming growth factor β (TGF-β), and these cytokines stimulate the overgrowth of synovial cells [3–6]. Because it forms pannus, a mass of synovial tissue, inflammation leads to destruction of the bone and cartilage [3–6].

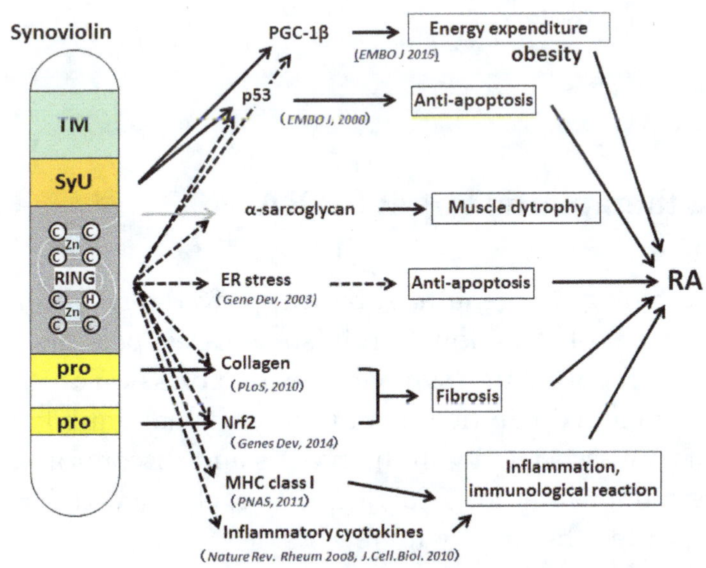

Figure 3. Synoviolin and its related disorders. The scientific summary of synoviolin function. Synoviolin is involved in a lot of disorders and would be a potential candidate for new drug of these disorders. Our compounds which inhibit the activity of synoviolin would be useful for these disorders. TM: transmembrane domain; SyU: SyU domain (amino acids, aa 236–270 of synoviolin); pro: prolin-rich region.

With regard to the relationship between synoviolin and inflammation, it was reported that IL-17 induction of synoviolin may contribute to RA chronicity [30], and synoviolin targets misfolded MHC class I heavy chains [31] and is a positive regulator of T-cell immunity [32]. Toh et al. demonstrated that synoviolin levels are elevated in circulating monocytes of RA patients [33]. It was reported that dual blockade of TNF and IL-17 decreased disease progression more effectively than when only one cytokine was blocked [34]. Therefore, it was suggested that synoviolin would be a potential candidate for new drug of chronic inflammation (**Figure 3**).

7. Synoviolin is also involved in fibrosis

Fibrosis is the terminal pathological feature of RA and results from excessive accumulation of the extracellular matrix (ECM) such as collagen and fibronectin [35]. Fibrosis is also major a pathological feature of chronic inflammatory disease. We previously demonstrated that synoviolin is upregulated in hepatic stellate cells (HSCs) of human cirrhosis, and synoviolin-heterozygous mice are resistant to CCl_4-induced hepatic injury [36]. Moreover, procollagen was abnormally accumulated in the ER of synoviolin-deficient mouse embryonic fibroblasts, suggesting the involvement of synoviolin in collagen secretion [36]. We also demonstrated that synoviolin expression and collagen secretion are enhanced in lung fibrosis using in vitro model, in which A549 human lung adenocarcinoma cells were transfected with exon-4 deleted surfactant protein C [37], which has been reported to induce ER stress [38, 39]. Li et al. demonstrated that synoviolin is involved in the renal fibrosis using the unilateral ureteral obstruction (UUO) model and plays an important role in the maturation of collagen [40]. These reports indicated that synoviolin plays an important role in fibrosis through the collagen expression and secretion (**Figure 3**).

8. Synoviolin as a therapeutic target for RA

During the past decade, biological agents have been approved for clinical use and dramatically have changed the treatment of RA. However, in some cases, patients fail to respond to the biologic treatment. It was reported that synoviolin overexpression of RA patients was associated with nonresponse to infliximab treatment (a monoclonal antibody against TNFα) [33]. Moreover, these agents are associated with high costs and discomfort arising from subcutaneous or intravenous administration. Thus, there is a clear need for the development of cheaper, orally administrated therapies with fewer side effects.

Since synoviolin is a pathogenic factor for chronic inflammation including RA and fibrosis (**Figure 3**), inhibition of synoviolin activity may be a useful therapeutic approach for the treatment of RA. Then, synoviolin is a drug-able molecule because: (1) synoviolin is an enzyme; (2) synoviolin localizes in cytoplasm; (3) the structure of synoviolin has been determined

(Nakajima T, unpublished data); and (4) specific substrates of synoviolin have been identified such as p53 [14]. Moreover, synoviolin may be a disease-modifying molecule because synoviolin may be involved in RA and fibrosis and may be implicated in some severe diseases such as interstitial pneumonia and systemic sclerosis. In making synoviolin a therapeutic target, downregulation of synoviolin and/or inhibition of its activity might be useful.

In order to reduce the amount of synoviolin, it is important to elucidate the transcriptional regulation of synoviolin. Establishing the mechanisms of transcriptional regulation of synoviolin should allow suppression of synoviolin transcription. We identified Ets binding site in the *synoviolin* proximal promoter as for crucial site of synoviolin expression. Moreover, the GA-binding protein (GABP) α/β complex is essential for its transcriptional regulation [41].

9. Development of synoviolin inhibitors

Next, in order to block the enzymatic activity of synoviolin, we performed high-throughput screening that inhibits the auto-ubiquitination activity of synoviolin. Over four million compounds from Pharmacopeia's compound collection were screened, and we found two unique compounds, termed LS-101 and LS-102 [42]. LS-101 and LS-102 demonstrated an inhibition of synoviolin auto-ubiquitination with IC_{50} of ~15 and 20 μM, respectively. LS-101 demonstrates stronger efficacy than LS-102, but less selectivity to synoviolin among other RING-type E3 ubiquitin ligases. Administration of either LS-101 or LS-102 also suppressed the clinical severity scores in mice collagen-induced arthritis (CIA) model. There was no difference in the protective effect between high dose of LS-101 and LS-102.

Moreover, it was also reported that LS-102 was able to suppress CCl_4-induced elevation of alanine aminotransferase (ALT) and restored normal liver morphology in CCl_4-induced liver cirrhosis mice model [43]. We also demonstrated that collagen secretion is suppressed by LS-102 in lung fibrosis using in vitro model [37]. Therefore, LS-102 is a novel potential drug for synoviolin inhibition. Thus, we proceed toward the optimization of LS-101 and LS-102 and get the derivative compounds from these compounds named LS-302 (Nakajima T, unpublished data). The arthritis scores of mice injected with LS-302 were also decreased. We hope our research will lead to the development of a new therapy for synoviolin-related diseases and serve as an example for the therapeutic benefit from E3 ligase inhibitors.

According to the UPS, a proteasome inhibitor has been developed. Bortezomib (BTZ) is the first proteasome inhibitor to gain the U.S. Food and Drug Administration (FDA) approval [44, 45]. BTZ induces apoptosis of a wide variety of cancer cells, and however, there are some patients who do not respond to therapy [44, 46]. There are second-generation proteasome inhibitors: carfilzomib [44, 47–49], ixazomib [44, 47, 48, 50], delanzomib [44, 47, 48, 51], oprozomib [44, 47, 48, 52], and marizomib [44, 48, 53]. These drugs are global inhibitors of the proteasome, and therefore, the associated toxicities prevent their use for the treatment of chronic disease such as RA. It is important to develop inhibitors of the UPS enzymatic cascade, and E3 ubiquitin ligase is suitable target given their large number and substrate specificity [54].

There is HDM2, the E3 ubiquitin ligase that regulates the degradation of p53 [55, 56], inhibitor currently in clinical trials [57, 58]. Then, synoviolin inhibitor would be a drug that follows a HDM.

Acknowledgements

This work was supported by JSPS KAKENHI Grant Number 20689019, 23659502, 26461478, 20249052, 20059033, 20013045, by grant from Takeda Science Foundation.

Author details

Naoko Yagishita[1], Satoko Aratani[2,3,4], Hidetoshi Fujita[2,3], Yoshihisa Yamano[1], Kusuki Nishioka[2] and Toshihiro Nakajima[1,2,3,4,5,6*]

*Address all correspondence to: marlin@tokyo-med.ac.jp

1 Department of Rare Diseases Research, Institute of Medical Science, St. Marianna University School of Medicine, Kawasaki, Kanagawa, Japan

2 Institute of Medical Science, Tokyo Medical University, Shinjuku-ku, Tokyo, Japan

3 Department of Future Medical Science, Institute of Medical Science, Tokyo Medical University, Shinjuku-ku, Tokyo, Japan

4 Physician, Student and Researcher Support Center, Tokyo Medical University, Shinjuku-ku, Tokyo, Japan

5 Integrated Genome Editing Section (iGES), Tokyo Medical University, Shinjuku-ku, Tokyo, Japan

6 Bayside Misato Medical Center, Niida, Kochi, Japan

References

[1] Harris ED. Rheumatoid arthritis. Pathophysiology and implications for therapy. N Engl J Med 1990; 322: 1277–1289.

[2] Feldmann M, Brennan FM, Maini RN. Rheumatoid arthritis. Cell 1996; 85: 307–310.

[3] Stanczyk J, Ospelt C, Gay RE, Gay S. Synovial cell activation. Curr Opin Rheumatol 2006; 18: 262–267.

[4] McInnes IB, Schett G. Cytokines in the pathogenesis of rheumatoid arthritis. Nat Rev Immunol 2007; 7: 429–442.

[5] McInnes IB, Schett G. The pathogenesis of rheumatoid arthritis. N Engl J Med 2011; 365: 2205–2219.

[6] Furst DE, Emery P. Rheumatoid arthritis pathophysiology: update on emerging cytokine and cytokine-associated cell targets. Rheumatology 2014; 53: 1560–1569.

[7] Amano T, Yamasaki S, Yagishita N, Tsuchimochi K, Shin H, Kawahara K, Aratani S, Fujita H, Zhang L, Ikeda R, Fujii R, Miura N, Komiya S, Nishioka K, Maruyama I, Fukamizu A, Nakajima T. Synoviolin/Hrd1, an E3 ubiquitin ligase, as a novel pathogenic factor for arthropathy. Genes Dev 2003; 17: 2436–2449.

[8] Bordallo J, Plemper RK, Finger A, Wolf DH. Der3p/Hrd1p is required for endoplasmic reticulum-associated degradation of misfolded lumenal and integral membrane proteins. Mol Biol Cell 1998; 9: 209–222.

[9] Shearer AG. Hampton, RY. Structural control of endoplasmic reticulum-associated degradation: effect of chemical chaperones on 3-hydroxy-3-methylglutaryl-CoA reductase. J Biol Chem 2004; 279: 188–196.

[10] Shearer AG. Hampton RY. Lipid-mediated, reversible misfolding of a sterol-sensing domain protein. EMBO J 2005; 24: 149–159.

[11] Hershko A, Ciechanover A. The ubiquitin system. Annu Rev Biochem 1998; 67: 425–479.

[12] Pickart CM. Mechanisms underlying ubiquitination. Annu Rev Biochem 2001; 70: 503–533.

[13] Morito D, Nagata K. Pathogenic hijacking of ER-associated degradation: is ERAD flexible? Mol Cell 2015; 59: 335–344.

[14] Yamasaki S, Yagishita N, Sasaki T, Nakazawa M, Kato Y, Yamadera T, Bae E, Toriyama S, Ikeda R, Zhang L, Fujitani K, Yoo E, Tsuchimochi K, Ohta T, Araya N, Fujita H, Aratani S, Eguchi K, Komiya S, Maruyama I, Higashi N, Sato M, Senoo H, Ochi T, Yokoyama S, Amano T, Kim J, Gay S, Fukamizu A, Nishioka K, Tanaka K, Nakajima T. Cytoplasmic destruction of p53 by the endoplasmic reticulum-resident ubiquitin ligase 'Synoviolin'. EMBO J 2007; 26: 113–122.

[15] Yagishita N, Yamasaki S, Nishioka K, Nakajima T. Synoviolin, protein folding and the maintenance of joint homeostasis. Nat Clin Pract Rheumatol 2008; 4: 91–97.

[16] Yagishita N, Ohneda K, Amano T, Yamasaki S, Sugiura A, Tsuchimochi K, Shin H, Kawahara K, Ohneda O, Ohta T, Tanaka S, Yamamoto M, Maruyama I, Nishioka K, Fukamizu A, Nakajima T. Essential Role of Synoviolin in Embryogenesis. J Biol Chem 2005; 280: 7909–7916.

[17] Ito E, Toki T, Ishihara H, Ohtani H, Gu L, Yokoyama M, Engel JD, Yamamoto M. Erythroid transcription factor GATA-1 is abundantly transcribed in mouse testis. Nature 1993; 362: 466–468.

[18] Ohneda K, Yamamoto M. Roles of hematopoietic transcription factors GATA-1 and GATA-2 in the development of red blood cell lineage. Acta Haematol 2002; 108: 237–45.

[19] Shimizu R, Takahashi S, Ohneda K, Engel JD, Yamamoto M. In vivo requirements for GATA-1 functional domains during primitive and definitive erythropoiesis. EMBO J 2001; 20: 5250–5261.

[20] Zon LI. Developmental biology of hematopoiesis. Blood 1995; 86: 2876–2891.

[21] Wekerle H, Ketelsen UP. Thymic nurse cells: Ia-bearing epithelium involved in T-lymphocyte differentiation? Nature 1980; 283: 402–404.

[22] Wekerle H, Ketelsen UP, Ernst M. Thymic nurse cells. Lymphoepithelial cell complexes in murine thymus: morphological and serological characterization. J Exp Med 1980; 151: 925–944.

[23] Witte PL, Robinson M, Henley A, Low MG, Stiers DL, Perkins S, Fleischman RA, Kincade PW. Relationships between B-lineage lymphocytes and stromal cells in long-term bone marrow cultures. Eur J Immunol 1987; 17: 1473–1484.

[24] Miyake K, Hasunuma Y, Yagita H, Kimoto M. Requirement for VLA-4 and VLA-5 integrins in lymphoma cells binding to and migration beneath stromal cells in culture. J Cell Biol 1992; 119: 653–662.

[25] Makrynikola V, Bianchi A, Bradstock K, Gottlieb D, Hewson J. Migration of acute lymphoblastic leukemia cells into human bone marrow stroma. Leukemia 1994; 8: 1734–1743.

[26] Iwagami S, Furue S, Toyosaki T, Horikawa T, Doi H, Satomi S, Itoh T, Sakata T, Suzuki R. Establishment and characterization of nurse cell-like clones from human skin. Nurse cell-like clones can stimulate autologous mixed lymphocyte reaction. J Immunol 1994; 153: 2927–2938.

[27] Shimaoka Y, Attrep JF, Hirano T, Ishihara K, Suzuki R, Toyosaki T, Ochi T, Lipsky PE. Nurse-like cells from bone marrow and synovium of patients with rheumatoid arthritis promote survival and enhance function of human B cells. J Clin Invest 1998; 102: 606–618.

[28] Nakagawa S, Toritsuka Y, Wakitani S, Denno K, Tomita T, Owaki H, Kimura T, Shino K, Ochi T. Bone marrow stromal cells contribute to synovial cell proliferation in rats with collagen induced arthritis. J Rheumatol 1996; 23: 2098–2103.

[29] Tomita T, Takeuchi E, Toyosaki-Maeda T, Oku H, Kaneko M, Takano H, Sugamoto K, Ohzono K, Suzuki R, Ochi T. Establishment of nurse-like stromal cells from bone marrow of patients with rheumatoid arthritis: indication of characteristic bone marrow

microenvironment in patients with rheumatoid arthritis. Rheumatology 1999; 38: 854–863.

[30] Toh ML, Gonzales G, Koenders MI, Tournadre A, Boyle D, Lubberts E, Zhou Y, Firestein GS, van den Berg WB, Miossec P. Role of interleukin 17 in arthritis chronicity through survival of synoviocytes via regulation of synoviolin expression. PLoS One 2010; 5: e13416.

[31] Burr ML, van den Boomen DJ, Bye H, Antrobus R, Wiertz EJ, Lehner PJ. MHC class I molecules are preferentially ubiquitinated on endoplasmic reticulum luminal residues during HRD1 ubiquitin E3 ligase-mediated dislocation. Proc Natl Acad Sci U S A. 2013; 110: 14290–14295.

[32] Xu Y, Zhao F, Qiu Q, Chen K, Wei J, Kong Q, Gao B, Melo-Cardenas J, Zhang B, Zhang J, Song J, Zhang DD, Zhang J, Fan Y, Li H, Fang D. The ER membrane-anchored ubiquitin ligase Hrd1 is a positive regulator of T-cell immunity. Nat Commun 2016; 15: 1–13.

[33] Toh ML, Marotte H, Blond JL, Jhumka U, Eljaafari A, Mougin B, Miossec, P. Overexpression of synoviolin in peripheral blood and synoviocytes from rheumatoid arthritis patients and continued elevation in nonresponders to infliximab treatment. Arthritis Rheum 2006; 54: 2109–2118.

[34] Koenders MI, Marijnissen RJ, Devesa I, Lubberts E, Joosten LA, Roth J, van Lent PL, van de Loo FA, van den Berg WB. Tumor necrosis factor-interleukin-17 interplay induces S100A8, interleukin-1β, and matrix metalloproteinases, and drives irreversible cartilage destruction in murine arthritis: rationale for combination treatment during arthritis. Arthritis Rheum 2011; 63: 2329–2339.

[35] Wynn TA, Ramalingam TR. Mechanisms of fibrosis: therapeutic translation for fibrotic disease. Nat Med 2012; 18: 1028–1240.

[36] Hasegawa D, Fujii R, Yagishita N, Matsumoto N, Aratani S, Izumi T, Azakami K, Nakazawa M, Fujita H, Sato T, Araya N, Koike J, Tadokoro M, Suzuki N, Nagata K, Senoo H, Friedman SL, Nishioka K, Yamano Y, Itoh F, Nakajima T. E3 ubiquitin ligase synoviolin is involved in liver fibrogenesis. PLoS One 2010; 5: e13590.

[37] Nakajima F, Aratani S, Fujita H, Yagishita N, Ichinose S, Makita K, Setoguchi Y, Nakajima T. Synoviolin inhibitor LS-102 reduces endoplasmic reticulum stress-induced collagen secretion in an in vitro model of stress-related interstitial pneumonia. Int J Mol Med 2015; 35: 110–116.

[38] Nogee LM. Genetics of the hydrophobic surfactant proteins. Biochim Biophys Acta 1998; 1408: 323–333.

[39] Mulugeta S, Nguyen V, Russo SJ, Muniswamy M, Beers MF. A surfactant protein C precursor protein BRICHOS domain mutation causes endoplasmic reticulum stress,

proteasome dysfunction, and caspase 3 activation. Am J Respir Cell Mol Biol 2005; 32: 521–530.

[40] Li L, Shen Y, Ding Y, Liu Y, Su D, Liang X. Hrd1 participates in the regulation of collagen I synthesis in renal fibrosis. Mol Cell Biochem 2014; 386: 35–44.

[41] Tsuchimochi K, Yagishita N, Yamasaki S, Amano T, Kato Y, Kawahara K, Aratani S, Fujita H, Ji F, Sugiura A, Izumi T, Sugamiya A, Maruyama I, Fukamizu A, Komiya S, Nishioka K, Nakajima T. Identification of a crucial site for synoviolin expression. Mol Cell Biol 2005; 25: 7344–7356.

[42] Yagishita N, Aratani S, Leach C, Amano T, Yamano Y, Nakatani K, Nishioka K, Nakajima T. RING-finger type E3 ubiquitin ligase inhibitors as novel candidates for the treatment of rheumatoid arthritis. Int J Mol Med 2012; 30: 1281–1286.

[43] Wu T, Zhao F, Gao B, Tan C, Yagishita N, Nakajima T, Wong PK, Chapman E, Fang D, Zhang DD. Hrd1 suppresses Nrf2-mediated cellular protection during liver cirrhosis. Genes Dev 2014; 28: 708–722.

[44] Dou QP, Zonder JA. Overview of proteasome inhibitor-based anti-cancer therapies: perspective on bortezomib and second generation proteasome inhibitors versus future generation inhibitors of ubiquitin-proteasome system. Curr Cancer Drug Targets 2014; 14: 517–536.

[45] Hou YC, Deng JY. Role of E3 ubiquitin ligases in gastric cancer. World J Gastroenterol 2015; 21: 786–793.

[46] Lü S, Wang J. The resistance mechanisms of proteasome inhibitor bortezomib. Biomark Res 2013; 1: 13

[47] Teicher BA, Tomaszewski JE. Proteasome inhibitors. Biochem Pharmacol 2015; 96: 1–9.

[48] Allegra A, Alonci A, Gerace D, Russo S, Innao V, Calabrò L, Musolino C. New orally active proteasome inhibitors in multiple myeloma. Leuk Res 2014; 38: 1–9.

[49] McBride A, Klaus JO, Stockerl-Goldstein K. Carfilzomib: a second-generation proteasome inhibitor for the treatment of multiple myeloma. Am J Health Syst Pharm 2015; 72: 353–360.

[50] Gentile M, Offidani M, Vigna E, Corvatta L, Recchia AG, Morabito L, Morabito F, Gentili S. Ixazomib for the treatment of multiple myeloma. Expert Opin Investig Drugs 2015; 24: 1287–1298.

[51] Berkers CR, Leestemaker Y, Schuurman KG, Ruggeri B, Jones-Bolin S, Williams M, Ovaa H. Probing the specificity and activity profiles of the proteasome inhibitors bortezomib and delanzomib. Mol Pharm 2012; 9: 1126–1135.

[52] Semren N, Habel-Ungewitter NC, Fernandez IE, Königshoff M, Eickelberg O, Stöger T, Meiners S. Validation of the 2nd generation proteasome inhibitor oprozomib for local therapy of pulmonary fibrosis. PLoS One 2015; 10: e0136188.

[53] Ma L, Diao A. Marizomib, a potent second generation proteasome inhibitor from natural origin. Anticancer Agents Med Chem 2015; 15: 298–306.

[54] Deshaies RJ, Joazeiro CA. RING domain E3 ubiquitin ligases. Annu Rev Biochem 2009; 78: 399–434.

[55] Haupt Y, Maya R, Kazaz A, Oren M. Mdm2 promotes the rapid degradation of p53. Nature 1997; 387: 296–299.

[56] Brooks CL, Gu W. p53 ubiquitination: Mdm2 and beyond. Mol Cell 2006; 21: 307–315.

[57] Issaeva N, Bozko P, Enge M, Protopopova M, Verhoef LG, Masucci M, Pramanik A, Selivanova G. Small molecule RITA binds to p53, blocks p53-HDM-2 interaction and activates p53 function in tumors. Nature Medicine 2004; 10: 1321–1328.

[58] Goldenberg SJ, Marblestone JG, Mattern MR, Nicholson B. Strategies for the identification of ubiquitin ligase inhibitors. Biochem Soc Trans 2010; 38: 132–136.

2

Molecular Imaging

Leszek Królicki and Adrian Michno

Abstract

Mechanisms responsible for the course of the rheumatic diseases have not been fully explained. Among the available tools that may help in studies of these mechanisms is molecular imaging—especially techniques emphasized by nuclear medicine. In contrast to CT, MRI or US examination that show only structural pathologies, radionuclide methods allow imaging of functional changes that occur in the course of the disease and usually are featured by a very high specificity. Recent advances in nuclear medicine allowed to develop target-specific agents making it possible to reveal molecular level disturbances that take place on the course of the ongoing disease. The fundamental radionuclide studies include PET, SPECT, and classic scintigraphy. Technological advances (especially hybrid modalities) allow obtaining images of much better resolution and allow combining both structural and functional data.

Keywords: PET, SPECT, markers of inflamation, radiotracers cordially

1. Introduction

Mechanisms responsible for the course of the rheumatic diseases have not been fully explained till today. Molecular imaging sits among the available tools that may help in studies of these mechanisms, particularly techniques emphasized by nuclear medicine.

In contrast to such imaging modalities as CT, US or MRI, that reveal only structural pathologies, radionuclide methods enable imaging of functional changes that occur in the course of the disease and more importantly are usually featured by a very high specificity. Radionuclide studies also make it possible to determine the changes in the molar concentration of specific chemical compounds up to 10^{-11} or even 10^{-3}–10^{-4} if an MRI is used. It means that radionuclide studies enable the performance of diagnosis of disorders in the molar concentration of the specific chemical compounds that take place in the course of the disease. It is important to note that the functional character of disorders should be the basis for the choice of treatment.

Over the last several decades, the introduction of new biological agents has greatly improved the effectiveness of treatment. Those agents influence the activity of specific receptor and metabolic pathways [1]. Along with the application of new agents, it has become necessary to introduce new diagnostic methods, which allow evaluation of the activity of those biological processes. Unfortunately, neither clinical examination nor laboratory tests nor conventional X-ray does not provide such findings. A clinical evaluation can be highly subjective; laboratory tests are frequently non-specific and inconsistent, while conventional X-ray shows structural changes only at the advanced stage of the disease.

It seems that the introduction of molecular imaging techniques may lift those limitations. The fundamental methods of molecular imaging are radionuclide studies. Recent advances in nuclear medicine allowed to develop target-specific agents making it possible to reveal molecular level disturbances that take place on the course of the ongoing disease [2]. The fundamental radionuclide studies include a PET, SPECT, and classic scintigraphy. Moreover, hybrid devices are used more frequently in diagnostics these days—these consist of gamma camera and CR/MRI. Thanks to hybrid techniques, it is possible to perform CT/MRI combined with scintigraphy (for example PET-CT, PET-MRI, and SPECT-CT). It is also important to mention that the combination of those techniques allows applying attenuation correction of the absorbed radiation that is being emitted by radioisotope, as well as making it possible to determine the exact location of the abnormal uptake of the radiopharmaceutical. Finally, the images obtained are of very high quality.

Technological advances allow obtaining images of much better resolution and allow combining both structural and functional data. Vogel et al. noted in his study that hybrid imaging technique ^{18}F-FDG PET-CT, apart from providing the capability of assessing the degree of inflammation localized in the tarsus of a rheumatoid arthritis (RA) patient, also allows precise localization of the disease activity in particular joints [3]. Neither physical examination nor X-ray can provide such relevant data. Furthermore, ^{18}F-FDG PET/CT allows to visualize and diagnose metabolically active subcutaneous nodules, activated lymph nodes or other affected joints in the course of the disease (such as those of the knee or atlantoaxial joints). This method allows better discrimination between juxtaarticular disease and articular processes as well as delineation of tendon sheath and bursal inflammation. Furthermore, this method makes it possible to delineate inflammation of the tendon sheaths and bursae. Miese et al. [4] also assessed the high suitability of PET/MRI apparatus in his work about the diagnosis of RA, in which he showed increased uptake of ^{18}F-FDG in the corresponding metacarpophalangeal joints that were affected by synovitis and tenovaginitis as identified on contrast-enhanced MRI.

MRI is second modern imaging modality that is very useful in the diagnosis of rheumatic diseases. This method features a very high resolution and similarly good contrast between the soft tissues. Thanks to the new sequences and specific contrast agents, and modern MRI allows imaging of vast amounts of pathologies.

Both of these methods provide the information about molecular pathological mechanisms that accompany the disease; thus allowing a better understanding of the pathophysiology of rheumatic diseases. Moreover, they allow a search of the new forms of molecular treatment that allow for an early and accurate prognosis as well as monitoring of therapy [5]. Beyond any doubts, another important feature of these methods is the capability of making the diagnosis at the subclinical phase of the disease, thanks to which a proper treatment can be started long before irreversible morphological changes occur.

Procedures offered by nuclear medicine meet the number of important expectations associated with the development of modern medical sciences, such as:

a. The capability of putting a considerably early diagnosis of pathological changes as well as the determination of their character, which is crucial to make an appropriate diagnosis before irreversible structural changes occur.

b. The ability of accurate determination of the degree of pathological changes.

c. The ability to predict the course of the disease and the subsequent introduction of personalized therapy.

d. The reduction of constantly increasing the costs of medical procedures by use of such evaluation tools that provide a good assessment of the effectiveness of the applied treatment.

e. The need of the determination of remission of the pathological changes as well as an early diagnosis of their relapse.

Taking these facts into account, it is clear that radionuclide studies and MRI have proven to be useful in solving all of the clinical issues. Moreover, it is important to note that it meets economic and pharmacological criteria for cost-effectiveness.

2. Radiopharmaceuticals

2.1. ^{18}F-FDG

The most commonly used radiopharmaceutical used in PET-CT studies is fluorodeoxyglucose (^{18}F-FDG), which is a structural glucose analog. Areas of increased tracer uptake indicate the intensification of metabolic processes associated with increased glucose demand. This feature can be found both in a tumor and inflammatory setting. Increased uptake of ^{18}F-FDG is associated with increased activity of the GLUT1 and GLUT3 transport mechanisms as well as the activity of hexokinase—these phenomena are typical for cells that undergo fast proliferation as well as other types of cells such as macrophages, neutrophils and young granulation tissue [6–8].

2.2. ^{11}C-choline

Choline is another tracer that features high sensitivity for proliferative processes that occur in the course of the disease. This tracer is uptaken by quickly dividing cells where it undergoes phosphorylation by choline kinase into phosphorylcholine. Choline is essential for phospholipids synthesis, especially phosphatidylcholine (also known as lecithin) which serves as the building block of the cell membranes. Increased uptake of choline depends on the mechanisms responsible for active transport via the cell membrane as well as on congestion-dependent passive diffusion. It has been found that increased uptake can be seen even in the early phase of the inflammation. Once present, its grade of accumulation corresponds with both the extent of the contrast-enhanced signal in an MRI study (with Gadovist as a tracer) and the accumulation of ^{18}FDG [9].

2.3. ^{67}Ga-citrate

This radiopharmaceutical has been used in both the diagnosis of cancer as well as acute and chronic foci of inflammation for several years. Gallium (administered via i.v. infusion) acts as an iron analog that binds to transferrin, ferritin, and leukocytes (primarily neutrophils) [10]. These molecules accumulate within the foci of inflammation secondary to increased capillary permeability. At the time when ^{67}Ga-bound macromolecules reach the inflammatory interstitial space, the isotope undergoes the process of transchelation into lactoferrin, ferritin and bacterial siderophores (if present). Moreover, lactoferrin is then being secreted by neutrophils that are present in the inflammatory foci caused by the disorders of the connective tissue [11]. Recently, ^{67}Ga-citrate is rarely used because of the vast availability of other—frequently much better—markers as well as other factors such as the unfavorable energetic profile of the emitted radiation, the long-lasting radioactivity of the blood (due to high affinity to the white blood cells) and relatively long half-life time. This results in significantly increased absorbed radiation dose in comparison to other radioisotopes, not to mention low quality of the obtained images. Another disadvantage of ^{67}Ga-citrate is the lack of specificity for inflammation because it accumulates similarly in neoplasms.

2.4. ^{99m}Tc and ^{111}In HIG

Both 99m-technetium and 111-indium can be used for labeling of human (polyclonal) immunoglobulins (HIG). HIG accumulate in the inflamed tissues because its mechanism of accumulation is related to the increased permeability of the vascular capillaries as well as increased blood flow to the inflamed area. This technique features very high sensitivity, not to mention that the grade of its accumulation highly corresponds to the severity of the inflammation, hence making it a useful prognostic tool. On the other hand, one of the disadvantages of this radiopharmaceutical includes lack of specificity [12].

2.5. ^{99m}Tc-diphosphonates

Similarly to gallium-67, ^{99m}Tc-diphosphonates are non-specific tracers used in the diagnosis of the inflammation—its mechanism of uptake relies on the metabolism of the osseous cells—its degree of uptake depends on the activity of osteoblasts (hence its perfect for imaging of the bone turnover). Bone scintigraphy is readily available and cheap method of evaluation of bones [13, 14]. As the severity of the inflammation progress, the uptake increases. In the setting of inflammation evaluation, the bone scan comes in the form of a triphasic examination, which consists of vascular, parenchymal, and late (bony) phase (**Figure 1**). Each phase presents a specific aspect of the pathology:

- Phase I—hyperemia,
- Phase II—increased volume of the vascular bed,
- Phase III—metabolic turnover and remodeling of the osseous tissue as a result of the ongoing pathology (inflammation and destruction of the cartilage).

This method is highly sensitive but features low specificity, which can be improved by hybrid SPECT-CT technique if one is available.

It is important to note that the accumulation of described radiopharmaceuticals in tissues affected by inflammation is non-specific because these tracers accumulate similarly in neoplastic foci. Due to that fact, there is recently ongoing research that aims to develop markers specific for inflammation occurring in the course of the rheumatic diseases.

2.6. Labeled leukocytes

Since the inflammation features the migration of leukocytes, there was an idea to use that mechanism in the diagnosis and localization of the inflammatory foci. Nuclear medicine has

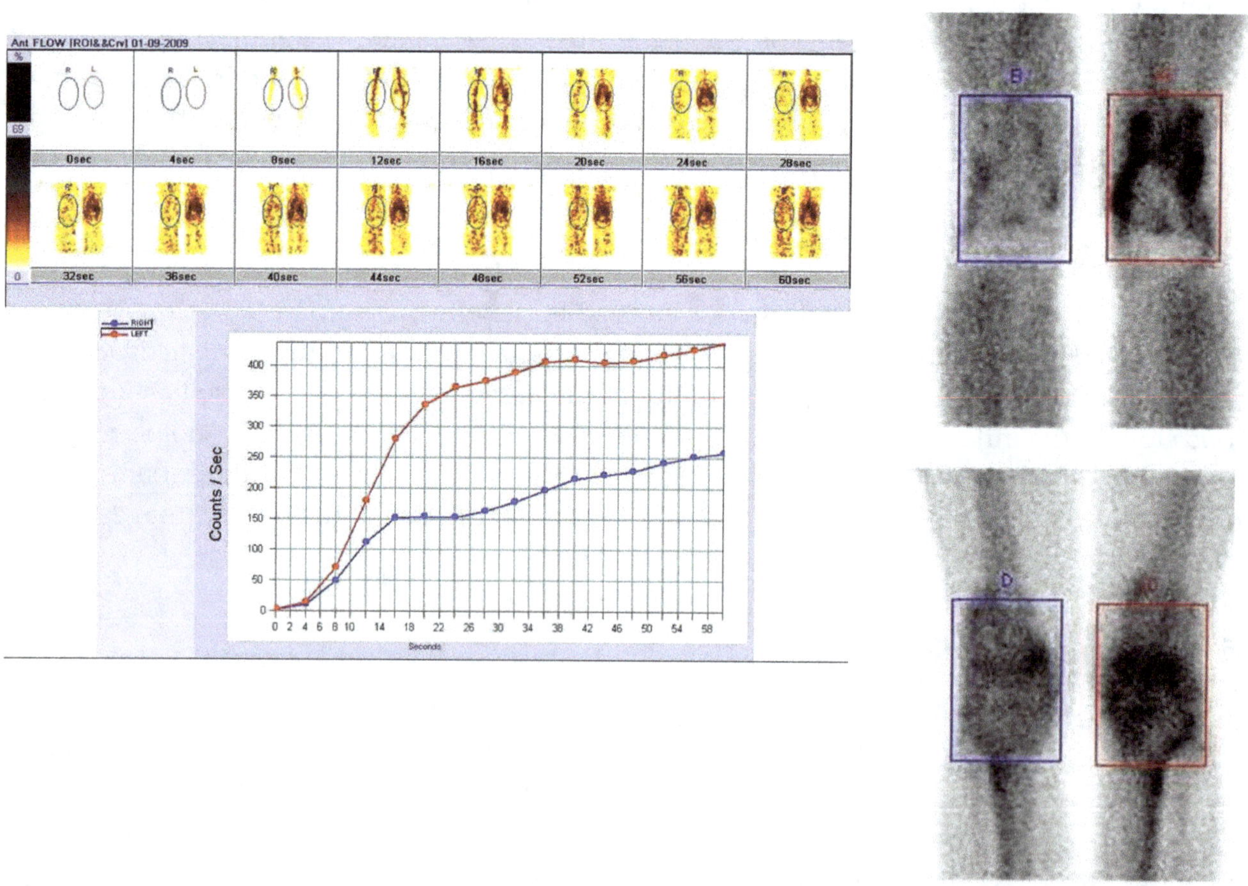

Figure 1. Triphasic bone scan after ^{99m}Tc-MDP administration in patient with RA shows increased blood flow (A), blood pool (B), and increased accumulation of the radiotracer in the bony phase (C) which indicates increased bony turnover in the affected left knee.

come to meet this need and has developed a radionuclide examination that makes it possible to label leukocytes of the patient (both in vitro and in vivo depending on the technique). In the setting of inflammation, neutrophils and monocytes are being recruited, and due to the phenomena of chemotaxis, they accumulate in the foci of inflammation. Thanks to this mechanism of accumulation, labeled leukocytes can be used in the diagnosis of RA as well as other inflammatory diseases. Labeled leukocytes emphasize two main techniques—in vivo and in vitro assay.

- *In vitro assay* is a technique that involves taking a blood sample, isolating a leukocyte suspension, labeling those leukocytes with ^{99m}Tc-HM-PAO or ^{111}In-oxine, and intravenous administration back to the patient. It is important to note that this procedure does not affect chemotaxis.
- *In vivo assay,* on the other hand, involves intravenous administration of ^{99m}Tc-labeled monoclonal antibodies against the specific NC-1 antigen that is present on the granulocyte cell membrane. In this procedure, the labeling process occurs directly in the blood of the patient. Moreland et al. [15] in his work have shown that there is a direct correlation between the foci of increased accumulation and the clinical picture in the course of rheumatoid arthritis. This examination may also be used as a tool to control anti-inflammatory treatment [15].

2.7. ^{11}C-PK11195

One of the proposals involved the introduction of ^{11}C-PK11195 isoquinoline carboxamide—this radiopharmaceutical binds to both monocytes and macrophages and serves as peripheral benzodiazepine receptor (PBR) antagonist also known as translocator protein (TSPO). This peptide is particularly active on the outer surface of the mitochondrial membrane of the activated macrophages, polymorphonuclear cells as well as nervous and lymphatic tissue [16–18]. It is responsible for the process of steroidogenesis, apoptosis, cell proliferation, and immune response. It has also been proved that this radiopharmaceutical is an effective marker in neuroinfection, due to the fact that peripheral benzodiazepine receptors can be typically found on activated glial cells.

2.8. ^{99m}Tc-J001X

Other noteworthy markers are those with the ability to label the macrophages. These kinds of cells are particularly active in inflammation based on the rheumatic disorders and play a major role in the inflammatory process. It was found that macrophages bind specifically to the proteoglycans of the bacteria. Hence a technique of proteoglycans labeling has been developed [19, 20].

Recently used tracer is called J001X—which is a poly-(1,3)-ᴅ-galactoside isolated from the cellular membrane of *Klebsiella pneumoniae.* This ^{99m}Tc labeled-substance allows tracing of the mononuclear phagocytes.

The effectiveness of this radiopharmaceutical in the diagnosis of RA-associated lung pathology appears to be promising, but until today there is no randomized study that would confirm its effectiveness. Lastly, this tracer was also used in imaging of sarcoidosis and scleroderma [21].

2.9. ^{99m}Tc-RP128

^{99m}Tc-RP128 is a peptide tracer used for imaging of leukocytes recruitment used for labeling of neutrophils and mononuclear phagocytes. ^{99m}Tc-RP128 is a pentapeptide tuftsin analog antagonist (TKPPR) that mediates the receptor-specific interaction and subsequently binds to tuftsin receptors. Tuftsin is an organic chemical compound consisting of amino acid residues such as threonine, lysine, proline, and arginine. It is produced by the spleen and its function is to stimulate macrophages and granulocytes to phagocytosis and chemotaxis. Tuftsin is derived from proteolytic cleavage of the Fc domain of the heavy chain of IgG. Tuftsin receptor's function is to mediate the immune functions; hence they represent important molecular targets. The mechanism of RP128 imaging is based on the upregulation of tuftsin receptors located in activated macrophages. Chaudhuri et al. [22] noted that the affinity of radiotracer is fourfold greater than their endogenous ligand. Despite that fact, this radiotracer was described only in a few works; thus there is a need for further research that would confirm its utility. Studies show that it accumulates in other organs to an only small extent (except kidneys). The grade of accumulation in healthy joints was moderate—in contrast to the affected joints, which featured a very high uptake. The sensitivity of the scan was 69% for swollen joints, 76% for painful joints, and 73% for joints with bone erosions [23].

2.10. ^{99m}Tc- and ^{111}In anti-E-selectin

Adhesion is another mechanism used in the diagnosis of the inflammation. Molecules responsible for this phenomena cause leukocytes to bind to the activated endothelial vessels resulting in their transendothelial migration. One of such molecules that are used in the diagnosis of the inflammation is E-selectin labeled with ^{99m}Tc or ^{111}In. E-selectin (CD62E, ELAM1) is a transmembrane glycoprotein that is transiently expressed on the luminal surface of activated vascular endothelium during a normal inflammatory response. E-selectin mediates the initial tethering and rolling of granulocytes, monocytes, and some lymphocytes via specific interactions with its carbohydrate-based ligands. It is then activated by interleukin-1 (IL-1), tumor necrosis factor-α (TNF-α), and bacterial LPS—it has to be noted that this may occur only in the setting of inflammation [24]. ^{111}In-1.2B6 monoclonal antibody (mAb) is another antibody that was used for imaging of selectin activity. Since this is a murine antibody, the administration of this radiopharmaceutical comes with a risk of developing human anti-mouse antibody (HAMA) response, a possibly life-threatening state that requires immediate medical attention. This fact limits the repetition of the study in patients in whom treatment control is necessary. Therefore, F(ab')2 fragments of 1.2B6 mAb—devoid of its Fc portions—were introduced [25].

2.11. Octreotide

Octreotide is a long-acting somatostatin analog that targets the activation of endothelium and macrophage recruitment at any of five identified G-protein-coupled somatostatin receptor subtypes (SST1–5). Hyper-expression of these receptors has been thoroughly documented in numerous pathological conditions hence it can be considered as a basis for octreotide imaging. The synovia of affected joints in RA patients features overexpression of somatostatin receptors—those that are targeted by octreotide. The SST2 expression on activated venule of endothelial cells and infiltrating mononuclear phagocytes have been identified in histological and immunochemistry examinations both in the affected synovia and fibroblast-like synovial cells. It is important to note that patients with favorable treatment results also show significantly lower expression of the somatostatin receptors; thus somatostatin scintigraphy may also be used in the prediction of the effectiveness of the treatment [26].

Somatostatin receptor expression also features a good correlation with the clinical data—its sensitivity estimates 75%. Vanhagen et al. [27] also noted that no radiotracer accumulation was observed in the joints of healthy individuals. Numerous works point that somatostatin analogs may be used in RA treatment as well. It has also been found that the administration of somatostatin analogs reduced the symptoms of the disease—presumably due to the inhibition of IL-6 and IL-8 production as well as inhibited proliferation that occurs in the affected synovium. Therefore, somatostatin scintigraphy may be used as a tool in the prediction of the somatostatin analog treatment effects, although until today there has been no randomized study to confirm it. Therefore, more research is required before its utility may be introduced to the guidelines [28].

2.12. Other radiopharmaceuticals

2.12.1. Anti-CD-3

Since mature T lymphocytes play a role in the development of RA, some radionuclide studies make it possible to label monoclonal antibodies against CD3 and T lymphocyte migration into the affected synovium. Recent advances allow Muromonab to be labeled with ^{99m}Tc and use it for imaging of rheumatic disease. It is essential to note that this examination correlates well with physical examination and patient history [29]. Moreover, scintigraphy with this tracer can be used in differential diagnosis of juvenile idiopathic arthritis and RA as well as other rheumatic diseases.

2.12.2. ^{99m}Tc-anti-CD4 mAb

Anti-CD4 imaging is also used for the evaluation of T lymphocyte infiltration. CD4 is expressed on the cell surface of mature T helper cells, thymocytes, and dendritic cells [30]. ^{99m}Tc-MAX.16H5, murine IgG1 was used in patients and showed affected joints in all RA patients. Studies indicate that the sensitivity of the ^{99m}Tc-MAX.16H5 scan is better than the bone scan.

2.12.3. ^{99m}Tc-Anti-CD20 mAb

Almost 95% of circulating normal and malignant B lymphocytes expresses CD20 antigen [31]. Furthermore, its expression is exclusive to B lymphocytes simultaneously featuring the lack of expression in the hematopoietic stem cells. Due to this fact, Rituximab as a mouse/human monoclonal antibody can be labeled with ^{99m}Tc and used for B cell infiltration imaging [32].

2.12.4. TNF-alpha

TNF plays an essential role in the development of RA [33]. The promising results have been described in studies which involved the use of ^{123}I-anakinra, infliximab (a monoclonal antibody that binds to membrane-bound and soluble TNF [34]) and ^{99m}Tc-Adalimumab.

3. Clinical application of radionuclide studies in the setting of rheumatoid arthritis and other inflammatory diseases

3.1. Rheumatoid arthritis

3.1.1. Diagnosis and disease progression

In vitro studies of Matsui et al. [35] has shown that in the setting of a murine model of collagen-induced arthritis, the peak of ^{18}F-FDG uptake occurs both at the stage of pannus creation and during the destruction of the bone caused by inflammation caused by proliferating fibroblasts. Another prominent role of macrophages includes the fact that their inactivated form accumulates ^{18}F-FDG merely to a small extent, while glucose demands after their hypoxia-induced activation increases significantly.

The degree of ^{18}F-FDG uptake in correlation to the disorder severity:

- Moderate uptake can be seen in the initial period of the disease progression, at which interstitial inflammatory cells recruitment, synovial cells hyperplasia, and edema can be seen.
- Uptake of ^{18}F-FDG noticeably increases as the bony destruction and pannus creation progresses.

It has been shown that the highest grade of ^{18}F-FDG accumulation not only is related to the proliferation of fibroblasts but also to the neutrophils as well. On the other hand, resting macrophages feature moderate accumulation of ^{18}F-FDG. In the setting of hypoxia, the activity of various inflammatory cells changes, while the activity of proinflammatory cytokines (such as TNF-alpha) increases. It has been observed that in these conditions there is increased ^{18}F-FDG uptake by macrophages and fibroblasts, while in the case of neutrophils, it remains at the background level. T cells accumulate ^{18}F-FDG to a small extent regardless of the microenvironment.

Summarizing, the degree of ^{18}F-FDG uptake correlates with the activity of proliferating fibroblasts as well as macrophages activated by hypoxia; hence allowing the ^{18}F-FDG study to be used in the evaluation of the disease severity.

Beckers et al. [36] assessed that the sensitivity of this technique in the setting of rheumatoid arthritis equals approx. 90%. Some works indicate that the study allows the identification of lesions in the subclinical phase of the disease as well as at the stage of its clinical remission. This fact plays a particularly important role in the treatment [37].

^{18}F-FDG PET-CT study also allows the assessment of the disease severity in other maladies, such as spondyloarthritis, polymyalgia rheumatica, Still's disease, polychondritis, IgG4-related disease, polymyositis, and dermatomyositis [38].

Some of the studies aimed to assess the usefulness of ^{11}C-choline as a marker for both the diagnosis and the severity assessment tool in rheumatic diseases. These indicated that it might be a good marker for the proliferation progress, which occur not only in the setting of tumors but also in the rheumatic conditions as well.

Roivainen et al. [39] made a comparison between ^{11}C-choline PET-CT to ^{18}F-FDG and gadolinium-enhanced MRI. The authors have shown that there is very high compliance between the pharmacokinetics of ^{18}F-FDG and ^{11}C-choline at the site of the affected joints. Regardless of the clinical symptoms of the inflammatory process, the accumulation of both markers occurred in the same joints that featured a clear contrast enhancement in the MR study. Moreover, authors state that ^{11}C-choline may be a very promising tracer for quantitative imaging of proliferative arthritis changes. However, to characterize the relationship of PET-CT results with the clinical and functional measures of inflammation, a subsequent prospective study involving a larger number of patients is necessary [39]. Among other radiopharmaceuticals, ^{11}C-(R)-PK11195 isoquinoline carboxamide is also being used for both the diagnosis of RA as well as an assessment of the disease severity. It was noted that this tracer tends to accumulate primarily in the activated macrophages and its degree of uptake highly corresponds to the severity of synovitis priorly assessed by histopathological examination. This examination turned out to be highly sensitive in both localizations of acute phase inflammation spots and the assessment of initial phase of the disease. It is considered that increased PET signal in inflamed joints occurs as a result of specific PBR-mediated uptake of ^{11}C-(R)-PK11195 caused by activated macrophages.

Van der Laken et al. [40] performed one of the first studies in the setting of the rheumatic disease. The authors concluded in their work that ^{11}C-(R)-PK11195 uptake on the PET scans was significantly higher in severely inflamed joints in comparison to those with moderate or mild signs of inflammation. Additionally, tracer uptake in contralateral, unaffected by inflammation knee joints of RA patients was significantly higher than in joints of healthy individuals from the control group (with no history of inflammatory joint disease or the presence of any subclinical disease activity). PET tracer uptake in the affected joints is highly correlated with PBR staining of sub-lining of synovial tissue, which also proves its correlation to CD68 staining of macrophages.

It is believed that this tracer may allow imaging of the ongoing pathology prior to its clinical manifestation due to the fact that macrophages infiltration into synovial joints is a common feature of asymptomatic synovitis in early RA [41, 42]. Furthermore, the application of ^{11}C-(R)-PK11195 imaging to RA may prove to be relevant to patient management since the presence and the number of macrophages in rheumatoid synovium strictly correlates with the progression of joint erosions that can be seen in the X-ray. Another use of this trace encompasses diagnosis of subclinical synovitis in patients with arthralgia. Last but not least, increased uptake of the tracer correlates with the progression of the disease.

3.1.2. Treatment control

Numbers of works indicate that ^{18}F-FDG is an excellent marker in the assessment of treatment effectiveness. The utility of ^{18}F-FDG as the marker in this assessment was suggested by Palmer et al. back in 1995 [43]. The authors in their work studied the influence of prednisolone and subsequent methotrexate treatment on findings in MRI and ^{18}F-FDG PET-CT. Results showed that as the volume of the pannus seen on MRI decreased, so did the uptake of ^{18}F-FDG—not to mention the improvement of the clinical picture (such as reduction of pain sensation, stiffness, and edema). However, none of the studied parameters correlated with the outcome of the treatment. Authors concluded that both morphological pictures visible in MRI study and the functional test of PET study allow the assessment of the quantitative effectiveness of the applied therapy.

Similar results were presented in 2004 by Beckers et al. who have shown a direct correlation between the clinical picture of a joint with the findings of an ultrasound examination and the degree of ^{18}F-FDG uptake in PET-CT [36]. Additionally, as it turned out, the degree of ^{18}F-FDG uptake in the affected joint highly correlates to the thickness of the synovial membrane priorly assessed in the ultrasound examination. Moreover, another correlation has been found between the number of joints with increased ^{18}F-FDG uptake (with consideration of their total uptake value) and the duration of the disease together with the degree of severity. In 2004, Brenner et al. indicated in his work that despite confirmed correlation between ^{18}F-FDG uptake and the effectiveness of the treatment, PET-CT is still not recommended as a routine evaluation tool due to its high costs and limited availability [44]. This technique would be more indicated if the findings could provide parameters that are not obtainable by other tests (such as MRI, bone scan or ultrasound examination). However, authors pinpoint few of such parameters, that is, the possibility of quantitative assessment of disease severity of each affected joint and the assessment of disease progression as well as monitoring of treatment effectiveness. Authors emphasize that further studies are necessary for the better determination of PET-CT study indications.

Beckers et al. [36] presented a noteworthy work which aimed to study the response to the anti-TNF-alpha treatment [44]. Authors in their work showed a significant correlation between the degree of ^{18}F-FDG uptake, MRI findings, synovial membrane thickness, and the concentration of matrix metalloproteinase (MMP)3 and CRP levels. Similarly, Elzinga et al. [45] showed in their work that decreased uptake of ^{18}F-FDG after application of anti-TNF therapy is an important prognostic factor that indicates the effectiveness of the treatment.

3.1.3. Prognosis

Elzinga et al. [45] concluded that decreased ^{18}F-FDG uptake in the metacarpophalangeal and wrist joints 2 weeks following the infliximab (anti-TNF-alpha) therapy allowed to predict the outcome of the treatment after 14 and 22 weeks. It was all possible to achieve that because of the presence of clear correlation between the fall of the tracer uptake and the severity of the disease, which has subsequently contributed to the development of disease activity score (DAS). However, this type of correlation was not found in later observations; thus it requires further research. Perhaps another radiopharmaceutical will turn out to be more useful in prognosis of anticipated outcomes of the given treatment.

3.2. Diagnosis of concomitant diseases

A PET-CT study is a useful tool in the diagnosis of concomitant neoplastic disorders in patients with lupus, systemic sclerosis, dermatomyositis/polymyositis or Sjögren syndrome. Epidemiological data in these groups of patients showed the occurrence is noticeably higher; especially lymphoma, pharyngeal, and pancreatic cancer [46–48].

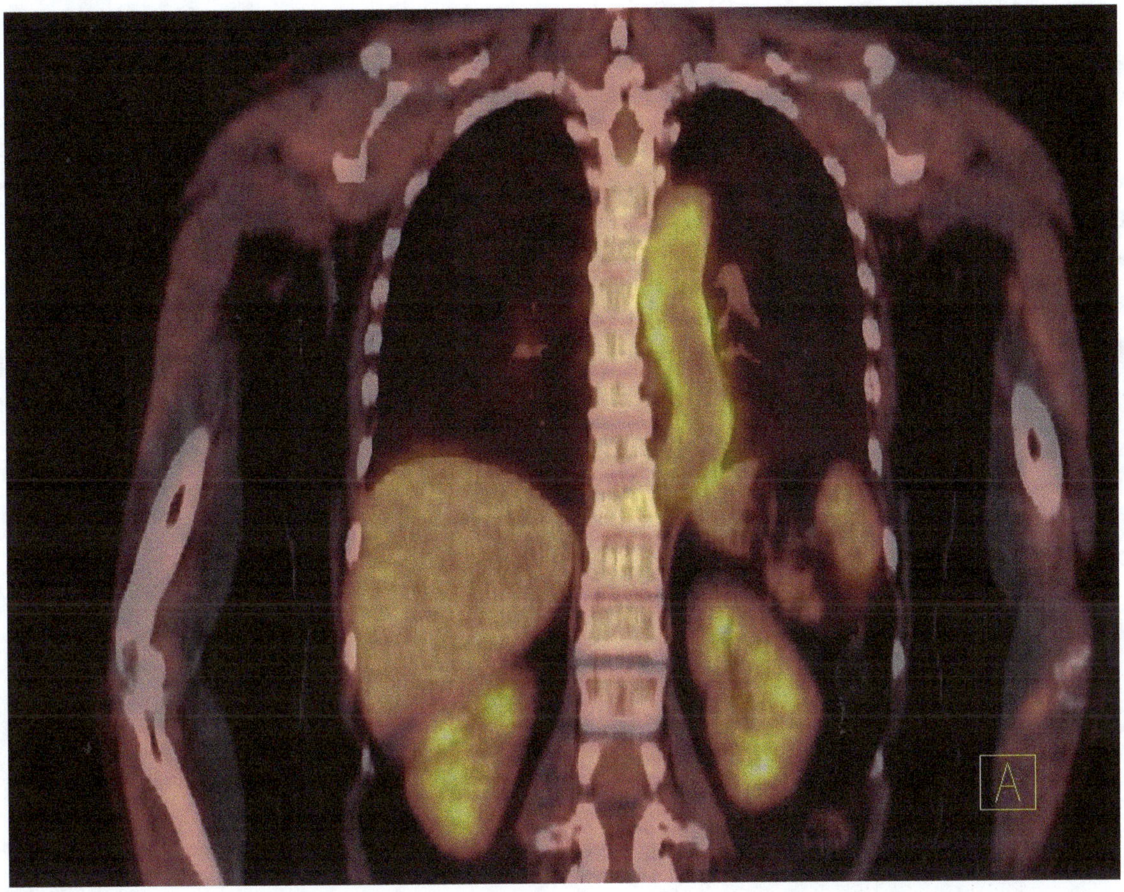

Figure 2. 18F-FDG PET-CT in patient with RA shows increased accumulation of the tracer in the wall of the aorta.

Autoimmune disease treatment involves the use of immunosuppressants, which aim to lower the immune response of the organism, simultaneously increasing the risk of infection (including a higher risk for relapse of tuberculosis) [49]. ^{18}F-FDG PET-CT study turns out to the most sensitive test for the diagnosis of infection. This examination can show abnormal focal uptake of the tracer in up to 90% of the patients suffering from autoimmune diseases; sensitivity and specificity in the diagnosis of neoplastic disorder equal 100 and 67%, respectively [50].

3.3. Fever of unknown origin

^{18}F-FDG PET-CT also showed to be promising in the diagnostic process in patients with the symptoms of FUO. In cases where other imaging studies showed to be inconclusive, ^{18}F-FDG PET-CT allows for the localization of pathological foci (either inflammation or a tumor based) in approx. 47% of the patients. Positive predictive value of this study has been assessed for 78% while negative predictive value—for 88% [51].

3.4. Vasculitis

Suspected large vascular vessels vasculitis is another indication for ^{18}F-FDG PET-CT. The term of vasculitis emphasizes the numbers of diseases, out of which Takayasu arteritis together with giant cell arteritis accounts for the most common types of vasculitis. Sensitivity and specificity of ^{18}F-FDG PET-CT in this setting equal 90%. In a meta-analysis performed by Balink et al. [52], the authors point out that sensitivity of this modality is higher than in any other imaging method (**Figure 2**).

4. Conclusion

Indeed, we can say that recently used studies such as MRI, CT or US in the setting of rheumatology are the marriage of convenience while radionuclide studies may be considered as a marriage of love. Such complex disease processes that occur in rheumatic diseases require comprehensive data that can be obtained only by procedures from the field of nuclear medicine.

Author details

Leszek Królicki[1*] and Adrian Michno[2]

*Address all correspondence to: leszek.krolicki@wum.edu.pl

1 Nuclear Medicine Department, Medical University of Warsaw, Warsaw, Poland

2 Department of Diagnostic Imaging, Bródno Hospital, Warsaw, Poland

References

[1] Smolen JS, Aletaha D, Koeller M, Weisman MH, Emery P. New therapies for the treatment of rheumatoid arthritis. Lancet. 2007;**370**:1861-1874

[2] Wunder A, Straub RH, Gay S, Funk J, Müller-Ladner U. Molecular imaging: Novel tools for visualizing rheumatoid arthritis. Rheumatology (Oxford). 2005;**44**:1341-1349

[3] Vogel WV, van Riel PL, Oyen WJ. FDG-PET/CT can visualise the extent of inflammation in rheumatoid arthritis of the tarsus. European Journal of Nuclear Medicine and Molecular Imaging. 2007;**34**:439

[4] Miese F, Scherer A, Ostendorf B, Heinzel A, Lanzman RS, Kropil P, Blondin D, Hautzel H, Wittsack HJ, Schneider M, Antoch G, Herzog H, Shah NJ. Hybrid 18F-FDG PET-MRI of the hand in rheumatoid arthritis: Initial results. Clinical Rheumatology. 2011;**30**:1247-1250

[5] Ladner U. Molecular imaging: Novel tools in visualizing rheumatoid arthritis. Rheumatology (Oxford). 2005;**44**:1341-1349

[6] Kubota R, Yamada S, Kubota K, Ishiwata K, Tamahashi N, Ido T. Intratumoral distribution of fluorine-18-fluorodeoxyglucose in vivo: High accumulation in macrophages and granulation tissues studied by microautoradiography. Journal of Nuclear Medicine. 1992;**33**:1972-1980

[7] Kubota K, Kubota R, Yamada S. FDG accumulation in tumour tissue. Journal of Nuclear Medicine. 1993;**34**:419-421

[8] Yamada S, Kubota K, Kubota R, Ido T, Tamahashi N. High accumulation of fluorine-18-fluorodeoxyglucose in turpentine-induced inflammatory tissue. Journal of Nuclear Medicine. 1995;**36**:1301-1306

[9] Roivainen A, Parkkola R, Yli-Kerttula T, Lehikoinen P, Viljanen T, Möttönen T, Nuutila P, Minn H. Use of positron emission tomography with methyl-11C-choline and 2-18F-fluoro-2-deoxy-D-glucose in comparison with magnetic resonance imaging for the assessment of inflammatory proliferation of synovium. Arthritis and Rheumatism. 2003;**48**:3077-3084

[10] Weiner R. The role of transferrin and other receptors in the mechanism of 67Ga localization. International Journal of Radiation Applications and Instrumentation. Part B. 1990;**17**:141-149

[11] Otsuki H, Brunetti A, Owens ES, Finn RD, Blasberg RG. Comparison of iron-59, indium111, and gallium-69 transferrin as a macromolecular tracer of vascular permeability and the transferrin receptor. Journal of Nuclear Medicine. 1989;**30**:1676-1685

[12] Pons F, Sanmarti R, Herranz R, Collado A, Piera C, Vidal-Sicart S, Muñoz-Gomez J, Setoain J. Scintigraphic evaluation of the severity of inflammation of the joints with 99Tcm-HIG in rheumatoid arthritis. Nuclear Medicine Communications. 1996;**17**:523-528

[13] Peepre K, Shah D, Solanki S, Tiwari AN, Pisal R. Clinical utility of nuclear medicine 99mTc-MDP bone scan in the early diagnosis of rheumatoid arthritis. The Turkish Journal of Pediatrics. 2008;**50**:194-195

[14] Rosenthall L. Nuclear medicine techniques in arthritis. Rheumatic Diseases Clinics of North America. 1991;**17**:585-597

[15] Moreland LW, Pratt PW, Mayes MD, Postlethwaite A, Weisman MH, Schnitzer T, Lightfoot R, Calabrese L, Zelinger DJ, Woody JN, Koopman WJ. Double-blind, placebo-controlled multicenter trial using chimeric monoclonal anti-CD4 antibody, cM-T412, in rheumatoid arthritis patients receiving concomitant methotrexate. Arthritis and Rheumatism. 1995;**38**:15811588

[16] Canat X, Carayon P, Bouaboula M, Cahard D, Shire D, Roque C, Le Fur G, Casellas P. Distribution profile and properties of peripheral type benzodiazepine receptors on human hemopoietic cells. Life Sciences. 1993;**52**:107-118

[17] Bazzichi L, Betti L, Giannaccini G, Rossi A, Lucacchini A. Peripheral-type benzodiazepine receptors in human mononuclear cells of patients affected by osteoarthritis, rheumatoid arthritis or psoriasic arthritis. Clinical Biochemistry. 2003;**36**:57-60

[18] Giusti L, Betti L, Giannaccini G, Mascia G, Bazzichi L, Lucacchini A. [3H]PK11195 binding sites in human neutrophils: Effect of fMLP stimulation and modulation in rheumatic diseases. Clinical Biochemistry. 2004;**37**:61-66

[19] Hmama Z, Kouassi E, Panaye G, Delassan S, Normier G, Binz H, Revillard JP. Binding of a bacterial acylpoly(1,3)galactoside to human blood leucocytes. Scandinavian Journal of Immunology. 1992;**36**:11-20

[20] Hmama Z, Normier G, Kouassi E, Flacher M, Binz H, Revillard JP. Binding of a membrane proteoglycan from *Klebsiella pneumoniae* and its derivatives to human leukocytes. Immunobiology. 1992;**186**:183-198

[21] Diot P, Diot E, Lemarie E, Guilmot JL, Baulieu JL, Asquier E, Valat C, Delarue A, Le Pape A. Imaging of pulmonary disease in scleroderma with J001X scintigraphy. Thorax. 1994;**49**:504508

[22] Chaudhuri MK, Konopinska D, Bump NJ, Najjar VA. The similarity between tuftsin (Thr-Lys-Pro-Arg) receptors and tuftsin antibody: A case of induced molecular mimicry. Annals of the New York Academy of Sciences. 1983;**419**:135-142

[23] Caveliers V, Goodbody AE, Tran LL, Peers SH, Thornback JR, Bossuyt A. Evaluation of 99mTc-RP128 as a potential inflammation imaging agent: Human dosimetry and first clinical results. Journal of Nuclear Medicine. 2001;**42**:154-161

[24] Koch AE, Burrows JC, Haines GK, Carlos TM, Harlan JM, Leibovich SJ. Immunolocalization of endothelial and leukocyte adhesion molecules in human rheumatoid and osteoarthritic synovial tissues. Laboratory Investigation. 1991;**64**:313-320

[25] Chapman PT, Jamar F, Keelan ET, Peters AM, Haskard DO. Use of a radiolabeled monoclonal antibody against E-selectin for imaging of endothelial activation in rheumatoid arthritis. Arthritis and Rheumatism. 1996;**39**:1371-1375

[26] Takeba Y, Suzuki N, Takeno M, Asai T, Tsuboi S, Hoshino T, Sakane T. Modulation of synovial cell function by somatostatin in patients with rheumatoid arthritis. Arthritis and Rheumatism. 1997;**40**:2128-2138

[27] Vanhagen PM, Markusse HM, Lamberts SW, Kwekkeboom DJ, Reubi JC, Krenning EP. Somatostatin receptor imaging. The presence of somatostatin receptors in rheumatoid arthritis. Arthritis and Rheumatism. 1994;**37**:1521-1527

[28] Paran D, Kidron D, Mayo A, Ziv O, Chowers Y, Caspi D, Yaron M, Paran H. Somatostatin analogue treatment attenuates histological findings of inflammation and increases mRNA expression of interleukin-1 beta in the articular tissues of rats with ongoing adjuvant-induced arthritis. Rheumatology International. 2005;**25**:350-356

[29] Marcus C, Thakur ML, Huynh TV, Louie JS, Leibling M, Minami C, Diggles L. Imaging rheumatic joint diseases with anti-T lymphocyte antibody OKT-3. Nuclear Medicine Communications. 1994;**15**:824-830

[30] Scoazec JY, Feldmann G. Both macrophages and endothelial cells of the human hepatic sinusoid express the CD4 molecule, a receptor for the human immunodeficiency virus. Hepatology. 1990;**12**:505-510

[31] Stashenko P, Nadler LM, Hardy R, Schlossman SF. Characterization of a human B lymphocyte-specific antigen. Journal of Immunology. 1980;**125**:1678-1685

[32] Malviya G, Laganà B, Milanetti F, Del Mastro C, Familiari D, Dierckx RA, Scopinaro F, D'Amelio R, Signore A. Use of 99m-technetium labelled Rituximab for imaging of patients with chronic inflammatory diseases. European Journal of Nuclear Medicine and Molecular Imaging. 2008;**35**(Suppl 2):S142-S143

[33] Tetta C, Camussi G, Modena V, Di Vittorio C, Baglioni C. Tumour necrosis factor in serum and synovial fluid of patients with active and severe rheumatoid arthritis. Annals of the Rheumatic Diseases. 1990;**49**:665-667

[34] Knight DM, Trinh H, Le J, Siegel S, Shealy D, McDonough M, Scallon B, Moore MA, Vilcek J, Daddona P, Ghrayeb J. Construction and initial characterization of a mouse-human chimeric anti-TNF antibody. Molecular Immunology. 1993;**30**:1443-1453

[35] Matsui T, Nakata N, Nagai S, Nakatani A, Takahashi M, Momose T, Ohtomo K, Koyasu S. Inflammatory cytokines and hypoxia contribute to 18F-FDG uptake by cells involved in pannus formation in rheumatoid arthritis. Journal of Nuclear Medicine. 2009;**50**:920-926

[36] Beckers C, Ribbens C, André B, Marcelis S, Kaye O, Mathy L, Kaiser MJ, Hustinx R, Foidart J, Malaise MG. Assessment of disease activity in rheumatoid arthritis with (18) F-FDG PET. Journal of Nuclear Medicine. 2004;**45**:956-964

[37] Brown AK, Conaghan PG, Karim Z, Quinn MA, Ikeda K, Peterfy CG, Hensor E, Wakefield RJ, O'Connor PJ, Emery P. An explanation for the apparent dissociation between clinical remission and continued structural deterioration in rheumatoid arthritis. Arthritis and Rheumatism. 2008;**58**:2958-2967

[38] Yamashita H, Kubota K, Mimori A. Clinical value of whole-body PET/CT in patients with active rheumatic diseases. Arthritis Research & Therapy. 2014;**16**:423

[39] Roivainen A, Yli-Kerttula T. Whole-body distribution of 11C-choline and uptake in knee synovitis. European Journal of Nuclear Medicine and Molecular Imaging. 2006; **33**:1372-1373

[40] van der Laken CJ, Elzinga EH, Kropholler MA, Molthoff CF, van der Heijden JW, Maruyama K, Boellaard R, Dijkmans BA, Lammertsma AA, Voskuyl AE. Noninvasive imaging of macrophages in rheumatoid synovitis using 11C-(R)PK11195 and positron emission tomography. Arthritis and Rheumatism. 2008;**58**:3350-3355

[41] Tak PP, Smeets TJ, Daha MR, Kluin PM, Meijers KA, Brand R, Meinders AE, Breedveld FC. Analysis of the synovial cell infiltrates in early rheumatoid synovial tissue in relation to local disease activity. Arthritis and Rheumatism. 1997;**40**:217-225

[42] Kraan MC, Versendaal H, Jonker M, Bresnihan B, Post WJ, t Hart BA, Breedveld FC, Tak PP. Asymptomatic synovitis precedes clinically manifest arthritis. Arthritis and Rheumatism. 1998;**41**:1481-1488

[43] Palmer WE, Rosenthal DI, Schoenberg OI, Fischman AJ, Simon LS, Rubin R, Polisson RP. Quantification of inflammation in the wrist with gadolinium-enhanced MR imaging and PET with 2-[F-18]-fluoro-2-deoxy-D-glucose. Radiology. 1995;**196**:647-655

[44] Brenner W. 18F-FDG PET in rheumatoid arthritis: There still is a long way to go. Journal of Nuclear Medicine. 2004;**45**:927-929

[45] Elzinga EH, van der Laken CJ, Comans EF, Boellaard R, Hoekstra OS, Dijkmans BA, Lammertsma AA, Voskuyl AE. 18F-FDG PET as a tool to predict the clinical outcome of infliximab treatment of rheumatoid arthritis: An explorative study. Journal of Nuclear Medicine. 2011;**52**:77-80

[46] Kiss E, Kovacs L, Szodoray P. Malignancies in systemic lupus erythematosus. Autoimmunity Reviews. 2010;**9**:195-199

[47] O'Byrne KJ, Dalgleish AG. Chronic immune activation and inflammation as the cause of malignancy. British Journal of Cancer. 2001;**85**:473-483

[48] Sela O, Shoenfeld Y. Cancer in autoimmune diseases. Seminars in Arthritis and Rheumatism. 1988;**18**:77-87

[49] Carter PH, Zhao Q. Clinically validated approaches to the treatment of autoimmune diseases. Expert Opinion on Investigational Drugs. 2010;**19**:195-213

[50] Oh JR, Song HC, Kang SR. The clinical usefulness of ^{18}F-FDG PET/CT in patients with systemic autoimmune disease. Nuclear Medicine and Molecular Imaging. 2011;**45**:177-184

[51] Ergül N, Çermik TF. FDG-PET or PET/CT in fever of unknown origin: The diagnostic role of underlying primary disease. International Journal of Molecular Imaging. 2011:318051

[52] Balink H, Bennink RJ, van Eck-Smit BLF, Verberne HJ. The role of ^{18}F-FDG PET/CT in large-vessel vasculitis: Appropriateness of current classification criteria? BioMed Research International. 2014;**2014**:687608

3

YKL-40: The Search for New Biomarkers in Rheumatoid Arthritis

Maria H. Kazakova and Victoria S. Sarafian

Abstract

There is a need for biomarkers to detect early joint inflammation and destruction of cartilage in different types of arthritis. YKL-40, a 39 kDa heparin- and chitin-binding secreted glycoprotein (also known as human cartilage gp39), has been recently discovered. Its exact biological function is still unclear. Specific receptors for YKL-40 have not been identified yet. The clinical significance of YKL-40 as a biomarker is discussed in different aspects. High level of YKL-40 is found in various human i`nflammatory and neoplastic diseases. We present a review highlighting the information available on YKL-40 and its significance in inflammatory joint diseases, like rheumatoid arthritis (RA). We also report original personal data on the topic concerning YKL-40 levels in serum and synovial fluid of patients with RA in comparison with ultrasonographic parameters and cytokine levels. The findings suggest that YKL-40 might be implicated in the pathogenesis of the disease and could indicate the level of joint inflammation.

Keywords: YKL-40, biomarkers, ultrasonography, cytokines, chitinases

1. Introduction

Identification of new biomarkers would be beneficial for improving biomedical research and drug development. Understanding the relationship between biological processes and clinical outcomes is significant for choosing optimal therapy [1].

A "biomarker" is "a characteristic that is objectively measured and evaluated as an indicator of normal biological processes, pathogenic processes, or pharmacological responses to a therapeutic intervention" [2]. The acceptance of novel biomarkers in clinical settings requires detailed validation process before they could be used in routine clinical practice.

Utility of new biomarkers depends on several aspects: whether the method for detection of the biomarker is a specific, sensitive, fast, and affordable, if the level of the biomarker provides new information about the disease, if the concentration of the biomarker could help the patient's treatment [3].

The current review summarizes our investigations and presents evidences for the role of YKL-40 in the diagnosis and prognosis monitoring of rheumatoid arthritis (RA).

2. YKL-40: gene, protein, regulation, and proposed functions

2.1. YKL-40: protein and gene

YKL-40 is a glycoprotein that is encoded by the *CHI3L1* gene and belongs to the mammalian chitinase-like proteins [4].

Chitinases are enzymes that digest chitin, providing cellular and tissue remodeling during homeostasis in fungi, helminths, insects, and crustaceans [5]. Mammals express both enzymatically active chitinases and enzymatically inactive chitinase-like proteins. The exact biologic role of chitinase-like proteins, such as human YKL-40 protein, is still unclear.

YKL-40 was found out in 1989 as the most abundant protein secreted by MG63 human osteosarcoma cell line [6]. It is also known as human cartilage glycoprotein-39 [4], chitinase 3-like-1 protein [7], chondrex [8], and breast regression protein 39 kDa [9].

The human *YKL-40* gene is located on chromosome 1q32.1 and consists of 10 exons [7]. The promoter sequence contains binding sites for several known factors. The Sp1-family transcription factor had a dominant role in controlling YKL-40 promoter activity [10]. It contains a single polypeptide chain, comprising 383 amino acids, where the three N-terminal amino acids are Y (tyrosine), K (lysine), and L (leucine) and had a molecular mass of 40 kDa [4]. Two mutations of the catalytic glutamic and aspartic acids to leucine and to alanine, respectively, are responsible for the lack of hydrolase activity of YKL-40 [10]. The crystallographic structure of human YKL-40 exhibits two globular domains, forming a groove which corresponds to the active cite of the protein [10].

2.2. YKL-40 ligands

Recent studies suggested different ligands for YKL-40. It was determined that the glycoprotein could facilitate the cross-link between syndecan-1 and integrin [11]. Syndecan-1 is a heparan sulfate proteoglycan acting as a transmembrane receptor. Its coupling with other receptors such as integrins might induce cell adhesion and angiogenesis [12]. It was suggested that YKL-40 could activate key signaling cascades—PI3K/AKT and MAPK/ERK resulting in high rate of cell proliferation and tumor cell survival [13, 14].

These signaling pathways could promote proliferation of synoviocytes and altered innate immunity in inflammatory arthritis [15, 16]. Kjaergaard et al. [17] suggested that another heparan sulfate proteoglycan, perlecan, might be a possible ligand for YKL-40. It was revealed that perlecan comprised distinct effects on angiogenesis dependent on integrin coupling [17, 18].

It was shown that lectin-glycan associations determined the organization of plasma membrane and modulated interactions between surface glycoproteins and receptors [19]. Recently, He et al. [20] identified the interleukin-13 subunit $\alpha2$ (IL-13Raα2) as a possible receptor for YKL-40. They found that the activation of YKL-40 was not dependent on interaction with IL-13Raα2, suggesting that a coreceptor should be considered. The authors supposed that IL-13, IL-13Raα2, and Chi3l1/YKL-40/formed a multimeric complex, but they did not provide details [20].

Still unanswered questions are as follows: how YKL-40 interacts with perlecan? how IL-13, YKL-40, and IL-13Rα2 cooperate? whether the glycoprotein binds to other receptors?

2.3. YKL-40 regulation

Studies focused on YKL-40 regulation revealed controversial data and diverse effects.

Insulin growth factor-I (IGF-I) and insulin growth factor-II (IGF-II) were shown to trigger YKL-40 secretion in guinea pig chondrocytes but not in human chondrocytes [21, 22]. The results might be due to differences in the investigated species.

Proinflammatory interleukins, such as IL-2, IL-6, IL-12, IL-13, IL-17, and IL-18, did not induce YKL-40 transcription in astrocytes [23], while IL-6 and IL-17 showed enhanced production in human primary chondrocyte culture [22, 24].

Different kinds of stressors (hypoxia, ionizating radiation, treatment with TNF-α, bFGF, p53 inhibition, serum depletion) were shown to influence YKL-40 induction on three human malignant glioma cell lines:U87, U118, and U373 [25]. It was found that corticosteroids inhibited YKL-40 protein and mRNA levels in subsets of macrophages (proinflammatory or classically activated macrophages) [26]. Zhang et al. determined that resveratrol inhibited YKL-40 expression by influencing its promoter activity and mRNA transcription levels in U87 cells in vitro [27].

Alterations in the extracellular microenvironment also alter YKL-40 synthesis. Microarray gene expression analysis showed that the gene was overexpressed in dedifferentiated human fetal chondrocytes in comparison with differentiated chondrocytes [28].

YKL-40 secretion is activated by cartilage resection or by replacement of chondrocytes from their native environment. The level of YKL-40 secreted by normal cartilage explants is low during the first day of culture and increases significantly after a few days [22].

A study on the expression of YKL-40 in normal mouse mammary gland development found that YKL-40 was upregulated in ductal epithelial cells. The glycoprotein had the ability to inhibit epithelial secretion and differentiation and to facilitate cell migration under hormone stimulation [29].

The available data regarding the regulation of YKL-40 are quite controversial. These results emphasize the differences in *in vitro* and *in vivo* effects of YKL-40 on cellular and systemic response. We could suggest that YKL-40 might play various roles depending on the cell type it is expressed by.

2.4. Proposed functions for YKL-40

Little is known about the functions of YKL-40 in normal conditions. The glycoprotein is detected during early human embryonic development which is related to rapid proliferation and morphogenetic changes [30].

There is no fixed reference value for YKL-40 in healthy people. It was determined that the level of the glycoprotein increased with age, and it was assumed to be used with an age-matched control group [31]. Johansen proposed serum YKL-40 concentration higher than 20% to be considered as elevated [32]. Published levels of YKL-40 in healthy individuals differ among populations [33–35] and are shown in **Table 1**. We could speculate that divergent YKL-40 levels could be explained with differences in sample collection and assays, genetic polymorphisms, or even epigenetics.

Researchers suggest that YKL-40 protects the extracellular matrix during tissue remodeling via suppression of different types of metalloproteinases [40]. Another study showed that the glycoprotein defined which cells to survive during mammary involution [41] and provided protection against apoptosis [42].

YKL-40 was supposed to induce signaling cascades in connective tissue and functioned as a growth factor for synovial cells and chondrocytes [32]. It was found that YKL-40 worked synergistically with insulin growth factor-1 (IGF-1) to induce fibroblasts growth [21]. YKL-40 was discussed as a differentiation marker for monocytes [7], mesenchymal stem cells [43], and chondrocytes [44].

YKL-40 functions as a migration and adhesion factor for vascular cells and helps the formation of branching tubules. Thus, the glycoprotein could play a role in angiogenesis [11].

A variety of independent investigations demonstrated that high levels of YKL-40 were related to metastasis and poor survival in different human carcinomas, such as breast cancer [11], colorectal cancer [45], ovarian cancer [46], high-grade glioma [47], and lymphoma [48], suggesting that YKL-40 might serve as a diagnostic, risk assessment, and prognostic biomarker. Other studies indicated that YKL-40 increased also in inflammatory disorders associated with tissue remodeling and destruction [24, 49].

	Population	Serum YKL-40 levels	References
1.	Danish	43	[33]
2.	French	59	[36]
3.	Chinese	61.1	[37]
4.	Bulgarian	84.19	[35]
5.	Japanese	101.7	[38]
6.	Turkish	114	[34]

Table 1. Mean serum YKL-40 levels (ng/ml) in healthy individuals from different populations [39].

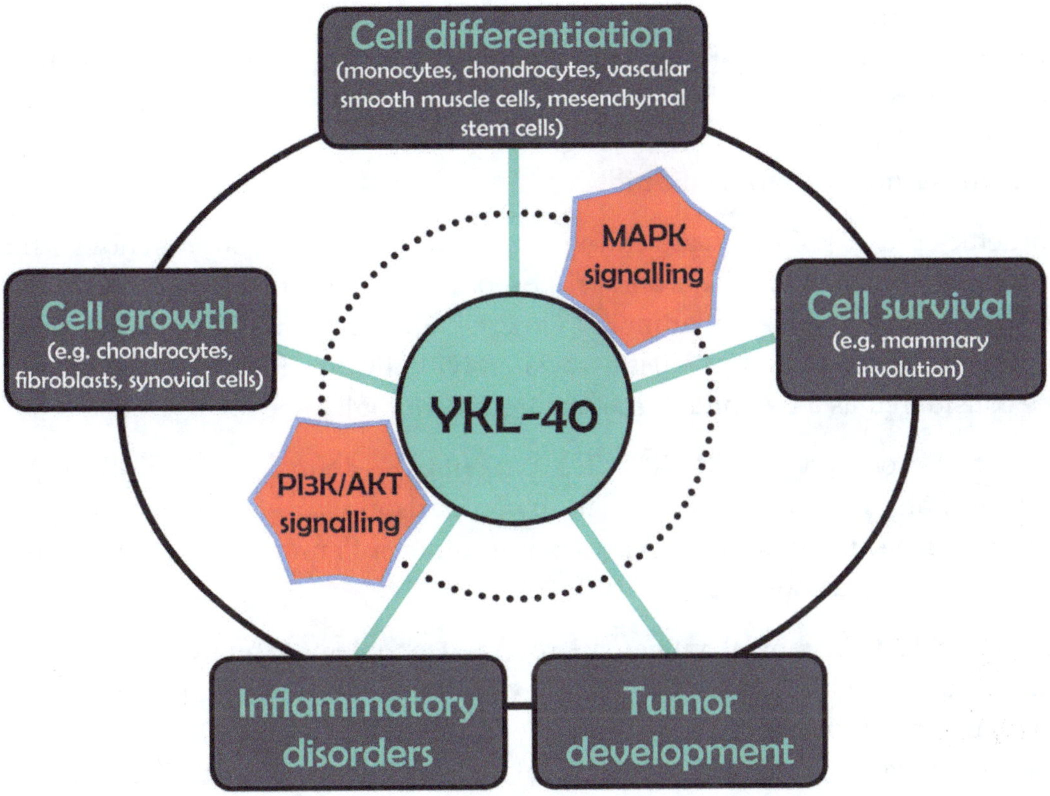

Figure 1. Biological functions of YKL-40. Involvement in cell growth and differentiation, cell survival, inflammatory disorders and tumor development; participation in two basic cell signaling cascades.

YKL-40 is a member of an evolutionary highly conserved protein family, described not only in humans [9, 30], proposing important biological role in normal and pathological conditions. The summarized functions of YKL-40 are presented in **Figure 1**.

3. YKL-40 and rheumatoid arthritis

It is believed that genetic and environmental factors are implicated in the etiology of RA. It is a chronic inflammatory disease which affects about 0.5–1% of the population. Patients suffer from chronic synovial inflammation, joint degradation, and functional disability [50]. Even though some clinical laboratory parameters are related to the risk of radiographic progression, they do not illustrate individual features in the pathogenesis of disease [51].

There is a lack of specific markers for early diagnosis, prognosis, and monitoring of effective treatment. Reliable biomarkers of joint inflammation and destruction in RA should be proteins produced by cells in the synovial fluid and leading to pathological alterations. YKL-40 is expressed and secreted by activated macrophages and neutrophils, fibroblast-like synovial cells, chondrocytes, and vascular smooth muscle cells [32]. Our immunocytochemical study also found that YKL-40 was present in polymorphonuclear cells in the synovial fluid of RA patients [52]. We suppose that it might reflect more precisely the local inflammatory process.

The investigations on the significance of serum YKL-40 as a novel inflammatory biomarker are polar. Some researchers show that it could be useful as an informative parameter in disease diagnosis and monitoring [53], and others state that it is merely a marker of joint inflammation [54].

3.1. YKL-40 in serum and synovial fluid

Johansen detected a 10-fold increase in the concentration of YKL-40 in synovial fluid compared to serum levels in RA patients and proposed that the level of YKL-40 might reflect cartilage degradation and synovial inflammation in RA [32]. These findings are in agreement with other studies, suggesting that YKL-40 is associated with the development of osteoarthritis and should be considered as a potential target for treatment [55].

Our observations focused on YKL-40 in RA patients also found significantly higher glycoprotein concentrations in the synovial fluid in comparison with serum levels [35]. However, we determined the same pattern of expression in other inflammatory joint diseases such as osteoarthritis, gout, and psoriatic arthritis [56].

Huber et al. established synovial antigen microarray technology to analyze antibody profile in RA patients. The synovial glycoprotein YKL-40 was one of the 225 peptides and proteins studied, and it was proved to generate autoantibody production [57]. YKl-40 was also detected as a target of T cells and as a specific and independent histologic marker in arthritic synovitis [58, 59].

There are a number of studies in which a multi-biomarker disease activity (MBDA) score is used to evaluate disease activity, prediction of radiographic progression, and prognosis in RA patients. MBDA score is estimated by measuring the concentrations of 12 serum biomarkers. YKL-40 is a part of the established panel of parameters [60, 61]. This fact confirms the potential significance of YKL-40 in the pathogenic route of RA.

The role of YKL-40 in inflammation still remains to be resolved. The question is whether YKL-40 is an active participant in the process of inflammation or is a result of the body response to it.

3.2. YKL-40 and conventional laboratory parameters

C-reactive protein (CRP) and erythrocyte sedimentation rate (ESR) are the best known and frequently used conventional parameters at the time of diagnosis of RA, but they are not considered as predictors of poor prognosis. Radiological progression of joint destruction could often appear despite normal values. This is a common event in early RA stages [62].

Several studies investigated the significance of YKL-40 in relation to CRP and ESR [53]. We also determined a strong association between YKL-40 levels in serum and synovial fluid and CRP and ESR [35]. Thus, YKL-40 could be regarded as an informative proinflammatory biomarker.

3.3. YKL-40 and ultrasonography

Angiogenesis is a major result of synovial inflammation and maintenance of the pannus in RA [63]. Conventional radiology and tomography could not provide direct visualization of the joint cartilage. The decreased in joint space is only an indirect evidence for joint destruction. Some authors use ultrasonograhy to measure and register early arthritic changes in joint thickness and to figure joint surfaces before they could be detected by routine radiologic methods [64]. We also applied ultrasonography as a sensitive technique for detecting synovial alteration. A relationship between ultrasonographic findings and YKL-40 was detected. Analysis of the data confirmed that the sonographic inflammation correlated with angiogenesis of the synovial membrane [35].

3.4. YKL-40 and angiogenesis

Vascular epidermal growth factor (VEGF) is a key factor in the pathogenesis of RA, serving both as a cell mitogen for endothelial cells and as a factor defining vascular permeability [65]. Several research groups revealed that secreted and expressed VEGF was related to the inflammatory response, to changes in the synovium, and to other conventional markers [65, 66].

YKL-40 also promotes attachment and migration of vascular endothelial cells, which indicates that the protein participates in angiogenesis [11]. Francescone et al. showed that YKL-40 induced VEGF expression in the U87 glioblastoma cell line and supposed that both molecules synergistically promoted endothelial cell angiogenesis [67].

VEGF was influenced by hypoxia, which contributed to RA development and altered response in arthritic synovium [64]. Similarly, YKL-40 was also upregulated by hypoxia in tumor cells [25]. It is assumed that the pathogenic features of arthritic synovium share the same characteristics with tumor cells.

3.5. YKL-40 and cytokines

Recent studies defined proinflammatory cytokines as major participants in RA pathogenesis resulting in identification of new molecular targets. It was shown that the production of tumor necrosis factor-alpha (TNF-α) is involved in the pathogenesis of RA [68], and biological inhibitors of this cytokine were approved for clinical use [69]. It was proved that levels of proinflammatory cytokines such as IL-1α, TNF-α, IL-6, and IFN-γ in the serum and synovial fluid of RA patients correlated with disease activity and progression [70]. Our investigations determined a strong link between serum and synovial levels of YKL-40 and serum TNF-α and IL-1β in patients with RA [71]. The cellular sources of TNF-α and IL-1β are circulating monocytes and macrophages [72]. It was shown that YKL-40 originated from the same cell types [32].

4. Conclusion

Investigations published so far determine YKL-40 as an important molecule in RA pathogenesis. It is assumed that circulating YKL-40 might reflect precisely the activity of local and systemic inflammation. The clinical utility of YKL-40 as diagnostic or prognostic marker in RA remains to be further clarified, but still it gives rise to serious expectations in the search of new promising biomarkers.

Acknowledgements

The studies are supported by Medical University–Plovdiv—Grants No-01/2009, NO-01/2010, DP-08/2012 and partially by DUNK 01/2009 from the Ministry of Education and Science—Bulgaria.

The authors thank Yana Feodorova, PhD for the help in the design of the figure.

Author details

Maria H. Kazakova and Victoria S. Sarafian*

*Address all correspondence to: victoriasarafian@gmail.com

Department of Medical Biology, Faculty of Medicine, Medical University-Plovdiv, Bulgaria

References

[1] Strimbu K, Tavel J. What are biomarkers? Curr Opin HIV AIDS. 2010;6:463–466. doi:10.1097/COH.0b013e32833ed177

[2] Atkinson AJ. Biomarkers and surrogate endpoints: preferred definitions and conceptual framework. Clin Pharmacol Ther. 2001;69:89–95.

[3] Morrow D, Cannon C, Jesse R, et al. Clinical characteristics and utilization of biochemical markers in acute coronary syndromes. Circulation. 2007;13:356–375.

[4] Hakala B, White C, Recklies AD. Human cartilage gp-39, a major secretory product of articular chondrocytes and synovial cells, is a mammalian member of a chitinase protein family. J Biol Chem. 1993;268:25803–25810.

[5] Chaplin D. Overview of the immune response. J Allergy Clin Immunol. 2010;125:S3–23. doi:10.1016/j.jaci.2009.12.9802012

[6] Johansen JS, Williamson MK, Rice JS, et al. Identification of proteins secreted by human osteoblastic cells in culture. J Bone Miner Res. 1992;7:501–512.

[7] Rehli M, Krause SW, Andreesen R. Molecular characterization of the gene for human cartilage gp-39(CHI3L1), a member of the chitinase protein family and marker for late stages of macrophage differentiation. Genomics. 1997;43:221–225.

[8] Harvey S, Whaley J, Eberhardt K. The relationship between serum levels of YKL-40 and disease progression in patients with early rheumatoid arthritis. Scand J Rheumatol. 2000;29:391–393.

[9] Morrison BW, Leder P. neu and ras initiate murine mammary tumors that share genetic markers generally absent in c-myc and int-2-initiated tumors. Oncogene. 1994;9:3417–3426.

[10] Fusetti F, Pijning T, Kalk KH, Bos E, Dijkstra BW. Crystal structure and carbohydrate-binding properties of the human cartilage glycoprotein-39. J Biol Chem. 2003;278:37753–37760.

[11] Shao R. YKL-40 acts as an angiogenic factor to promote tumor angiogenesis. Front Physiol. 2013;4:122.

[12] McQuade KJ, Beauvais DM, Burbach BJ, Rapraeger AC. Syndecan-1 regulates alphav-beta5 integrin activity in B82L fibroblasts. J Cell Sci. 2006;119:2445–2456.

[13] Faibish M, Francescone R, Bentley B, Yan W, Shao R. A YKL-40-neutralizing antibody blocks tumor angiogenesis and progression: a potential therapeutic agent in cancers. Mol Cancer Ther. 2011;10:742–751. doi:10.1158/1535-7163.MCT-10-0868

[14] Kim H, Lee B, Song Y, et al. Potential association between coronary artery disease and the inflammatory biomarker YKL-40 in asymptomatic patients with type 2 diabetes mellitus. Cardiovasc Diabetol. 2012;11:84. doi:10.1186/1475-2840-11-84

[15] Malemud Ch. Intracellular signaling pathways in rheumatoid arthritis. J Clin Cell Immunol. 2013. doi:10.4172/2155-9899.1000160

[16] Wisler BA, Dennis JE, Malemud CJ. New organ-specific pharmacological strategies interfering with signaling pathways in inflammatory disorders/autoimmune disorders. Curr Signal Transduct Ther. 2011;6:279–291.

[17] Kjaergaard A, Johansen J, Bojesen S, Nordestgaard B. Role of inflammatory marker YKL-40 in the diagnosis, prognosis and cause of cardiovascular and liver diseases. Crit Rev Clin Lab Sci. 2016. doi:10.1080/10408363.2016.1190683

[18] Clarke DN, Al Ahmad A, Lee B, et al. Perlecan domain V induces VEGf secretion in brain endothelial cells through integrin $\alpha5\beta1$ and ERK-dependent signaling pathways. PLoS One. 2012;7:e45257.

[19] Rabinovich D, Croci G. Regulatory circuits mediated by lectin-glycan interactions in autoimmunity and cancer. Immunity. 2012;36:322–335.

[20] He C, Lee CG, Cruz C, Lee CM, Zhou Y,Ahangari F, et al. Chitinase 3-like 1 regulates cellular and tissue responses via IL-13 receptor $\alpha2$. Cell Rep. 2013;4(4):830–841. doi:10.1016/j.celrep.2013.07.032

[21] De Ceuninck F, Gaufillier S, Bonnaud A, Sabatini M, Lesur C, Pastoureau P. YKL-40 (Cartilage gp-39) induces proliferative events in cultured chondrocytes and synoviocytes and increases glycosaminoglycan synthesis in chondrocytes. Biochem Biophys Res Commun. 2001;285:926–931.

[22] Johansen JS, Olee T, Price PA, Hashimoto S, Ochs RL, Lotz M. Regulation of YKL-40 production by human articular chondrocytes. Arthritis Rheum. 2001;44:826–837.

[23] Bonneh-Barkay D, Bissel S, Kofler J, Starkey A, Guoji Wang G, Clayton A. Wiley Astrocyte and macrophage regulation of YKL-40 expression and cellular response in neuroinflammation. Brain Pathol. 2012;22:530–546. doi:10.1111/j.1750-3639.2011.00550.x

[24] Väänänen T, Koskinen A, Paukkeri E, et al. YKL-40 as a novel factor associated with inflammation and catabolic mechanisms in osteoarthritic joints. Mediat Inflamm. 2014. doi:10.1155/2014/215140

[25] Junker N, Johansen JS, Hansen LT, Lund EL, Kristjansen PEG. Regulation of YKL-40 expression during genotoxic or microenvironmental stress in human glioblastoma cells. Cancer Sci. 2005;96:183–190.

[26] Kunz L, Wout E, Schadewijk A, Postma D, Kerstjens, Sterk P, Hiemstra P. Regulation of YKL-40 expression by corticosteroids: effect on pro-inflammatory macrophages in vitro and its modulation in COPD in vivo. Respir. Res. 2015;16:154–164.

[27] Zhang W, Kawanishi M, Miyake K et al. Association between YKL-40 and adult primary astrocytoma. Cancer. 2010;116:2688–2697.

[28] Stokes DG, Liu G, Coimbra IB, Piera-Velazquez S, Crowl RM, Jimenez SA. Assessment of the gene expression profile of differentiated and dedifferentiated human fetal chondrocytes by microarray analysis. Arthritis Rheum. 2002;46:404–419.

[29] Scully S, Yan W, Bentley B, Cao Q, Shao R. Inhibitory activity of YKL-40 in mammary epithelial cell differentiation and polarization induced by lactogenic hormones: a role in mammary tissue involution. PLoS One. 2011;6:e25819. doi:10.1371/journal.pone.0025819

[30] Johansen JS, Høyer PE, Larsen LA, Price PA, Møllgård K. YKL-40 protein expression in the early developing human musculoskeletal system. J Histochem Cytochem. 2007;55:1213–1228.

[31] Bojesen SE, Johansen JS, Nostegaard BG. Plasma YKL-40 levels in healthy subjects from the general population. Clin Chim Acta. 2011. doi:10.1016/j.cca.2011.01.022

[32] Johansen JS. Studies on serum YKL-40 as a biomarker in diseases with inflammation, tissue remodelling, fibroses and cancer. Dan Med Bull. 2006;53:172–209.

[33] Johansen JS, Lottenburger T, Nielsen HJ, Jensen JE, Svendsen MN, Kollerup G, Christensen IJ. Weekly, and long-time variation in serum concentrations of YKL-40 in healthy subjects. Cancer Epidemiol Biomarkers Prev. 2008:2603–2608.

[34] Gungen G, Ardic F, Findikoglu G, Rota S. The effect of mud pack therapy on serum YKL-40 and hsCRP levels in patients with knee osteoarthritis. Rheumatol Int. 2009. doi:10.1007/s00296-010-1727-4

[35] Kazakova M, Batalov A, Deneva T, Mateva N, Kolarov Z, Sarafian V. Relationship between sonographic parameters and YKL-40 levels in rheumatoid arthritis. Rheumatol Int. 2013;33:341–346.

[36] Conrozier Th, Carlier M-C, Mathieu P, Colson F, Debard AL, Richard S, et al. Serum levels of YKL-40 and C reactive protein in patients with hip osteoarthritis and healthy subjects: a cross sectional study. Ann Rheum Dis. 2000;59:828–831.

[37] Zou X, Zhang W. The efficacy of YKL-40 and CA125 as biomarkers for epithelial ovarian cancer. Braz J Med Biol Res. 2010;43:1232–1238.

[38] Yamamori H, Hashimoto R, Ohi K, Yasuda Y, Fukumoto M, Kasahara E, et al. A promoter variant in the chitinase 3-like 1 gene is associated with serum YKL-40 level and personality trait. Neurosci Lett. 2012;513:204–208.

[39] Kazakova M, Sarafian V. YKL-40 in health and disease: a challenge for joint inflammation. Biomed Rev. 2013;24:49–56.

[40] Ling H, Recklies AD. The chitinase 3-like protein human cartilage glycoproein 39 inhibits cellular responses to the inflammatory cytokines interleukin-1 and tumor necrosis factor-alpha. Biochem J. 2004;380:651–659.

[41] Malinda KM, Ponce L, Kleinman HK, et al. Gp38k, a protein synthesized by vascular smooth muscle cells, stimulates directional migration of human umbilical vein endothelial cells. Exp Cell Res 1999;250:168–173.

[42] Lee CG, Hartl D, Lee GR, Koller B, Matsuura H, Da Silva CA, Sohn MH, Cohn L, Homer RJ, Kozhich AA, et al. Role of breast regression protein 39 (BRP-39)/chitinase 3-like-1 in Th2 and IL-13-induced tissue responses and apoptosis. J Exp Med. 2009;206:1149–1166.

[43] Hoover D, Zhu V, Chen R, Briley, Rameshwar P, et al. Expression of the chitinase family glycoprotein YKL-40 in undifferentiated, differentiated and trans-differentiated mesenchymal stem cells. PLoS One. 2013;8. doi:info:doi/10.1371/journal.pone.0096230

[44] Imabayashi H, Mori T, Gojo S, Kioyono T, Sugiyama T, Irie R, Isoga T, Hata J, Toyama Y, Umezawa A. Redifferentiation of dedifferentiated chondrocytes and chondrogenesis of human bone marrow stromal cells via chondrosphere formation with expression profiling by large-scale cDNA analysis. Exp Cell Res 2003;288:35–50.

[45] Johansen JS, Christensen IJ, Jørgensen L, Olsen J, Rahr H, Nielsen K, Laurberg S, Brünner N, Nielsen H. Serum YKL-40 in risk assessment for colorectal cancer: a prospective study of 4,496 subjects at risk of colorectal cancer. Cancer Epidemiol Biomarkers Prev. 2015;3:621–626. doi:10.1158/1055-9965.EPI-13-1281

[46] Chiang YC, Lin HW, Chang CF, Chang MC, Fu CF, Chen TC, et al. Overexpression of CHI3L1 is associated with chemoresistance and poor outcome of epithelial ovarian carcinoma. Oncotarget. 2015;6:39740–39755.

[47] Steponaitis G, Skiriute D, Kazlauskas A, Golubickaite I, Stakaitis R, Tamašauskas A, Vaitkiene P. High CHI3L1 expression is associated with glioma patient survival. Diagn Pathol. 2016;11:42. doi:10.1186/s13000-016-0492-4

[48] Hottinger A, Iwamoto F, Karimi S, Riedel E, Dantis J, Park J, et al. YKL-40 and MMP-9 as serum markers for patients with primary central nervous system lymphoma. Ann Neurol. 2011;70:163–169. doi:10.1002/ana.22360

[49] Létuvé S, Kozhich A, Arouche N, Grandsaigne M, Reed J, Dombret MC, et al. YKL-40 is elevated in patients with chronic obstructive pulmonary disease and activates alveolar macrophages. J Immunol. 2008;181:5167–5173.

[50] Mclnnes I, Schett G. The pathogenesis of rheumatoid arthritis. N Engl J Med. 2011;365:2205-2219.

[51] Liao KP, Weinblatt ME, Cui J, et al. Clinical predictors of erosion-free status in rheumatoid arthritis: a prospective cohort study. Rheumatology (Oxford). 2011;50:1473–1479.

[52] Kazakova M, Batalov A, Kolarov Z, Sarafian V. Serum and synovial YKL-40 levels in psoriatic arthritis. Sci Technol. 2012;2:60–63.

[53] Kassem I, Mahmoud L, Salah W. Study of resistin and YKL-40 in rheumatoid arthritis. J Am Sci. 2010;6:1004–1012.

[54] Syversen SW, Goll GL, Heijde D, Landeve R, Lie BA, Odegard S, et al. Prediction of radiographic progression in rheumatoid arthritis and the role of antibodies against mutated citrullinated vimentin: results from a 10-year prospective study. Ann Rheum Dis. 2009;69:345–351. doi:10.1136/ard.2009.113092

[55] Szychlinska M, Trovato F, Di Rosa M, Malaguarnera L, Puzzo L, Leonardi R, Castrogiovanni P, Musumeci G. Co-expression and co-localization of cartilage glycoproteins CHI3L1 and lubricin in osteoarthritic cartilage: morphological, immunohistochemical and gene expression profiles. Int J Mol Sci. 2016:17:359. doi:10.3390/ijms17030359

[56] Kazakova M, Batalov A, Mateva N, Kolarov Z, Sarafian V. Comparative significance of YKL-40 in different types of arthritis. In: Front. Immunol. Conference 15th International Congress of Immunology (ICI); 22-28 August 2013; Milan. Italy: doi:10.3389/conf.fiL

[57] Hueber W, Kidd B, Tomooka B, Lee B, Bruce B, Fries J, et al. Antigen microarray profiling of autoantibodies in rheumatoid arthritis. Arthritis Rheum. 2005;52:2645–2655. doi::10.1002/art.21269

[58] Cope A, Sonderstrup G. Evaluating candidate autoantigens in rheumatoid arthritis. Springer Semin Immunopathol. 1998;20:23–39.

[59] Baeten D, Steenbakkers PG, Rijnders AM, Boots AM, Veys EM, de Keyser F. Detection of major histocompatibility complex/human cartilage gp-39 complexes in rheumatoid arthritis synovitis as a specific and independent histologic marker. Arthritis Rheum. 2004;50:444–451.

[60] Bakker M, Cavet G, WG Jacobs J, Bijlsma J, Haneym D, Shen Y, Hesterberg L, et al. Performance of a multi-biomarker score measuring rheumatoid arthritis disease activity in the CAMERA tight control study. Ann Rheum Dis. 2012;71:1692–1697.

[61] Hambardzumyan K, Bolce R, Saevarsdottir S, Cruickshank S, Sasso E, et al. Pretreatment multi-biomarker disease activity score and radiographic progression in early RA: results from the SWEFOT trial. Ann Rheum Dis. 2015;74:1102–1109.

[62] Emery P, Salmon M. Early rheumatoid arthritis: time to aim for remission? Ann Rheum Dis. 1995;54:944–947.

[63] Paleolog E. The vasculature in rheumatoid arthritis: cause or consequence? Int J Exp Pathol. 2009;90:249–261.

[64] Batalov A, Kuzmanova S, Penev D. Ultrasonographic evaluation of knee joint cartilage in rheumatoid arthritis patients. Folia Med. 2000;4:23–26.

[65] Lee S, Joo Y, Kim W, et al. Vascular endothelial growth factor levels in the serum and synovial fluid of patients with rheumatoid arthritis. Clin Exp Rheumatol. 2001;19:321–324.

[66] Sone H, Sakauchi M, Takahashi A, et al. Elevated levels of vascular endothelial growth factor in the sera of patients with rheumatoid arthritis correlation with disease activity. Life Sci. 2001;69:1861–1869.

[67] Francescone RA, Scully S, Faibish M, et al. Role of YKL-40 in the angiogenesis, radioresistance, and progression og glioblastoma. J Biol Chem. 2011. doi:10.1074/jbc.M110.212514

[68] Feldmann M, Maini R. Discovery of TNF-alpha as a therapeutic target in rheumatoid arthritis: preclinical and clinical studies. Joint Bone Spine. 2002;69:12–18.

[69] Maini R, Taylor P. Anti-cytokine therapy for rheumatoid arthritis. Annu Rev Med. 2000;51:207–229.

[70] Kolarov Z, Altunkova I, Baleva M, Martinova F, Monov S, Shumnalieva R. Relation between serum and synovial fluei levels of IL-1-alpha, TNF-alpha, IL-6, IFN-gamma and sIL-6r and clinical, immunological and genetic factors in rheumatoid arthritis patients. In: Ann. Rheum. Dis Annual European Congress of Rheumatol. EULAR 2015; 10-13 June 2015; Italy: p. 914.

[71] Kazakova-Velinova M. Immunobiological studies on YKL-40 in inflammatory joint and tumor processes [PhD thesis]. Medical University, Plovdiv; 2013.

[72] Arleevskaya M, Gabdoulkhakova A, Filina J, et al. Mononuclear phagocytes in rheumatoid arthritis patients and their relatives-family similarity. Open Rheumatol J. 2011;5:36–44.

4

MicroRNAs in Rheumatoid Arthritis: From Pathogenesis to Clinical Utility

Agnieszka Paradowska-Gorycka and
Barbara Stypińska

Abstract

Emerging evidence suggests that microRNAs (miRNAs) play a key role in the regulation of immunological functions including innate and adaptive immune responses, development and differentiation of immune cells, and the prevention of autoimmunity. The current state of our knowledge in this area is far from being complete, and continued investigations will be needed to reveal a better understanding of the miRNA network that is involved in the pathogenesis of rheumatoid arthritis (RA). In RA, miRNA plays an important role in many different cellular processes. It has been shown that they modulate inflammatory responses, proliferation of synoviocytes, and production of metalloproteinases in rheumatoid joins and affect the development, differentiation, effector, and regulatory functions of T and B cells and cytokine production. The specific circulating miRNA species may also be useful for the diagnosis, classification, and prognosis of diseases and prediction of the therapeutic response.

Keywords: pathogenesis, epigenetics, microRNA, function of miRNAs, polymorphisms

1. Introduction

Rheumatoid arthritis (RA) is an autoimmune, polygenic disease, which affects millions of people worldwide [1]. Human genetic and epigenetic studies have shown that causal factors of disease include contributions from at least 40 different genes and the effect of environmental factors. Epigenetics represents a new aspect in autoimmunity, which regulates gene expression without alternating DNA sequence. The epigenetic mechanisms are implicated in the final interpretation of the encoded genetic information by regulating gene expression, and alterations in their profile influence the activity of the immune system. Although there are controversies regarding the involvement of genetic and epigenetic factors in RA etiology, it is becoming obvious that the two systems (genetic and epigenetic) interact with each other and are ultimately responsible for RA development.

Recently, the list of molecules important for RA pathogenesis has been extended to microRNAs (miRNAs), which play a central role in regulating both adaptive and innate immune response, development and differentiation of immune cells, and the prevention of autoimmunity [2]. miRNAs regulate protein expression at the posttranscriptional level through reduction of mRNA stability and inhibition of translation [3]. Human miRNA genes are located on all chromosomes except the chromosome Y, are mainly observed in introns (70%), constitute only 3% of the human genome, and regulate about 90% of different genes [4, 5]. These molecules participate in the regulation of the expression of genes involved in the fundamental biological processes related to development, proliferation, and apoptosis, as well as pathological processes including autoimmunity [6, 7].

Although we are still at a very early stage in understanding their impact on immunity, miRNAs are changing the way we think about the development of the immune system and regulation of immune functions. While characterization of miRNA expression patterns in RA patients can have potential diagnostic use, new discoveries in cell type-specific miRNA expression profile, during the disease progression, may provide further understanding of RA pathogenesis. Because miRNAs are stable in plasma or serum, they may be use as biomarkers for the prediction of the disease activity, the differentiation of RA from other rheumatic diseases, or the monitoring of current therapy.

2. Biogenesis

Mature miRNAs are single-stranded, small, noncoding RNAs about 22 nt long. The biogenesis of miRNAs is under tight temporal and spatial control. It starts in nucleus where long primary miRNAs (pri-miRNAs) are transcribed by RNA polymerase II. miRNA sequences are located within various genomic contexts including both intronic and exonic regions. Pri-miRNA transcription is regulated by transcription factors like p53, MYC, ZEB1, ZEB2, and myoblast determination protein 1 (MYOD1). Additionally, epigenetic factors (DNA methylation and histone modifications) regulate this process. The resulting transcript is capped with a specially modified nucleotide at the 5' end (MGpppG) and polyadenylated with a poly(A) tail at 3' end. Pri-miRNA is subsequently cleaved by the so-called microprocessor complex and forms a precursor hairpin miRNA (pre-miRNA). Microprocessor complex is composed of RNase III enzyme—Drosha and of the RNA-binding protein DGCR8 (also known as Pasha). In the next step, pre-miRNA is exported from the nucleus to the cytoplasm in a process involving exportin-5 (Exp-5) and GTP-binding nuclear protein RAN•GTP. Following translocation to the cytoplasm, the pre-miRNA is cleaved, by the cytoplasmic RNase III enzyme Dicer, into 19- to 23-nucleotide mature miRNA duplexes. Although either strand of the duplex may potentially act as a functional miRNA, only one is usually loaded into the RNA-induced silencing complex (RISC) where the miRNA and its mRNA target interact (reviewed by Ref. [8]). miRNA guides RISC complex to the 3'-untranslated region (3'-UTR) of target mRNA to prevent translation of the mRNA into protein. The other (termed the passenger) strand is degraded or released from the cell. There are few different mechanisms of miRNA export from the cell. miRNAs may be released from the cell by exosomes or microvesicles. Moreover, miRNAs can form complexes with high-density lipoproteins or RNA-binding proteins such as Ago2 and in that form circulate outside the cell. Exact mechanism of how these complexes are transported from the cell still remains unknown. They may be released passively, after cell death, or actively through specific membrane channels or proteins. Interestingly, other pathways for miRNA biogenesis are also emerging. Examples include those that are independent of Drosha or Dicer, "mirtrons"—some small nucleolar RNAs (snoRNAs) and endogenous short hairpin RNAs (shRNAs) [8–10].

3. Mechanism of action

Small noncoding miRNA has the potential to broadly influence various molecular pathways via suppression of unwanted mRNA transcripts. These highly conserved ~22-nucleotide long miRNAs recognize its mRNA target through "seed region" that is located at the 5' end of miRNA and span from nucleotide positions 2–7. It binds to mRNAs' complementary sequence usually located within 3'-untranslated region (3'-UTR). miRNAs silence its target expression via various mechanisms leading to mRNA degradation or preventing mRNA from being translated [11]. After specific mRNA sequence recognition, argonaute (AGO) protein recruits factors that induce translational repression or mRNA degradation. Target mRNA destination depends probably on the sequence complementarity level with miRNA—complete complementarity leads to mRNA degradation and partial complementarity to translational inhibition, although there are exceptions to this rule. Interestingly, some target mRNAs can be exclusively repressed by degradation or translational inhibition, but often it occurs by combination of these two processes (reviewed in Refs. [9, 12]).

3.1. Inhibition of translation

There are still many unknowns around mechanism of translational repression of target mRNA. It is not clear whether miRNA represses translation at the step of translational initiation or posttranslational level [13]. Significant number of studies support model of repression at posttranslational level (protein degradation) or at late stage of translation (premature termination or impaired elongation). These studies demonstrated that miRNA-repressed mRNAs maintained the same distribution pattern across polyribosomes compared with nonrepressed mRNAs [14, 15]. However, other studies showed contradictory results, indicating that repression occurs at the translational initiation step. There are many models proposing mechanism of this process.

Almost all proposed models consider GW182 interaction with one of the Ago proteins as a first step of translational repression. In first model, GW182 disrupts the association between eIF4G and poly-A-binding protein (PABP) and prevents the circularization required for efficient translation. In the second model, formation of the mRNA 40S preinitiation complex occurs, but miRISC complex prevents 60S ribosome from joining it, resulting in translation repression. The third scenario assumes that ribosome is detached earlier leading to premature translation termination. Another possible proposed mechanism assumes that target mRNA is accumulated in so-called processing bodies (P-bodies) that prevents from interaction with translational machinery [12, 16].

3.2. Destabilization of target mRNA

There are two mechanisms of miRNA-mediated mRNA degradation-specific cleavage and non-cleavage mRNA degradation. mRNA degradation by miRNA requires Ago, GW182, and the cellular decapping and deadenylation machinery. miRNA sufficient complementarity to target mRNA leads to its specific cleavage. The process is facilitated through Ago protein slicer activity. Ago cleavage site is determined by miRNA sequence, not mRNA paring residues, and occurs within mRNA pairing site to the 10th and 11th residues of miRNA. Therefore, the degree of complementarity at the 3' end of miRNA is more important than at the 5' end. After cleavage miRNA remains intact and is able to mediate another mRNA silencing [17, 18]. Non-cleavage degradation of target mRNA involves GW182. GW182 forms a bridge between RISC and CCR4-NOT deadenylase complex leading to mRNA deadenylation and decapping [19, 20].

4. Biological function of microRNAs

MicroRNAs as endogenous regulatory molecules are present in plant, animal, and human cells, and they are essential for proper development and functioning of the organism. Their main role is associated with posttranscriptional regulation of the expression of numerous genes in both pathogenic and pathological aspects of diseases (**Figure 1**) [21, 22]. miRNAs together with Argonaute (AGO) proteins, forming a core of the miRNA-induced silencing complex (miRISC) which mediates gene silencing [23]. Each miRNA has several different targets, and many of mRNAs are subject to regulation by more than one miRNA [24]. Over 60% of human genes are controlled by miRNAs, which indicates the great importance of these molecules [23].

The continuous miRNA-mRNA interaction is essential for miRNA function. miRNA genes are present either as independent transcription units or located in introns and exons of other genes. Gene silencing can be done either through degradation of a specific mRNA or as a result of the inhibiting of the transcript translation. Furthermore, the mechanisms by which miRNA complementarity to its target mediates repression are varied [25, 26]. In some cases the miRNA binds with complementarity in the seed region (nucleotides 2–8 of the miRNA) within the 3'-untranslated region (UTR) of mRNA and leads to inhibit target gene translation or less commonly within the 5'-UTR region that enhancement of translation [25, 27]. But on the other hand, the miRNA-mRNA interaction occurs in the central region (bases ~9 to 12) leading to the mRNA cleavage and subsequent degradation [26]. Generally, miRNAs do not act to completely silence their targets, but rather decrease expression. However, the identification of the type of interaction between miRNA and mRNA remains a very important focus to understand control in gene expression [26, 27].

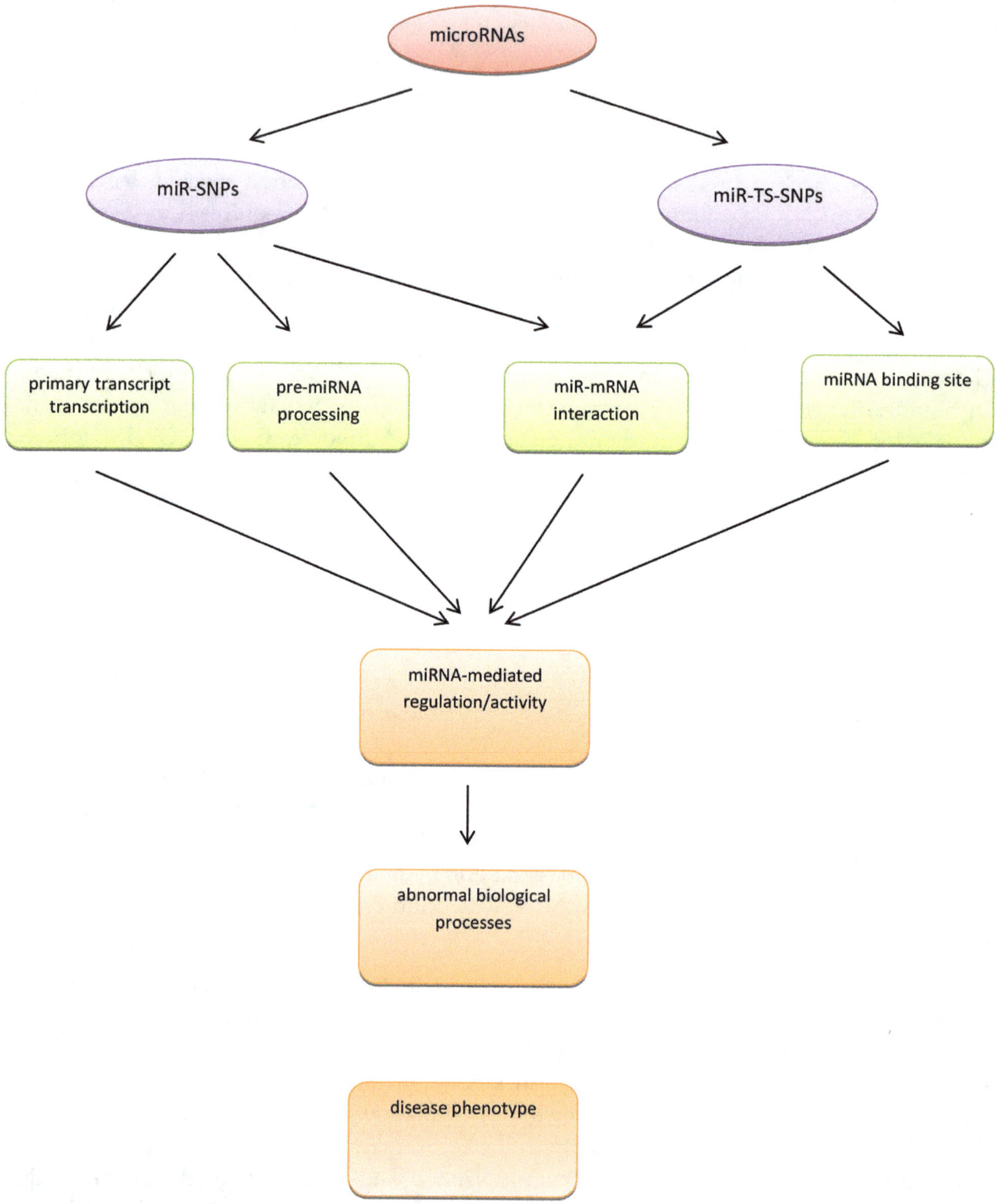

Figure 1. Biological functions of microRNAs.

In the last years, a large number of studies examined cellular miRNA profiles, where expression changes under stress conditions, in cancer, and in other diseases. Distortion of miRNA expression may result in abnormalities in the course of numerous cellular processes, such as development, differentiation, proliferation, inflammation, cell fate determination, apoptosis, signal transduction, organ development, hematopoietic lineage differentiation, host-viral interactions, osteogenesis, and stem cell and germ line proliferation [22, 24, 25, 27–30]. These discoveries may help to clarify molecular mechanisms of diseases and based on this knowledge and may help to develop new drugs. However, since the amount of miRNA may be differ, its total quantity in the different type of cells and gene silencing efficiency depends on the concentration of mRNA targets interpretation of miRNA expression, as well as profiles, including clinical studies, should be performed with attention.

While the majority of miRNAs are found intracellularly, miRNAs may also function beyond RISC, as an extracellular, in virtually all known body fluids [31, 32]. The extracellular miRNAs are secreted into exosomes or microvesicles [26]. However, little is known about the origin of body fluid miRNAs in both healthy and disease conditions or what factors affect their levels in serum/plasma [31]. One hypothesis suggests that blood cells are the major contributors to extracellular miRNAs in the serum or plasma, but another hypothesis speculates that organs may also contribute to extracellular miRNAs because tissue-enriched miRNAs (e.g., miR-122 in the liver, miR-133 in the muscle, miR-208 in the heart, and miR-124 in the brain) are also detected in serum or plasma [31]. Independently of existing hypotheses, explanation of the origin of the extracellular miRNA would increase our understanding of their potential pathophysiological significance. In addition, regardless of their origin, extracellular miRNAs are extremely stable, and their concentration did not significantly change with prolonged incubation of blood plasma at room temperature [23]. The level and composition of extracellular miRNAs in body fluids, such as serum or plasma, are correlated with several pathological conditions, including cancer, diabetes, inflammatory diseases, as well as tissue injury [31]. Moreover, expression patterns of miRNAs are also different between disease state and normal tissue [26] and appear to be tissue specific [21]. However, current knowledge about the biological function of extracellular miRNAs is in its infancy stage. Nevertheless, it seems that extracellular miRNAs may act as signaling molecules and mediate distant cell-cell communication. Cross talk mediated by these miRNAs may provide new insights into the understanding of the mechanisms underlying various dysfunctional conditions. Cross talk through these miRNAs may provide new look at the understanding of the mechanisms underlying the various dysfunctional states [31].

5. Rheumatoid arthritis as a chronic civilization disease

Rheumatoid arthritis is one of the most prevalent chronic inflammatory diseases and is characterized by progressive joint inflammation, by destruction of articular cartilage and underlying bone, and by synovial hyperplasia. RA can affect any joint, with a joint cavity lined by synovial membrane (SM) [33, 34]. The disease process is highly variable, with periods of exacerbation and remission, and uncontrolled inflammation leads to progressive joint damage, pain, long-term disability, and reduced quality of life in many patients [34, 35].

Although RA affects people all over the world, women are affected three times more than men with the peak of incidence between 35 and 55 years of age [33, 36–38]. The incidence of rheumatoid arthritis is relatively constant in most European and North-American populations and is estimate between 0.5% and 1%. RA incidence decreases from north to south and from urban to rural areas. A positive family history increased the risk of RA, and we can see that the familial RA occurrences are about 10–30% of patients, whereas the concordance rate is 12–15% in monozygotic twins and 3–4% in dizygotic twins [39].

RA is pathologically heterogeneous and it is classified among systemic autoimmune disorders because of the presence of rheumatoid factor (RF) and other autoantibodies such as anticitrullinated protein autoantibodies (ACPAs) [35, 40, 41]. RF is present in about 60–85% patients with RA; ACPAs appear to be equally sensitive (75%) and highly specific: 94% for the established disease and 61% for early RA, which may be able to serve as an early diagnostic marker and prognostic factor of joint destruction [42].

Although the exact etiology remains an active area of worldwide research, it is generally accepted that the RA is a multifactorial disease of which pathogenesis is defined by genetic and environmental factors [21]. Genetic predisposition is responsible for 50–60% of the risk of developing RA [43, 44]. A genetic link to RA was established through the observation of familial clustering of RA and large-scale genome-wide association studies (GWAS) [45]. Moreover, it is suggested that only the specific combination of genetic factors in an individual might determine the outcome of the disease [7]. HLA-DRB1 alleles, which share a common sequence, known as the "shared epitope" account for approximately 30% to 50% of overall genetic susceptibility to RA. Probably some other genes associated with components of the innate and adaptive immune system and other mechanisms such as epigenetics may also play a role in the pathogenesis of RA. Epigenetic mechanisms are engaged in the final interpretation of the genetic information by regulation of the gene expression, and changes in their profile influence the activity of the immune system [46]. The change in epigenetic mechanisms is implicated in the final interpretation of the encoded genetic information by regulating gene expression; on the other hand, genetic mutations in epigenetic regulators may alter the epigenetic profile. Consequently, epigenetics and genetics can be two sides of the same coin, as has been determined in the field of rheumatoid arthritis research [46]. Future challenges are understanding and leveraging of the role of genetics and epigenetic modifications, as well as their functional characteristics in RA pathogenesis and translation of fundamental discoveries into clinical practice [47].

6. miRNAs in the pathogenesis of rheumatoid arthritis

Up to date about 2,500 different miRNAs were discovered in humans. From all of these miRNAs, some may play an important role in the regulation of the innate and adaptive immune responses in patients with RA. Increasing number of studies has shown that abnormal miRNA expression in different fluids or cells from RA patients may lead to inflammation, cytokine signaling, bone degradation, and invasive behavior of resident cells [6]. In addition, there is growing evidence that miRNAs as crucial mediators of inflammation may also regulate the plasticity and the effector functions of differentiated Th-cell subsets [24, 48]. miRNAs on the one hand have an important role in defining and maintaining the gene expression programmer of differentiated Th17 cells, but on the other hand, the miRNA expression in regulatory T cells (Treg cells) is important for the maintenance of self-tolerance. And as we know, abnormally activated inflammatory Th cells and defective Treg cells play primary role in the pathogenesis of RA. Moreover, miRNA expression may be also diverse in the different stages of RA progression, allowing miRNAs to help monitor disease activity and help to understand its pathogenesis [6]. Understanding the potential link between miRNAs and the pathogenesis of RA may lead to future insights into disease diagnosis and treatment [4, 22].

The first evidence that miRNAs may be involved in the molecular mechanisms of RA arose in 2007 with the recognition, in the serum of RA patients, of autoantibodies directed against GW bodies that are cytoplasmic structures for storage and/or degradation of mRNA [4]. The first miRNAs that shown abnormal expression within the inflamed joints of RA patients includes miR-16, miR-146a, and miR-155 [4, 49]. These multifunctional miRNAs play a central role in the inflammatory response and immune dysfunction, in response to microbial components, and are upregulated after immune cell maturation [4]. miR-16 and miR-146a play a role in the regulation of the tumor necrosis factor alpha (TNF-α) signaling, which is one of the key cytokines involved on the pathogenesis of RA [2, 50]. Furthermore, miR-155 could suppress matrix metalloproteinases (MMPs) through the interaction with proinflammatory cytokines and Toll-like receptor (TLR) ligands and lead to modulation of joint inflammation [2, 51]. miR-146a and miR-155 are responsible for the maintenance of immune homeostasis, and their expression changes in RA may alert cytokine secretion from different immune cells [30]. Moreover, "miR-146a and miR-155 are considered the 'yin and yang' of inflammation as these miRNAs are negative and positive regulators of inflammatory responses, respectively" [30]. miR-155 promotes T-cell–mediated tissue inflammation by the regulation of the Th1- and Th17-cell response, and it also through the targeting of SOCS1, a negative regulator of IL-2 signaling, controls Treg cell homeostasis [24]. Like miR-155, miR-146a is highly expressed in Treg cells. Furthermore, in contrast to miR-155, miR-146a required for the suppressive activity of Treg cells is essential for the ability of Treg cells to restrain IFN-γ-mediated pathogenic Th1 responses and associated inflammation [24, 50]. Whereas miR-146a rather reduces the proinflammatory immune responses, miR-155 enhances inflammatory processes [48]. The main advantage of the detection of miR-16 and miR-146a in serum/plasma is that this opens the possibility to test as a biomarker to monitoring disease activity/course, because both have shown positive correlation with C-reactive protein (CRP) and disease activity score in 28 joints (DAS28) [4, 48].

Other tissue and/or extracellular miRNAs have been also shown to be associated with RA (**Table 1**), and those miRNAs can regulate specific cytokine pathways, thus leading to inflammation [27]. Characteristics of miRNA profile in patients with RA suggest putative functions of these factors in cytokine secretion and signaling during chronic inflammatory processes in the joints. The miR-10a, miR-16, miR-23b, and miR-203 may serve to fine-tune cytokine signaling, and they may be responsible for the induction of autoimmune inflammation [24, 50]. Upregulation of miR-16 and miR-203 in synovium of RA patients is responsible for the regulation of the TNF-α signaling and for increased matrix metalloproteinases (MMPs), as well as

IL-6 production, respectively, thus indicating that these miRNAs may plays a role as proinflammatory and joint destructive factors [27, 50]. In contrast, miR-10a and miR-23b, which are downregulated in RA synovial tissue, regulate signaling pathway of proinflammatory cytokines such as IL-1β, TNF-α and IL-6, IL-8, and IL-17, as well as MCP-1 and MMPs, and they may be a strong pathological factors that play a critical role in the onset and progression of RA [50, 52]. The cytokines are also a key regulator of Th17/Treg imbalance, which participate in the immune dysfunction. The immune dysfunction in RA patients is found to be induced by decreased expression of miR-21, which may suppress Treg development while promoting Th17 differentiation. Moreover, this miRNA may serve as a novel regulator of Th17/Treg balance in autoimmune diseases including RA [53]. Another miRNA, which participate in the balance between Th17 and Treg cells, is miR-10a, which exhibits high expression in natural Treg cells, limiting the conversion of inducible Treg cells into follicular helper T cells (Tfh cells) and inhibiting Th17 differentiation [54].

miRNAs	Localization	Target gene	Changes	Function
miR-10a	PBMCs, DCs, nTreg cells	STAT - Signal transducer and activator of transcription Foxp3, Bcl-6, Ncor2	Downregulation	- Control IL-6 and IL-21 signaling - Regulate the stability of Treg cells - Limit the conversion of iTreg cells into Tfh cells - Inhibit Th17 differentiation
miR-16	PBMCs, plasma, synovial fluid	TNF-α	Upregulation	- Marker of disease activity
miR-17-92	RASFs, FLS, B cells	MMP-1, IL-6, IL-8, MCP-1, RANTES	Downregulation	- Modulate apoptosis, proliferation - Joint inflammation and destruction - Regulated proinflammatory cytokine production
miR-21	plasma, PBMCs, $CD4^{+}T$	Foxp3 STAT3	Upregulation	- Regulate th17/Treg balance
miR-22	RASFs	CYR61	Downregulation	- Synovial tissue hyperplasia - Th17 differentiation
miR-23b	ST	IL-1β TNF-α IL-17	Downregulation	- Induction of autoimmune inflammation
miR-24	plasma	TGF - transforming growth factor-β1	Upregulation	- Marker of disease activity - Enhance the inflammation
miR-26a	PBMCs, plasma		Upregulation	- Diagnostic biomarker
miR-30a	ST	BECN1 - beclin 1	Downregulation	- Reduce apoptosis

miRNAs	Localization	Target gene	Changes	Function
miR-34a	RASFs	XIAP	Downregulation	- Contribute to apoptosis
miR-124a	RASFs, synoviocytes	CDK-2 MCP-1 VEGF	Downregulation	- Regulator of RASFs and autoimmune inflammation - Contribute to angiogenesis
miR-125b	serum, blood	NF-κB	Downregulation	- Induce of excessive inflammation
miR-146	SF, ST, RASFs, PBMCs, blood, serum, T cells, B cells, monocytes, macrophages	TLR4, NOX4 - NADPH oxidase 4,	Upregulation	- Marker of disease activity - Inhibit Th1-mediated responses - Suppress activity of Treg cells - Modulated apoptosis
miR-155	ST, SF, RASFs, PBMCs, blood, serum, macrophages	SHIP-1, SOCS-1MyD88, MAP3K10 - Mitogen-Activated Protein Kinase Kinase Kinase 10	Upregulation	- Regulate cytokine expression - Require for homeostasis and function of Treg cells
miR-203	RASFs	MMP-1, NF-κB	Upregulation	- Participate in joint inflammatory state
miR-223	PBMCs, RASFs, ST, plasma, macrophages, monocytes, T cells		Upregulation	- Regulate osteoclastogenesis
miR-451	T cells, neutrophils	p38 MAPK - mitogen-activated protein kinases, CPNE3 - copine 3	Downregulation	- Role in inflammation

PBMCs, peripheral blood mononuclear cells; RASFs, RA synovial fibroblasts; FLS, fibroblast-like synoviocytes; MMP-1, matrix metalloproteinase-1; MCP-1, monocyte chemoattractant protein-1; RANTES, regulated on activation, normal T cell expressed and secreted; ST, synovial tissue; XIAP, X-linked inhibitor of apoptosis protein; CDK-2, cyclin-dependent kinase 2; VEGF, vascular endothelial growth factor; SF, synovial fluid; SHIP-1, Src homology 2-containing inositol phosphatase-1

Table 1. Candidate miRNAs for the RA pathogenesis.

Several of different cells, such as T cells, B cells, or macrophages, have been identified as the sources leading to local joint deformation [55]. These cells are the sources of some miRNAs that, through the regulation of the osteoclastogenesis and differentiation of articular chondrocytes, are implicated in the renewal of cartilage and bone degradation [50]. The best known miRNAs involved in joint destruction are miR-146a and miR-155. However, recently marked expression of other miRNAs, miR-223 and miR-19a/b, have been shown within inflamed joint in patients with RA [3, 4, 51, 56]. miR-223 overexpression suppressed the production of osteoclasts and expression of osteoclast-marked genes [50]. Moreover, an inverse correlation between the plasma miR-223 levels and the tender join count was observed [4]. The expression of the miR-19 was downregulated in RA fibroblast-like synoviocytes (FLS), and this plays a role in joint destruction, in response to TLR stimulation [57]. miR-19a and miR-19b negatively regulate the synthesis of IL-6 and regulate the expression of MMP3, suggesting a role of both these miRNAs in protecting patients with RA from joint inflammation and consequently destruction [57].

The above-addressed miRNAs are not only important positive/negative regulators of inflammatory response and immune dysfunction, but they also may be useful for the prediction of the disease course and identification of early pathological events, as well as beneficial for the development of new therapeutic strategies [50].

7. Therapeutic potential of miRNA in treatment of rheumatoid arthritis

The discovery of the miRNA as regulators of gene expression was followed by a wave of interest and intensive studies for elucidating their role both in physiological and pathological conditions. The obtained results raised hopes for the possibility of developing a number of therapeutic uses of these molecules. miRNAs are characterized by many features that make them excellent candidates for biomarker drug entity. These molecules are small with sequence well-known and often conserved among species, which are very attractive features from a drug development standpoint.

Some alterations of miRNA expression have been associated with many human disorders including autoimmune diseases, metabolic disorders, and genetic diseases. By targeting cells affected with improper miRNA expression, the normal balance of the expression can be restored. Novel systems to achieve targeted modulation of specific miRNA in vivo were developed. By controlling the miRNA that regulate mRNAs in cells, they can be used for therapeutic treatment for certain cellular disorders. Individual miRNAs can be targeted using specifically modified antisense oligonucleotides—anti-miRNAs. By virtue of specific modifications, anti-miRNAs gain improved binding affinity, nuclease resistance, and in vivo delivery. For example, 2′-O-methoxyethyl phosphorothioate (MOE) or N,N-diethyl-4-(4-nitronaphthalen-1-ylazo)-phenylamine (ZEN) oligonucleotide modifications were generated to improve binding affinity and block exonuclease degradation. Other examples are anti-miRNAs conjugated to cholesterol to improve its uptake into the cell through the membrane. Furthermore, the great potential seems to lie in the ability of individual miRNAs to regulate the expression of many related genes, which could lead to the regulation of whole signaling pathways or metabolic modulation using one or more miRNA molecules. On the other hand, effect on multiple targets also involves high risk due to the unexpected side effects. Nevertheless, important role of microRNA in regulation of all cellular processes and constant tissue-specific expression indicates its high potential for diagnostic and therapeutic usage [9]. Moreover, miRNA properties and characteristics indicate their excellent potential to be clinical biomarkers. It is well-known that perfect biomarker should be stable in a sample, easy to assess, specific, and sensitive to relevant changes, and miRNA fulfil these criteria. Although cell endogenous miRNA is not very stable and easily degraded, it was discovered that miRNA detected in the blood [21] (plasma, platelets, nucleated blood cells) and synovial fluid [32] is stable and in the case of miRNA in the blood even resistant to harsh condition like high temperature, high and low pH, or multiple freeze-thaw cycles. miRNAs require this surprising stability due to microparticles (exosomes, microvesicles, and apoptotic bodies), RNA-binding proteins (like Ago2), or lipoprotein complexes [high-density lipoprotein (HDL)] that protect them from degradation. The value of miRNA as molecular biomarkers for diagnosis, prognosis, and prediction of therapeutic response is widely documented in cancer. Another advantage that raises interest in the use of circulating miRNAs as clinical biomarkers is fact that there are highly sensitive and specific miRNA detection methods in a quantitative manner, such as real-time PCR, sequencing, and microarrays. In that respect, circulating miRNAs offer many features to make them an attractive class of biomarkers [10].

7.1. miRNA as potential therapeutic agent for RA treatment

The involvement in the pathophysiology of RA coupled with specific characteristics of miRNAs has triggered the scientific community to start exploring the possibilities of viewing miRNAs as therapeutic entities. Especially the potential of a single miRNA to modulate several genes and affect multiple distinct disease-regulatory pathways simultaneously makes miRNAs particularly attractive candidate targets for chronic inflammatory disease as RA. However, only a limited number of groups have explored the therapeutic potential of miRNAs in RA.

Among many approaches considering belief that one miRNA is able to control several genes and pathways, targeting miR-155 represents the most encouraging miRNA-based therapeutic strategy today.

Currently available data clearly show that miR-155 is crucial for the development of arthritis by increasing production of proinflammatory cytokines and promoting differentiation of antigen-specific T cells and antigen-specific antibodies. Interestingly Kurowska-Stolarska et al. observed that miR-155 deficiency is protective against development of collagen-induced arthritis (CIA) in mice. Inhibition of miR155 was associated with impaired production of proinflammatory cytokines, development of the autoreactive Th17 cells, production of anti-collagen II antibodies, and lack of articular inflammation. MiR-155-deficient mice display reductions in both joint inflammation and bone erosion [58]. Beside miR-155, several miRNAs have been implicated in diseases that affect cartilage or have been identified as essential in cartilage homeostasis or repair. For example, the expression of miR-26a was shown to be reduced in splenic cells isolated from rats with induced arthritis. Treatment with methotrexate restored the expression miR-26a to levels comparable to those of non-arthritic controls, and repeated miR-26a injections stabilized disease severity and reduced synovitis, but had no effect on joint destruction [59]. miR-26a can affect bone formation, through angiogenesis and osteogenesis-positive regulation. Overexpression of miR-26a resulted in enhanced bone regeneration coordinated with improved vascularization in mouse, leading to complete repair of the defect [60]. Nakasa et al. demonstrated in vivo and in vitro that miR146a is also able to prevent bone/cartilage destruction. They observed that in $CD14^+$ human cells transfected by dsmiR-146a and treated with M-CSF and TNFα or Receptor Activator for Nuclear Factor κ B Ligand (RANKL) for osteoclastogenesis induction—tumor necrosis factor receptor-associated factor 6 (TRAF6) protein levels—and the number of Tartrate-resistant acid phosphatase (TRAP)-positive cells were significantly reduced compared to cells transfected with nonspecific dsRNA. Also osteoclast function was significantly inhibited in those cells. Furthermore they tested the efficacy of ds miR-146a inhibition of bone destruction in vivo and observed that the extent of bone and cartilage destruction was reduced in arthritic mice injected with ds miR-146a compared to mice treated with nonspecific dsRNA. However, despite the inhibition of bone/cartilage destruction by ds miR-146a injection, there was no significant difference in the arthritis score between the ds miR-146a-treated group and the nonspecific dsRNA-treated group suggesting that administration of ds miR-146a alone may not be a sufficient treatment for RA [61]. Another group that observed underexpression of miR-451 in neutrophils isolated from patients with RA used a systemic administration to restore normal expression level of miR-451 in mice with monogenic model of autoimmune arthritis (SKG mice). This approach led to reduction in the number of neutrophils in synovium, by suppressing their migration. This "miR-451" treatment resulted in reduced severity of arthritis in SKG mice suggesting its potential as therapeutic agent in RA [62]. miR-124 was also found to negatively regulate osteoclastogenesis of mouse bone marrow macrophages. In rats with adjuvant-induced arthritis (AIA), miR-124 expression level was significantly decreased. Nakamachi et al. observed that injection of miR-124 into rat AIA joints reduces disease severity. It is probably due to miR-124-mediated targeting of NFATC1, a master transcription factor of osteoclast differentiation. This suggests a potential of miR-124 as future therapeutic entity used for arthritis amelioration [63, 64].

Studies on miRNA-based treatment strategies are rare, but we can expect that these therapies will be developed in the near future. Although mentioned above preclinical studies demonstrate the potential of delivering therapeutic miRNAs, numerous challenges still remain in designing effective and safe delivery of these agents in a cell- or tissue-specific manner. We are still lacking evidence of similar miRNA deregulation in human RA and of the ex vivo correction of disease phenotypes in patient-derived cell or tissue samples. Furthermore, the cellular mechanisms that could explain observed clinical benefits of miRNA therapies still need to be characterized in depth.

7.2. miRNA as RA diagnostic biomarkers

The knowledge about potential value of miRNA as molecular biomarkers for diagnosis, prognosis, and prediction of therapeutic response in RA has been expanded. Several abnormally expressed miRNAs in circulation or inflamed joints in RA have been identified. That suggests theirs potential to be used as biomarkers that help to establish or confirm a diagnosis, monitor the degree of immunologic activity or inflammation, or provide prognostic information regarding disease progression and severity. There are few studies that referred the possibility to use plasma and synovial miRNAs as diagnostic biomarkers that distinguish healthy people from patients with RA or another disease with similar symptoms. For example, upregulation of miR-146a, miR-155, and miR-223 has been shown in various compartments such as serum, blood, synovial fluid, and tissues in patients with RA. Many studies observed elevated levels of expression of miR-146a in different tissues from RA patients; some of them confirm that miR146a level is correlated with disease activity that highlights its significance in RA pathogenesis and diagnostic biomarker potential [51, 65–67]. Elsayed et al. confirmed significant upregulation of miR-146a expression in the whole blood of patients with RA and that miR-146a in diagnostic performance was better than anti-CCP and RF. miR-146a expression level allowed for distinguishing RA patients from healthy controls (HCs) with high sensitivity and specificity (96 and 100%, respectively). Moreover, its expression level was positively correlated with disease activity [68]. It is important to note that these studies are limited by a relatively small number of patients and were conducted in patients from different races and ethnicities. Similarly Kriegsmann et al. observed that miR-146a, miR-155, and miR-223 were significantly elevated in RA compared to osteoarthritis (OA) synovial tissues. The sensitivity and specificity for the detection of RA were 0.76/0.80 for miR-146a, 0.80/0.95 for miR-155, and 0.86/0.81 for miR-223. In combination these miRNAs gave even better results as RA diagnostic biomarker with a sensitivity and specificity of 0.84/0.91, respectively [69]. Murata et al. performed comprehensive array study to find out which miRNAs in plasma samples significantly differentiate patients with RA (patients with high disease activity, who had never received any biological therapy such as the anti-TNF agents) from HCs. They tested eleven preselected candidate miRNAs in 102 patients with RA and 104 HCs and found out that miR-125a-5p, miR-26a, and miR-24 expression levels gave the best results. For miR-24, miR-26a, and miR-125a-5p, the values of sensitivity and the specificity were 63.7 and 89.5%, 53.9 and 94.3%, 64.7 and 89.5%, respectively. These results suggest that plasma miR-24, miR-26a, and miR-125a-5p can be diagnostic biomarkers with high specificity. The combinations of miR-24, miR-30a-5p, and miR-125a-5p (termed ePRAM for "estimated probability of RA by plasma miRNAs") with sensitivity 78.4% and specificity 92.3% are more efficient for RA differentiation and have higher diagnostic significance as biomarkers in RA. These selected miRNAs correlate with disease activity (besides miR-125a-5p) erythrocyte sedymentiation rate (ESR), CRP, RF, ACPA, or DAS28 and not only can be markers for diagnosis of RA but also for disease activity of RA [70]. In a small study, Murata et al. assessed the diagnostic usefulness of plasma miR-132 for patients with RA or OA. They showed that plasma miR-132 differentiate RA and OA patients from healthy controls (83.8% of sensitivity and 80.7% of specificity for RA and 84.0% of sensitivity and 81.2% of specificity for OA) but failed to distinguish them from each other. Interestingly they observed that miRNAs in synovial fluid (miR-16, miR-146a, miR-155, and miR-223) from RA patients were significantly higher than those of patients with OA, suggesting that synovial fluid miRNAs could be a useful tool for diagnosis of RA from OA; however, they did not correlate with clinical variables of RA including DAS28 [32].

Although, evidence that supports the therapeutic potential of miRNA-based strategies is growing, further investigations are required to find suitable miRNAs for utilizing as biomarkers for diagnosis, predicting drug efficacy in order to plan optimal management of RA patients.

7.3. miRNA as response to treatment biomarkers

Almost all newly diagnosed RA patients enter their treatment with methotrexate monotherapy. If it fails (and it is ineffective in 66% of patients), other disease-modifying antirheumatic drugs (DMARD) and then one of biologic agents are prescribed. Considering that each type of biology treatment targets different inflammatory mechanisms, sometimes it may take some time to find the best therapy for a patient. Although biological medicines significantly improved RA treatment, there are still some stumbling blocks to be overcome. The major problems of the treatment with biologics are serious potential side effects and high cost of biologics. Currently clinical and serological markers that sufficient predict disease outcome are unavailable. Therefore one of the most challenging issues is the identification of biomarkers that will predict therapeutic outcome and thus would improve patient care and medical cost-effectiveness. Potential value of miRNAs as molecular biomarker for prognosis treatment response is still unexplored in RA. However, there are several reports demonstrating possibility to use them as therapy outcome predictors [6, 71]. Duroux-Richard and Jorgensen proposed hsa-miR-23a-3p and hsa-miR-223-3p as predictors of therapy response and biomarkers of response to anti-TNFα/DMARDs combination therapy. Strong increase in hsa-miR-23a-3p and hsa-miR-223-3p expressions indicated good response to treatment. Moreover those changes significantly correlated with clinical and inflammatory parameters (such as DAS28, CRP, or ESR). Most importantly expression level of these miRNAs showed its potential to predict therapy outcome. hsa-miR-23-3p and hsa-miR-223-3p levels were predictors of nonresponse to anti–TNF-α/DMARD combination treatment with a sensitivity of 62.5 and 57.1% and a specificity of 86.4 and 90.2%, respectively. The combination of these two miRNAs demonstrated an increase in both the sensitivity (62.5%) and specificity (91.5%) in relation to those given by each miRNA alone [6].

Another circulating miRNAs suggested to be a potential predictive biomarker of response to RA treatment was miR-125b. Duroux-Richard et al. observed that miR-125b expression significantly distinguish RA patients from healthy donors and OA patients but not from patients with other rheumatic disorders like tumor necrosis factor receptor-associated periodic syndrome (TRAPS) or spondyloarthritis (SpA). Results obtained in this study also showed that high expression of miR-125b was associated with good response to rituximab therapy. Serum expression levels of tested miRNA before treatment were significantly higher in good responders than in nonresponders. However, it was not correlated with disease activity parameters. These data suggest miR-125b might be considered as a biomarker that predicts therapy response but is not useful as disease activity marker [72].

The realization of personalized medicine requires comprehensive understanding of genetic and nongenetic factors that may be responsible for drug response. Although several miRNAs appear to be attractive molecular biomarkers, discovery of perfect biomarkers for RA diagnosis and prediction of treatment outcome is still in the future. Better understanding of the role of miRNAs in RA pathogenesis and identification of specific miRNA expression patterns in RA may provide novel molecular prognostic and diagnostic biomarker markers and new gene therapy strategies for treating RA.

8. miRNA polymorphisms

As mentioned, RA is a common, but heterogeneous, disease with the heritability about 60 % [73]. As genetic variants are present at birth, genetic studies can help us identify the key genes and pathways that contribute to both occurrence and severity of disease [74]. The last 60 years provided evidence for the genetic basis of rheumatoid arthritis by identifying genetic susceptibility variants. Three basic approaches were applied to recognize these susceptibility loci: candidate single nucleotide polymorphisms (SNPs), linkage, and genome-wide association studies (GWAS), which genotype thousands to millions of SNPs in large human samples. However, more than 10 years after the completion of the human genome sequencing project and numerous GWA studies, we still do not fully understand the genetic basis of RA [74, 75].

Since miRNAs are an important class of regulators of gene expression, genetic polymorphisms located in miRNA genes (miR-SNPs) and/or in miRNA binding sites of target genes (miR-TS-SNPs) can act as regulatory SNPs through modifying the activity of miRNAs to affect the susceptibility to and/or severity of disease (**Figure 2**) [76, 77]. The miR-SNPs are thought to affect function in one of three ways. First, genetic alternation in miRNA genes affects its expression through the transcription of the primary transcript; second, via altering pri-miRNA and pre-miRNA processing; and third, by affecting the miRNA-mRNA interactions [77–79]. In contrast to SNPs in miRNA genes, the miR-TS-SNPs, which are present at or near a miRNA binding site in 3'-untranslated region (UTR) of the target gene, are abundant in the human genome [80]. These SNPs can potentially alter miRNA function by creating as well as destroying a miRNA binding site [78]. Moreover, the functional impact of miR-TS-SNPs on disease phenotype largely depends on whether the corresponding miRNA is expressed in a particular tissue and the expression of other possibly compensatory miRNAs [77]. Prediction of SNPs that could alter the expression of a miRNA or its complementarily with the target genes, and as a result the normal function of the involved molecular pathway, seems to be of great importance [79]. Moreover, the polymorphisms associated with miRNAs may have a more important role in RA disease onset and progression than originally suspected. However, to date only a limited number of studies have identified miR-SNPs and/or miR-TS-SNPs relevant to RA (**Table 1**) [81, 82]. In a genome-wide interaction analysis, miR-146a and miR-499 have received much attention in this field. Up today, miR-146a, the most studied miRNAs in patients with RA, is encoded by chromosome 5q33 and can bind to the 3'-UTR of many target mRNAs, including interleukin-1 receptor-associated kinase 1 (IRAK-1), tumor necrosis factor receptor-associated factor 6 (TRAF-6), and other transcripts associated with inflammatory signaling [83, 84]. The common miR-146a polymorphism [85, 85], which may affect the stability of the miRNA, thereby influencing its expression level [82, 86], is not associated with susceptibility to RA [81, 85, 87], but the miRNA-146a rs2910164 variant might increase the risk of RA in the female population and may influence disease activity [84]. Moreover, it remains unclear which allele is associated with a significantly higher level of mature miR-146a. On the other hand, miR-499, the gene of which is located on 20q11.22 chromosome, targets IL-17 receptor B (IL-17RB), IL-23a, IL-2 receptor B (IL-2Rβ), IL-6, IL-2, B- and T-lymphocyte attenuator, IL-18 receptor (IL-18R), IL-21, peptidyl arginine deiminase type 4 (PADI4), and regulatory factor X 4 (influences human leukocyte antigen class II expression) [83, 84]. The miR-499 polymorphism at position rs3746444T > C, located within the stem region of the miR-499 gene is closely associated with the inflammation of RA and can serve a potential diagnostic biomarker for RA [81, 84]. To date, very little is known about the role of miRNA SNPs in the pathogenesis of RA, and even less is known about whether it could affect miRNA-mRNA interactions. That way, the mechanism by which sequence variations—due to genetic or posttranscriptional changes—in miRNAs and/or in their target genes that modulate miRNA binding characteristics or miRNA expression can affects the inflammatory processes requires further functional studies. With the development of large-scale RNA-sequencing methods, a new light could be shed on these mechanisms [80].

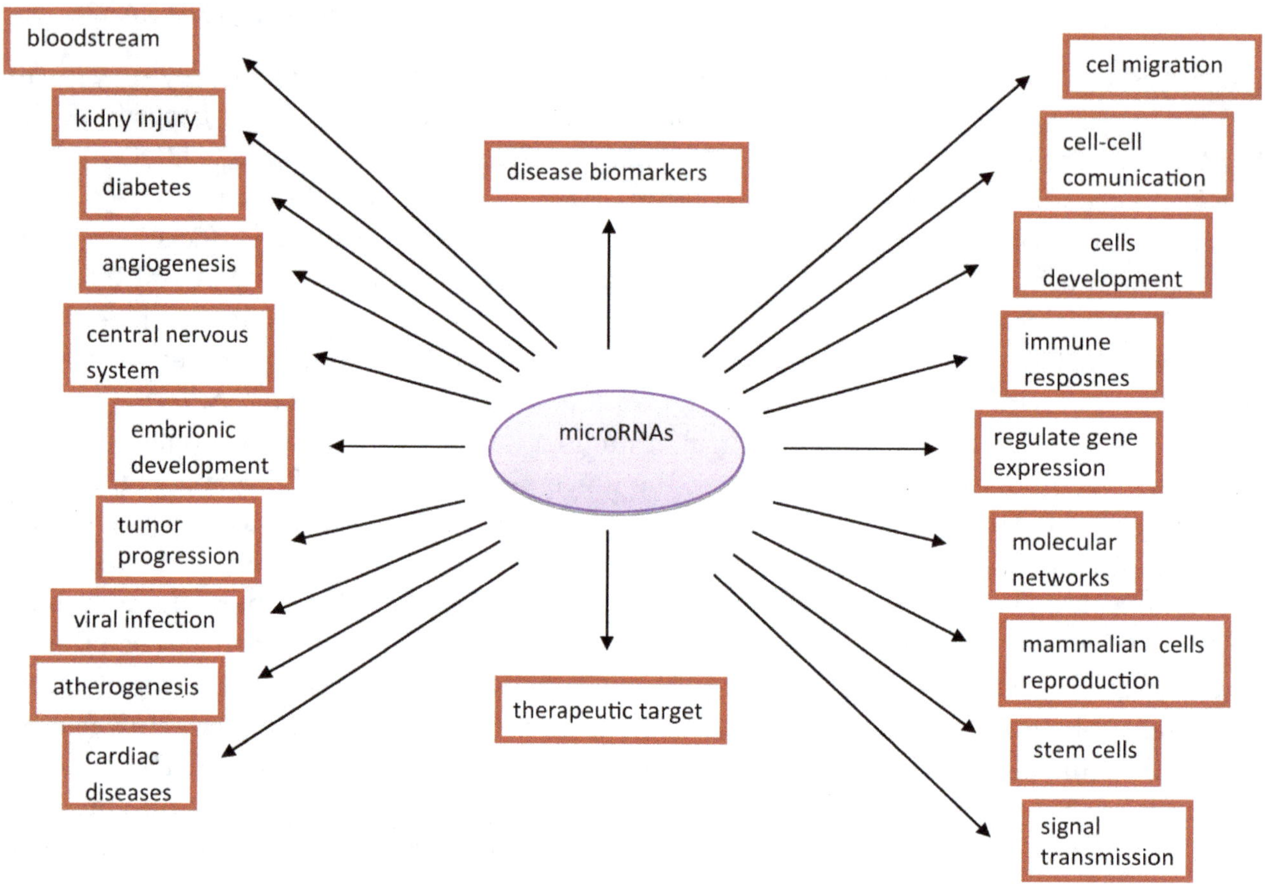

Figure 2. Single nucleotide polymorphisms located in miRNAs.

9. Conclusion

RA is a syndrome in which many different elements of the immune system become activated. A growing number of GWAS demonstrated that genetic polymorphisms, the standard genetic marker to identify associated alleles, make a substantial but incomplete contribution to the risk of RA developing. Now it is widely accepted that epigenetic mechanisms such as miRNAs, a class of powerful and major gene regulators, are also involved in the coordination of the immune processes in the rheumatoid arthritis. Both tissue and extracellular miRNAs are not only key molecules in the molecular mechanisms of the disease but also are very important biomarkers for several pathological conditions and represent a promising therapeutic approach in future. Circulating miRNAs may be suitable for clinical use as they are stable present in body fluids such as plasma or serum. Recent evidence has suggested that miRNA levels in serum or plasma are often higher than in the synovial fluid. In addition, miRNA expression profiles in synovial fluids were similar to those in synovial tissues. These findings demonstrated that synovial tissues and infiltrating cells are the primary source of synovial fluid miRNAs. In contrast, miRNAs that are presented in the serum or plasma are released by several tissues and cells different from those in synovium [32]. Because rheumatoid arthritis is a systemic disease which can have not only a joint involvement but also other organs may be affected, cell-free circulating miRNA signature in serum or plasma is of great interest.

Acknowledgements

This work was supported by a grant from the Polish National Science Center (2015/19/B/NZ5/00247).

Author details

Agnieszka Paradowska-Gorycka* and Barbara Stypińska

*Address all correspondence to: paradowska_aga@interia.pl

Department of Biochemistry and Molecular Biology, National Institute of Geriatrics, Rheumatology and Rehabilitation, Warsaw, Poland

References

[1] Klein K, Gay S. Epigenetic modifications in rheumatoid arthritis, a review. Curr Opin Pharmacol. 2013;13(3):420-425. doi:10.1016/j.coph.2013.01.007.

[2] Salehi E, Eftekhari R, Oraei M, Gharib A, Bidad K. MicroRNAs in rheumatoid arthritis. Clin Rheumatol. 2015;34(4):615-628. doi:10.1007/s10067-015-2898-x.

[3] Filková M, Aradi B, Senolt L, et al. Association of circulating miR-223 and miR-16 with disease activity in patients with early rheumatoid arthritis. Ann Rheum Dis. 2014;73(10):1898-1904. doi:10.1136/annrheumdis-2012-202815.

[4] Duroux-Richard I, Jorgensen C, Apparailly F. What do microRNAs mean for rheumatoid arthritis? Arthritis Rheum. 2012;64(1):11-20. doi:10.1002/art.30651.

[5] Singh RP, Massachi I, Manickavel S, et al. The role of miRNA in inflammation and autoimmunity. Autoimmun Rev. 2013;12(12):1160-1165. doi:10.1016/j.autrev.2013.07.003.

[6] Castro-Villegas C, Pérez-Sánchez C, Escudero A, et al. Circulating miRNAs as potential biomarkers of therapy effectiveness in rheumatoid arthritis patients treated with anti-TNFα. Arthritis Res Ther. 2015;17(1):49. doi:10.1186/s13075-015-0555-z.

[7] Smigielska-Czepiel K, van den Berg A, Jellema P, et al. Comprehensive analysis of miRNA expression in T-cell subsets of rheumatoid arthritis patients reveals defined

signatures of naive and memory Tregs. Genes Immun. 2014;15(2):115-125. doi:10.1038/gene.2013.69.

[8] Ha M, Kim VN. Regulation of microRNA biogenesis. Nat Rev Mol Cell Biol. 2014;15(8):509-524. doi:10.1038/nrm3838.

[9] Bhaskaran M, Mohan M. MicroRNAs: history, biogenesis, and their evolving role in animal development and disease. Vet Pathol. 2014;51(4):759-774. doi:10.1177/0300985813502820.

[10] Creemers EE, Tijsen AJ, Pinto YM. Circulating microRNAs: novel biomarkers and extracellular communicators in cardiovascular disease? Circ Res. 2012;110(3):483-495. doi:10.1161/CIRCRESAHA.111.247452.

[11] Kawano S, Nakamachi Y. The role of miRNA, in Rheumatoid Arthritis. Rheum Arthritis – Etiol Consequences Co-Morbidities. 2012. doi:10.5772/25861.

[12] Gu S, Kay MA, Carthew R, et al. How do miRNAs mediate translational repression? Silence. 2010;1(1):11. doi:10.1186/1758-907X-1-11.

[13] Bartel DP. MicroRNAs: genomics, biogenesis, mechanism, and function. Cell. 2004;116(2):281-297. doi:10.1016/S0092-8674(04)00045-5.

[14] Petersen CP, Bordeleau M-E, Pelletier J, Sharp PA. Short RNAs repress translation after initiation in mammalian cells. Mol Cell. 2006;21(4):533-542. doi:10.1016/j.molcel.2006.01.031.

[15] Nottrott S, Simard MJ, Richter JD. Human let-7a miRNA blocks protein production on actively translating polyribosomes. Nat Struct Mol Biol. 2006;13(12):1108-1114. doi:10.1038/nsmb1173.

[16] Wahid F, Shehzad A, Khan T, Kim YY. MicroRNAs: synthesis, mechanism, function, and recent clinical trials. Biochim Biophys Acta – Mol Cell Res. 2010;1803(11):1231-1243. doi:10.1016/j.bbamcr.2010.06.013.

[17] Hutvágner G, Zamore PD. A microRNA in a multiple-turnover RNAi enzyme complex. Science. 2002;297(5589):2056-2060. doi:10.1126/science.1073827.

[18] Llave C, Xie Z, Kasschau KD, Carrington JC. Cleavage of Scarecrow-like mRNA targets directed by a class of Arabidopsis miRNA. Science. 2002;297(5589):2053-2056. doi:10.1126/science.1076311.

[19] Behm-Ansmant I, Rehwinkel J, Doerks T, Stark A, Bork P, Izaurralde E. mRNA degradation by miRNAs and GW182 requires both CCR4:NOT deadenylase and DCP1:DCP2 decapping complexes. Genes Dev. 2006;20(14):1885-1898. doi:10.1101/gad.1424106.

[20] Wu L, Fan J, Belasco JG. MicroRNAs direct rapid deadenylation of mRNA. Proc Natl Acad Sci U S A. 2006;103(11):4034-4039. doi:10.1073/pnas.0510928103.

[21] Mitchell PS, Parkin RK, Kroh EM, et al. Circulating microRNAs as stable blood-based markers for cancer detection. Proc Natl Acad Sci U S A. 2008;105(30):10513-10518. doi:10.1073/pnas.0804549105.

[22] Huang R-Y, Li L, Wang M-J, Chen X-M, Huang Q-C, Lu C-J. An exploration of the role of microRNAs in psoriasis: a systematic review of the literature. Medicine (Baltimore). 2015;94(45):e2030. doi:10.1097/MD.0000000000002030.

[23] Makarova JA, Shkurnikov MU, Wicklein D, et al. Intracellular and extracellular microRNA: an update on localization and biological role. Prog Histochem Cytochem. 2016;51:33–49. doi:10.1016/j.proghi.2016.06.001.

[24] Baumjohann D, Ansel KM. MicroRNA-mediated regulation of T helper cell differentiation and plasticity. Nat Rev Immunol. 2013;13(9):666-678. doi:10.1038/nri3494.

[25] Miao C-G, Xiong Y-Y, Yu H, et al. Critical roles of microRNAs in the pathogenesis of systemic sclerosis: New advances, challenges and potential directions. Int Immunopharmacol. 2015;28(1):626-633. doi:10.1016/j.intimp.2015.07.042.

[26] Mohr AM, Mott JL. Overview of microRNA biology. Semin Liver Dis. 2015;35(1):3-11. doi:10.1055/s-0034-1397344.

[27] Ceribelli A, Nahid MA, Satoh M, Chan EKL. MicroRNAs in rheumatoid arthritis. FEBS Lett. 2011;585(23):3667-3674. doi:10.1016/j.febslet.2011.05.020.

[28] Huang C, Geng J, Jiang S. MicroRNAs in regulation of osteogenic differentiation of mesenchymal stem cells. Cell Tissue Res. 2016. doi:10.1007/s00441-016-2462-2.

[29] Gao Y, Peng J, Ren Z, et al. Functional regulatory roles of microRNAs in atherosclerosis. Clin Chim Acta. 2016;460:164-171. doi:10.1016/j.cca.2016.06.044.

[30] Vicente R, Noël D, Pers Y-M, Apparailly F, Jorgensen C. Deregulation and therapeutic potential of microRNAs in arthritic diseases. Nat Rev Rheumatol. 2016;12(4):211-220. doi:10.1038/nrrheum.2015.162.

[31] Liang H, Gong F, Zhang S, Zhang C-Y, Zen K, Chen X. The origin, function, and diagnostic potential of extracellular microRNAs in human body fluids. Wiley Interdiscip Rev RNA. 5(2):285-300. doi:10.1002/wrna.1208.

[32] Murata K, Yoshitomi H, Tanida S, et al. Plasma and synovial fluid microRNAs as potential biomarkers of rheumatoid arthritis and osteoarthritis. Arthritis Res Ther. 2010;12(3):R86. doi:10.1186/ar3013.

[33] Tanaka Y. Current concepts in the management of rheumatoid arthritis. Korean J Intern Med. 2016;31(2):210-218. doi:10.3904/kjim.2015.137.

[34] Mimori T. Clinical significance of anti-CCP antibodies in rheumatoid arthritis. Intern Med. 2005;44(11):1122-1126. http://www.ncbi.nlm.nih.gov/pubmed/16357447. Accessed August 25, 2016.

[35] Paradowska A, Maśliński W, Grzybowska-Kowalczyk A, Łacki J. The function of interleukin 17 in the pathogenesis of rheumatoid arthritis. Arch Immunol Ther Exp (Warsz). 55(5):329-334. http://www.ncbi.nlm.nih.gov/pubmed/18219763. Accessed August 25, 2016.

[36] Kelly M. Robert BRIDGES: pioneer in rheumatology. Med Hist. 1961;5:297-299. http://www.ncbi.nlm.nih.gov/pubmed/13752390. Accessed August 25, 2016.

[37] Cobb S, Kasl S V. The epidemiology of rheumatoid arthritis. Am J Public Health Nations Health. 1966;56(10):1657-1663. http://www.ncbi.nlm.nih.gov/pubmed/5951485. Accessed August 25, 2016.

[38] Williams EA, Fye KH. Rheumatoid arthritis. Targeted interventions can minimize joint destruction. Postgrad Med. 2003;114(5):19-28. http://www.ncbi.nlm.nih.gov/pubmed/14650090. Accessed August 25, 2016.

[39] Reveille JD. Genetic studies in the rheumatic diseases: present status and implications for the future. J Rheumatol Suppl. 2005;72:10-13. http://www.ncbi.nlm.nih.gov/pubmed/15660456. Accessed August 25, 2016.

[40] Romagnani S. Human Th17 cells. Arthritis Res Ther. 2008;10(2):206. doi:10.1186/ar2392.

[41] Layh-Schmitt G, Colbert RA. The interleukin-23/interleukin-17 axis in spondyloarthritis. Curr Opin Rheumatol. 2008;20(4):392-397. doi:10.1097/BOR.0b013e328303204b.

[42] Sakaguchi S, Yamaguchi T, Nomura T, Ono M. Regulatory T cells and immune tolerance. Cell. 2008;133(5):775-787. doi:10.1016/j.cell.2008.05.009.

[43] Awasthi A, Kuchroo VK. Th17 cells: from precursors to players in inflammation and infection. Int Immunol. 2009;21(5):489-498. doi:10.1093/intimm/dxp021.

[44] Bax M, van Heemst J, Huizinga TWJ, Toes REM. Genetics of rheumatoid arthritis: what have we learned? Immunogenetics. 2011;63(8):459-466. doi:10.1007/s00251-011-0528-6.

[45] Viatte S, Plant D, Raychaudhuri S. Genetics and epigenetics of rheumatoid arthritis. Nat Rev Rheumatol. 2013;9(3):141-153. doi:10.1038/nrrheum.2012.237.

[46] Glant TT, Mikecz K, Rauch TA. Epigenetics in the pathogenesis of rheumatoid arthritis. BMC Med. 2014;12:35. doi:10.1186/1741-7015-12-35.

[47] Bottini N, Firestein GS. Epigenetics in rheumatoid arthritis: a primer for rheumatologists. Curr Rheumatol Rep. 2013;15(11):372. doi:10.1007/s11926-013-0372-9.

[48] Zhou Q, Haupt S, Kreuzer JT, et al. Decreased expression of miR-146a and miR-155 contributes to an abnormal Treg phenotype in patients with rheumatoid arthritis. Ann Rheum Dis. 2015;74(6):1265-1274. doi:10.1136/annrheumdis-2013-204377.

[49] Kim T-H, Choi SJ, Lee YH, Song GG, Ji JD. Gene expression profile predicting the response to anti-TNF treatment in patients with rheumatoid arthritis; analysis of GEO datasets. Joint Bone Spine. 2014;81(4):325-330. doi:10.1016/j.jbspin.2014.01.013.

[50] Churov A V, Oleinik EK, Knip M. MicroRNAs in rheumatoid arthritis: altered expression and diagnostic potential. Autoimmun Rev. 2015;14(11):1029-1037. doi:10.1016/j.autrev.2015.07.005.

[51] Stanczyk J, Pedrioli DML, Brentano F, et al. Altered expression of microRNA in synovial fibroblasts and synovial tissue in rheumatoid arthritis. Arthritis Rheum. 2008;58(4):1001-1009. doi:10.1002/art.23386.

[52] Mu N, Gu J, Huang T, et al. A novel NF-κB/YY1/microRNA-10a regulatory circuit in fibroblast-like synoviocytes regulates inflammation in rheumatoid arthritis. Sci Rep. 2016;6:20059. doi:10.1038/srep20059.

[53] Dong L, Wang X, Tan J, et al. Decreased expression of microRNA-21 correlates with the imbalance of Th17 and Treg cells in patients with rheumatoid arthritis. J Cell Mol Med. 2014;18(11):2213-2224. doi:10.1111/jcmm.12353.

[54] Takahashi H, Kanno T, Nakayamada S, et al. TGF-β and retinoic acid induce the microRNA miR-10a, which targets Bcl-6 and constrains the plasticity of helper T cells. Nat Immunol. 2012;13(6):587-595. doi:10.1038/ni.2286.

[55] Chen X-M, Huang Q-C, Yang S-L, et al. Role of microRNAs in the pathogenesis of rheumatoid arthritis: novel perspectives based on review of the literature. Medicine (Baltimore). 2015;94(31):e1326. doi:10.1097/MD.0000000000001326.

[56] Lu M-C, Yu C-L, Chen H-C, Yu H-C, Huang H-B, Lai N-S. Increased miR-223 expression in T cells from patients with rheumatoid arthritis leads to decreased insulin-like growth factor-1-mediated interleukin-10 production. Clin Exp Immunol. 2014;177(3):641-651. doi:10.1111/cei.12374.

[57] Philippe L, Alsaleh G, Suffert G, et al. TLR2 expression is regulated by microRNA miR-19 in rheumatoid fibroblast-like synoviocytes. J Immunol. 2012;188(1):454-461. doi:10.4049/jimmunol.1102348.

[58] Kurowska-Stolarska M, Alivernini S, Ballantine LE, et al. MicroRNA-155 as a proinflammatory regulator in clinical and experimental arthritis. Proc Natl Acad Sci U S A. 2011;108(27):11193-11198. doi:10.1073/pnas.1019536108.

[59] Jiang C, Zhu W, Xu J, et al. MicroRNA-26a negatively regulates toll-like receptor 3 expression of rat macrophages and ameliorates pristane induced arthritis in rats. Arthritis Res Ther. 2014;16(1):R9. doi:10.1186/ar4435.

[60] Li Y, Fan L, Liu S, et al. The promotion of bone regeneration through positive regulation of angiogenic-osteogenic coupling using microRNA-26a. Biomaterials. 2013;34(21):5048-5058. doi:10.1016/j.biomaterials.2013.03.052.

[61] Pauley KM, Cha S. miRNA-146a in rheumatoid arthritis: a new therapeutic strategy. Immunotherapy. 2011;3(7):829-831. doi:10.2217/imt.11.70.

[62] Murata K, Yoshitomi H, Furu M, et al. MicroRNA-451 down-regulates neutrophil chemotaxis via p38 MAPK. Arthritis Rheumatol (Hoboken, NJ). 2014;66(3):549-559. doi:10.1002/art.38269.

[63] Nakamachi Y, Ohnuma K, Uto K, Noguchi Y, Saegusa J, Kawano S. MicroRNA-124 inhibits the progression of adjuvant-induced arthritis in rats. Ann Rheum Dis. 2016;75(3):601-608. doi:10.1136/annrheumdis-2014-206417.

[64] Lee Y, Kim HJ, Park CK, et al. MicroRNA-124 regulates osteoclast differentiation. Bone. 2013;56(2):383-389. doi:10.1016/j.bone.2013.07.007.

[65] Niimoto T, Nakasa T, Ishikawa M, et al. MicroRNA-146a expresses in interleukin-17 producing T cells in rheumatoid arthritis patients. BMC Musculoskelet Disord. 2010;11(1):209. doi:10.1186/1471-2474-11-209.

[66] Pauley KM, Satoh M, Chan AL, Bubb MR, Reeves WH, Chan EK. Upregulated miR-146a expression in peripheral blood mononuclear cells from rheumatoid arthritis patients. Arthritis Res Ther. 2008;10(4):R101. doi:10.1186/ar2493.

[67] Abou-Zeid A, Saad M, Soliman E. MicroRNA 146a expression in rheumatoid arthritis: association with tumor necrosis factor-alpha and disease activity. Genet Test Mol Biomarkers. 2011;15(11):807-812. doi:10.1089/gtmb.2011.0026.

[68] Elsayed HMA, Khater WS, Ibrahim AA, Hamdy MSE, Morshedy NA. MicroRNA-146a expression as a potential biomarker for rheumatoid arthritis in Egypt. Egypt J Med Hum Genet. 2016. doi:10.1016/j.ejmhg.2016.07.001.

[69] Kriegsmann M, Randau TM, Gravius S, et al. Expression of miR-146a, miR-155, and miR-223 in formalin-fixed paraffin-embedded synovial tissues of patients with rheumatoid arthritis and osteoarthritis. Virchows Arch. 2016;469(1):93-100. doi:10.1007/s00428-016-1939-4.

[70] Murata K, Furu M, Yoshitomi H, et al. Comprehensive microRNA analysis identifies miR-24 and miR-125a-5p as plasma biomarkers for rheumatoid arthritis. PLoS One. 2013;8(7):e69118. doi:10.1371/journal.pone.0069118.

[71] Duroux-Richard I, Jorgensen C, Apparailly F. miRNAs and rheumatoid arthritis – promising novel biomarkers. Swiss Med Wkly. 2011. doi:10.4414/smw.2011.13175.

[72] Duroux-Richard I, Pers Y-M, Fabre S, et al. Circulating miRNA-125b is a potential biomarker predicting response to rituximab in rheumatoid arthritis. Mediators Inflamm. 2014;2014:342524. doi:10.1155/2014/342524.

[73] Kurkó J, Besenyei T, Laki J, Glant TT, Mikecz K, Szekanecz Z. Genetics of rheumatoid arthritis – a comprehensive review. Clin Rev Allergy Immunol. 2013;45(2):170-179. doi:10.1007/s12016-012-8346-7.

[74] Raychaudhuri S. Recent advances in the genetics of rheumatoid arthritis. Curr Opin Rheumatol. 2010;22(2):109-118. doi:10.1097/BOR.0b013e328336474d.

[75] Sethupathy P, Collins FS. MicroRNA target site polymorphisms and human disease. Trends Genet. 2008;24(10):489-497. doi:10.1016/j.tig.2008.07.004.

[76] Gong J, Tong Y, Zhang H-M, et al. Genome-wide identification of SNPs in microRNA genes and the SNP effects on microRNA target binding and biogenesis. Hum Mutat. 2012;33(1):254-263. doi:10.1002/humu.21641.

[77] Dole NS, Delany AM. MicroRNA variants as genetic determinants of bone mass. Bone. 2016;84:57-68. doi:10.1016/j.bone.2015.12.016.

[78] Ryan BM, Robles AI, Harris CC. Genetic variation in microRNA networks: the implications for cancer research. Nat Rev Cancer. 2010;10(6):389-402. doi:10.1038/nrc2867.

[79] Jin Y, Lee CGL. Single nucleotide polymorphisms associated with microRNA regulation. Biomolecules. 2013;3(2):287-302. doi:10.3390/biom3020287.

[80] Pivarcsi A, Ståhle M, Sonkoly E. Genetic polymorphisms altering microRNA activity in psoriasis – a key to solve the puzzle of missing heritability? Exp Dermatol. 2014;23(9):620-624. doi:10.1111/exd.12469.

[81] Yang B, Chen J, Li Y, et al. Association of polymorphisms in pre-miRNA with inflammatory biomarkers in rheumatoid arthritis in the Chinese Han population. Hum Immunol. 2012;73(1):101-106. doi:10.1016/j.humimm.2011.10.005.

[82] Chatzikyriakidou A, Voulgari P V, Georgiou I, Drosos AA. miRNAs and related polymorphisms in rheumatoid arthritis susceptibility. Autoimmun Rev. 2012;11(9):636-641. doi:10.1016/j.autrev.2011.11.004.

[83] Xu HY, Wang ZY, Chen JF, et al. Association between ankylosing spondylitis and the miR-146a and miR-499 polymorphisms. PLoS One. 2015;10(4):e0122055. doi:10.1371/journal.pone.0122055.

[84] El-Shal AS, Aly NM, Galil SMA, Moustafa MA, Kandel WA. Association of microRNAs genes polymorphisms with rheumatoid arthritis in Egyptian female patients. Joint Bone Spine. 2013;80(6):626-631. doi:10.1016/j.jbspin.2013.03.005.

[85] Zhou X, Zhu J, Zhang H, Zhou G, Huang Y, Liu R. Is the microRNA-146a (rs2910164) polymorphism associated with rheumatoid arthritis? Association of microRNA-146a (rs2910164) polymorphism and rheumatoid arthritis could depend on gender. Joint Bone Spine. 2015;82(3):166-171. doi:10.1016/j.jbspin.2014.12.009.

[86] Apparailly F. Looking for microRNA polymorphisms as new rheumatoid arthritis risk loci? Joint Bone Spine. 2010;77(5):377-379. doi:10.1016/j.jbspin.2010.06.002.

[87] Li K, Tie H, Hu N, et al. Association of two polymorphisms rs2910164 in miRNA-146a and rs3746444 in miRNA-499 with rheumatoid arthritis: a meta-analysis. Hum Immunol. 2014;75(7):602-608. doi:10.1016/j.humimm.2014.05.002.

5

Longitudinal Growth in Rheumatologic Conditions: Current and Emerging Treatments of Growth Delay in Children with Chronic Autoimmune Diseases

Hulya Bukulmez

Abstract

Chronic rheumatologic, inflammatory diseases of childhood, such as juvenile idiopathic arthritis (JIA), Crohn's disease (CD), and systemic lupus erythematosus (SLE), affect both trabecular bone formation and remodeling and longitudinal bone growth resulting in short stature and causing bone developmental deformities. Inflammation alone or together with poor nutritional intake and chronic glucocorticoid therapy are major factors in growth retardation seen in children with chronic inflammatory diseases. When the growing process is continuous, acute or chronic inflammation causes dysregulation of both central endocrine and local paracrine secretion of the growth factors and hormones, impairing bone growth in children. In this chapter, we review major growth factors such as growth hormone that affect longitudinal growth and how they are affected by inflammation in childhood rheumatologic diseases. We also review a recently described growth factor, CNP, and its potential therapeutic role in chronic inflammatory diseases.

Keywords: juvenile idiopathic arthritis, natriuretic peptides, dwarfism, growth factor, atrial natriuretic peptide, B-type natriuretic peptide, C-type natriuretic peptide, natriuretic peptide receptor 1, −2, −3

1. Introduction

Longitudinal growth is a continuous process under the influence of multiple complex factors starting from prenatal life until end of puberty. Major factors that control longitudinal growth can be summarized as genetic background, nutrition, and endocrine growth factors. Major endocrine factors that control longitudinal growth are growth hormone (GH) and insulin-like growth factor (IGF), thyroid stimulating hormone (TSH), parathyroid hormone (PTH), insulin, and sex steroids. There are also multiple growth factors in the growth plates and other organs that are involved in processing the growth factors in the regulation of longitudinal bone growth. Some of these growth factors are found and secreted by the growing cartilage and bone tissue and under the influence of the endocrine hormones. These are insulin-like growth factor 1 (IGF-1), insulin-like growth factor-binding protein 3 (IGFBP-3), fibroblast growth factors (FGF), Indian hedgehog (Ihh), parathyroid hormone-like receptor protein (Pthrp), and C-type natriuretic peptide (CNP).

1.1. How do growth hormones and factors affect longitudinal skeletal growth?

Skeletal growth and development follows two different pathways: chondrogenesis and osteogenesis (both endochondral and membranous bone growth). Longitudinal growth is mainly controlled by endochondral ossification which is orchestrated by a complex network of endocrine and paracrine growth hormones and factors that control growth plate cartilage and bone tissue.

While membranous bone such as those in our skull forms as a result of direct mechanism of mesenchymal cell differentiation into osteoblasts, endochondral osteogenesis follows an initial mesenchymal stem cell differentiation into chondrocytes, and the chondrogenesis process is later replaced by bone tissue [1–4]. During endochondral growth, mesenchymal cells (See **Figure 1**) first condense in the growth plate and then with interactions between cells via local transcription factors such as Sox9 and other extracellular molecules such as collagen II differentiate gradually into chondrocytes. Chondrocytes proliferate and organize in columns making stacks which are perpendicular to gravity. They gradually stop proliferating and become pre-hypertrophic with increased matrix synthesis (**Figure 1**) [5, 6]. Eventually, these cells stop proliferating and start terminally differentiating into hypertrophic chondrocytes. Finally, the hypertrophic zone of the growth plate becomes mineralized. Then the vascular system merges into this hypertrophic chondrocyte region and with more signaling the mineralized tissue is possibly resorbed by osteoclasts that originate from hematopoietic stem cells. Eventually, mineralized tissue is replaced by bone tissue which is made by osteoblasts that differentiate from mesenchymal cells. Thus, endochondral bone growth combines together chondrogenesis, extracellular matrix formation, mineralization, and osteogenesis process. These processes are synchronized by a series of systemic growth hormones such as growth hormone (GH), thyroid-stimulating hormone (TSH), glucocorticoids and local growth factors such as parathyroid hormone-related peptide (Pthrp) and members of the transforming growth factor β (TGF- β), fibroblast growth factors (FGF), Indian hedgehog (Ihh), and Wnt's [7, 8] (**Figure 1**). Intracellular pathways that are activated by the orchestra of factors are yet to be determined. Sox9 and Runx2, transcription factors, have been shown to regulate chondrogenesis and hypertrophic differentiation [9, 10].

During linear growth, endocrine hormones such as GH, IGF-1, glucocorticoids, and thyroid stimulating hormone first interact at the level of hypothalamus and pituitary [11, 12] and

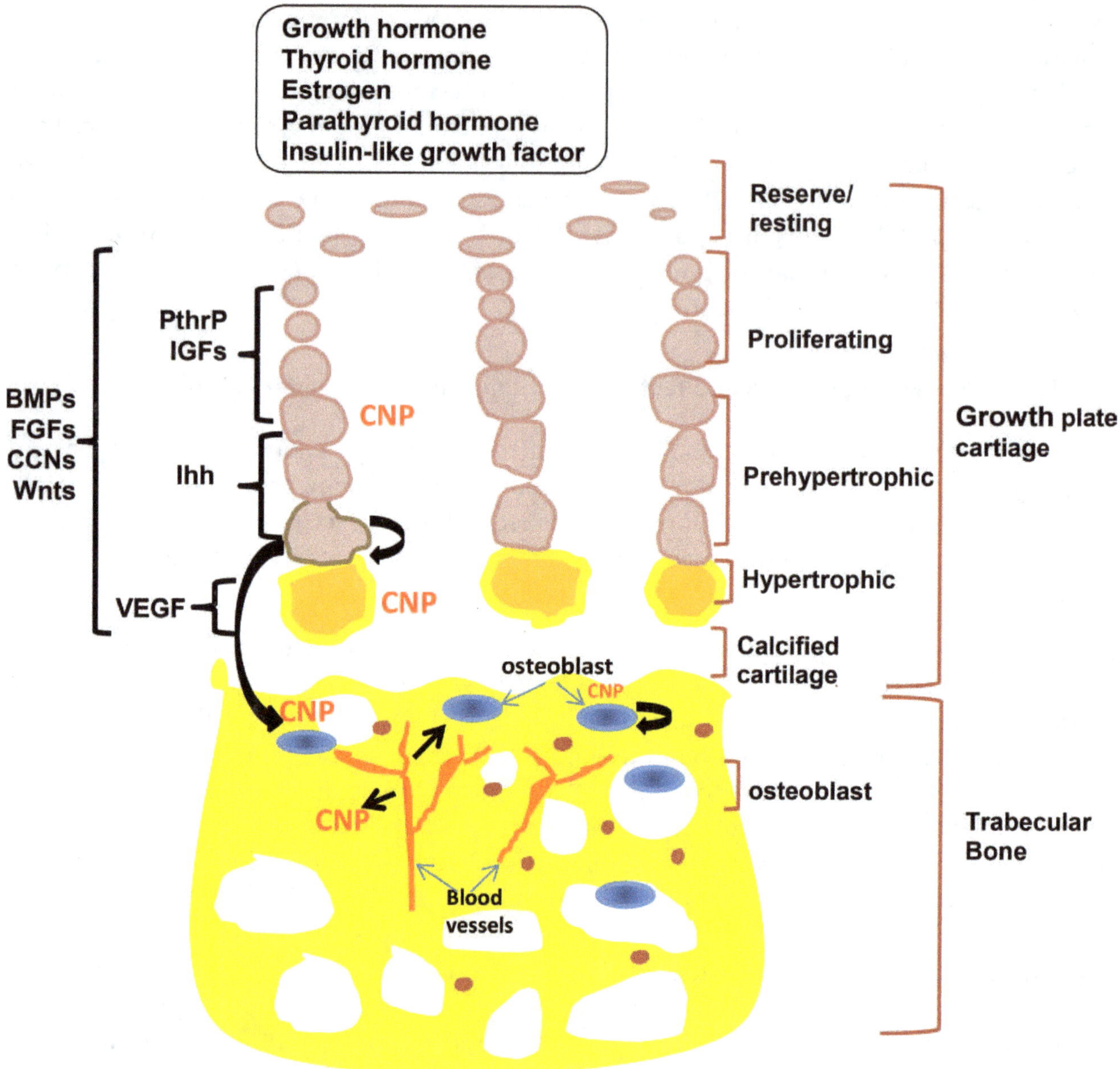

Figure 1. Longitudinal growth is regulated by multiple systemic (in bubble) and local growth factors expressed differentially in the proliferating, hypertrophic chondrocyte zones of the growth plate (black text on the left of the figure). CNP seems to be expressed and plays a role in the growth plate cartilage, in the osteoblasts and in the endothelial cells of vessel walls.

then, they act directly on peripheral target tissues, such as liver [13, 14], heart [15], kidney and growth plates [14, 16].

GH action regulates growth plates using both direct and indirect mechanisms. While GH directly stimulates chondrocyte proliferation on the growth plate [17], it indirectly stimulates the production of IGF-1 that promotes chondrocyte hypertrophy, which in turn exerts its effects directly on the growth plate.

Various danger signals or stimuli, such as TNF-α, LPS, or low-oxygen tension, increase the expression of IGF-1, vascular endothelial growth factor (VEGF), and FGF-2 with mechanisms dependent on NF-κB activation and result in bone resorption, osteopenia [11]. Excess of TNF-α during systemic arthritis has been found to be responsible for periarticular osteopenia most probably due to the same mechanism. GH action has both direct and indirect effects on the growth plate. GH acts indirectly, stimulating the production of IGF-1 that promotes chondrocyte hypertrophy, which in turn exerts its effects on the growth plate. The direct effect of GH on the growth plate stimulates chondrocyte proliferation [18]. Most recently, nitric oxide (NO) and C-type natriuretic peptide (CNP) have been identified as new regulators of endochondral bone growth, as they both stimulate chondrogenesis and both act through a common mediator, cyclic guanosine monophosphate (cGMP) [19].

While it is important to study anabolic effects of growth factors and hormones that promote chondrogenic differentiation in the growth plate, it is also very important to recognize the effects of factors that play roles in remodeling such as factors that control osteoclastic differentiation or activity. Osteoclasts are major cells that degrade bones for remodeling. The balance between bone degradation and bone building is critical for physiological bone homeostasis. Factors such as NF-κB and cytokines that are controlled by this factor may cause an imbalance during systemic inflammatory diseases such as JIA [20, 21]. NF-κB activation is a relevant component for osteoclast development, differentiation, and survival, cooperating with other pro-inflammatory cytokines [22]. Loss of NF-κB signaling prevents osteoclastogenesis [23]. NF-κB knockout mice showed severe osteopetrosis [24].

2. Growth delay in chronic inflammatory diseases

In chronic inflammatory childhood diseases such as inflammatory bowel diseases, mainly Crohn's disease, juvenile idiopathic arthritis, systemic lupus erythematosus, or other diseases in which there are excess number of circulating cytokines, it is suggested that growth hormone signaling pathways are disrupted [25–27].

Out of all factors that affect growth during chronic inflammatory diseases, growth hormone GH/IGF axis has been studied the most. Multiple steps of the growth hormone and its effector IGF-1 axis may be interrupted; these are poor signal transduction of growth hormone in the liver and in the growth plate and diminished IGFBP concentrations, which directly affect the growth plate and suppress the sensitivity of IGF-1.

After the growth hormone is secreted by the pituitary gland, it stimulates the hepatic tissue to generate IGF-1 which increases the growth plate chondrocyte proliferation.

Pro-inflammatory cytokines play a critical role in the disruption of the IGF-1/GH axis. Many studies have shown that pro-inflammatory cytokines such as IL-6, TNF-α, and IL-1β interact with the IGF-1/GH system. Transgenic mice for IL-6 develop low serum level IGF-1 and develop severe growth delay [25]. There is also evidence that suggests a role for suppressors of the cytokine signaling (SOCS) family proteins in IL-6 dysregulation [26]. The KxB/N transgenic mouse model for arthritis has also been described to have growth delay during our studies [27]. KxB/N mouse has increased serum levels of IL-1β and TNF-α and they develop systemic inflammatory arthritis [28]. Thus, high levels of any pro-inflammatory cytokine are sufficient to arrest the growth process in developing organisms with open growth plates.

The IGF-1 signaling pathway is altered in chondrocytes during chronic inflammatory conditions by pro-inflammatory cytokine activities (TNF-α, IL-6, and IL-1). These pro-inflammatory mediators work via disruption of intracellular MAPK/extracellular signal-regulated kinases (ERKs) and phosphoinositide 3-kinase (PI3K) [29, 30].

Besides the inhibition of the MAPK pathway, there are also debates about the potential of disrupted miRNA effect on overexpression of proteins involved in the regulation of GH/IGF-1 axis. miRNA deregulation previously has been reported during childhood chronic inflammatory diseases such as IBD and JIA [21, 31].

In juvenile idiopathic arthritis (JIA), bone growth abnormalities are seen as either or both short stature and bone deformities. The prevalence of juvenile rheumatoid arthritis is as high as 20 per 100,000 people per year. Growth delay in generalized linear growth occurs predominantly in the systemic onset juvenile arthritis population and to a lesser degree in those with poly-articular onset JIA associated with RF positivity [32]. During active disease in JIA, elevated serum levels of cytokines may modify target cell's sensitivity by down-regulating the GH receptor (GHR) gene expression, leading to short stature as an adult [33]. Therefore, the shortcoming of GH function during JIA is explained more as resistance to growth hormones than deficiency in growth hormone secretion.

Growth hormone (GH) treatment by providing excess GH in the circulation can overcome growth hormone resistance and improve growth velocity and prevent development of short stature in children affected from JIA.

Recent studies suggest that early initiation of GH treatment helps in maintaining normal growth in children with JIA [34, 35]. Thus, recombinant growth hormone treatment has been the mainstream since no other medications that induce skeletal growth are available to be used in pediatrics [36, 37]. Nevertheless, even with GH treatment, catch-up growth is variable and is more dependent on the severity of the inflammatory state, duration, and additional corticosteroid treatment [34, 37–41].

Another childhood disease studied for its growth delay complication is Crohn's disease, an inflammatory bowel disease (IBD). Almost, one-third of the children affected by Crohn's disease (CD) develop longitudinal growth delay. Unlike JIA, Crohn's disease patients do not develop bony deformities since the major inflammatory target is not the joint cartilage but the intestinal system. Additional to the pro-inflammatory cytokine excess that directly affects the growth plate during active disease in Crohn's disease, other factors such as malnutrition, mal-absorption of the nutrients, and central nervous system were also blamed for longitudinal growth delay. Especially those patients affected more with jejunum inflammation have poor nutrition and severe deficiency in energy metabolism as well as a chronic inflammation state which contributes to the growth delay [42]. In Crohn's disease it has been suggested that chronic inflammation interferes with both central and peripheral growth hormone/factor secretion causing hormonal deficiency and/or resistance. While inflammatory cytokines directly affect appetite centers, they also disrupt growth hormone signal transduction and proteolyze IGFBP-3 and inhibit the IGF-1 expression in the growth plate [43].

3. Other growth factors that affect longitudinal growth: C-type natriuretic peptide

C-type natriuretic peptide NP is anabolic in the growth plate, articular cartilage, and in bone tissue: We and others have shown that CNP is anabolic in the growth plate and that CNP/natriuretic peptide receptor-B (NPR-B)/cyclic guanosine monophosphate (cGMP) signaling regulates linear bone growth/endochondral bone formation through the cGMP-dependent protein kinase II (cGK-2). CNP induces chondrocyte proliferation, differentiation, and extracellular matrix (ECM) production.

We have recently shown that transgenic mice that overexpress CNP under the control of the type-II collagen promoter had increased endochondral bone growth with thick and matrix-rich articular joint cartilage. Most importantly, we have also shown that in an animal model of inflammatory arthritis, CNP overexpression in chondrocytes protects the articular cartilage integrity and prevents subchondral bone defects [27]. Our transgenic mice that overexpressed CNP on cartilage developed dense trabeculation under the subchondral bone supporting in vitro experiments showing increased matrix secretion by osteoblastic cells [44]. In addition, there is data about CNP enhancing ECM secretion in cultured articular chondrocytes seeded on a type-II collagen-coated scaffold [45]. CNP has a unique dual anabolic effect on chondrocytes and osteoblasts for matrix synthesis. Together, these findings suggest that CNP is an ideal growth factor to be used in TE for osteochondral defects since it may promote both cartilage and bone regeneration.

CNP improves vasculogenesis and graft survival: Vascular endothelial cells also express and secrete CNP, and CNP has a major role in embryonic vasculogenesis and graft vasculogenesis [46, 47].

Angiogenesis is essential for bone formation during embryonic life and after fracture, indicating a further role in bone fracture healing for CNP.

3.1. CNP signaling pathway

Natriuretic peptides are one of the main classes of cGMP inducers which are known as atrial natriuretic peptide (ANP), brain natriuretic peptide (BNP), and C-type natriuretic peptide (CNP). Natriuretic peptides are secreted proteins that control cell behavior through activation of two major transmembrane receptors, natriuretic peptide receptor 1 and 2 (NPR1 and NPR2) [48–50]. Receptors NPR1 and NPR2 have guanylyl cyclase activity and synthesize cGMP in response to ligand binding. ANP and BNP signal mainly through NPR1/GC-A, while CNP predominantly activates NPR2/GC-B. All three ligands also bind to a third receptor, NPR3, which is known as the clearance receptor that does not have an intracellular signaling part from the molecule and limits ligand availability once attached and limits natriuretic peptide signaling.

Once CNP gene and its signaling were disrupted in mice, those mice suffered from postnatal dwarfism [51]. While CNP knock-out mice developed normal membranous ossification, endochondral ossification was severely impaired and all long bones and vertebrae were significantly shorter. About 70% of null mice die in the first 100 days after birth. When crossed with transgenic mice that overexpressed CNP in cartilage, knock-out mice phenotype was completely rescued.

Further organ culture experiments (femur) confirmed CNP's effect as the potent stimulator of endochondral bone growth. Other mice models were present in which Npr2 was knocked out and similar dwarf phenotype was observed, thus further confirming the importance of CNP signaling pathways. A loss-of-function mutation in the cGMP-dependent protein kinase II (cGKII gene) has also recently been identified as the cause of dwarfism in mice which is a downstream effector of CNP. When Npr3 is knocked out, an opposite phenotype of skeletal over growth is observed [52, 53].

All natriuretic peptides (ANP, BNP, and CNP) have the ability to bind NPRA, NPRB, and NPRC, while CNP has the most affinity to bind NPRB which seems to control endochondral bone growth the most. Mice deficient for ANP, BNP, or NPR1 genes were reported not to develop dwarfism or abnormal skeletal phenotypes [54, 55], suggesting that these genes play only minor supportive roles during endochondral bone formation. Overexpression of BNP in transgenic mice developed skeletal overgrowth, but this was explained as overstimulation of NPR2 by excess levels of BNP [56, 57].

4. CNP's role in cartilage homeostasis

Transgenic mice that overexpress CNP (CNPcol2a1TG) in cartilage develop skeletal overgrowth and increased bone density: in order to further study the effects of CNP in skeletal growth and bone architecture in vivo, we generated transgenic mice by cloning human CNP cDNA (450 bp) into a construct that contained mouse collagen type II (Col2a1) promoter (GenBank #m65161) to specifically overexpress CNP in chondrocytes. Growth plates of CNPcol2a1TG mice showed increased numbers of proliferative chondrocytes measured by BrdU uptake ($p < 0.05$) and increased numbers of enlarged hypertrophic chondrocytes

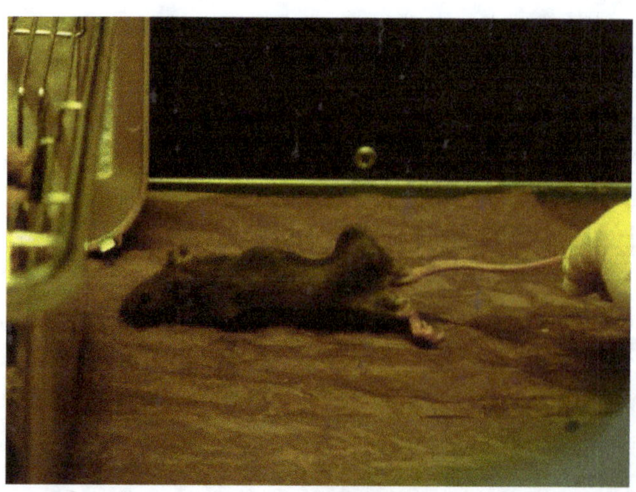

Figure 2. 20 weeks old male CNPcol2a1TG mice with kyphosis and excess growth of longitudinal and vertebral bones.

with increased proteoglycan deposition as evidenced by strong Safranin-O staining [27]. CNPcol2a1TG mice developed increased endochondral bone growth (30%) and developed kyphosis due to vertebral overgrowth by 18 weeks (**Figure 2**). In the skeletal histomorphology of CNPcol2a1TG mice, the most intriguing finding was the increased trabecular bone formation in proximity to the growth plate cartilage, subchondral (juxta-articular) bones, and in vertebrae.

5. CNP's role in bone homeostasis

C-type natriuretic peptide (CNP) has dual anabolic effects on cartilage and bone tissues. We have recently shown that CNP is a major contributor to post-natal skeletal growth in humans by its effects on the growth plate cartilage [58]. CNP also has an anabolic effect on bone morphogenesis [59]. Previous reports of in vitro experiments suggest that the CNP signaling system is an autocrine/paracrine regulator of osteoblast growth and differentiation, and CNP plays a role in bone remodeling [60, 61].

Although it is one of the major regulators of endochondral bone growth with its impact on cartilage tissue and its homeostatic role in the growing bone tissue, CNP's role in adult bone is unclear. Recent research in ewes (adult female sheep) showed that when estrogen was given CNP, content was increased the most in the estrogen-responsive trabecular bones (vertebrae and iliac bones) more than the longitudinal bones (tibia). The same study suggested that dexamethasone injections to ewes did not change the content of CNP in bone tissue, while plasma CNP peptides and bone alkaline phosphatase levels were significantly decreased.

Dwarf mice, that is. Npr2 knockout or Nppc KO, have not been reported for the lack of their bone mineral content or bone mineral density. Our observation in the CNPcol2a1TG mice that overexpressed CNP, particularly in the cartilage tissue, was that both vertebral bones and the metaphysis/epiphysis of long bones, around the growth plates, develop significantly increased trabeculation and mineralization [59, 62]. This may be because Nppc overexpression was more significant in the growth plate cartilage and somewhat in the joint cartilage in our CNPcol2a1TG mice. Others using different promoters that caused increased production of CNP (SAP-CNP-Tg mice) in serum showed the effect of CNP on bone turnover microcomputed tomography (CT) analysis revealed increased trabeculation and dense bones lumber vertebrae in contrast to long bones such as femur. However, the fracture model showed that there is increased bone turnover and fracture healing in the SAP-CNP-Tg mice even in long bones with less trabecular ratio. Bone histomorphometric analysis of the tibiae from SAP-CNP-Tg mice showed that stabilized femoral fracture healing is advanced in SAP-CNP-Tg mice supporting the hypothesis that CNP regulates bone homeostasis and contributes to remodeling [63].

Osteoblastic cell culture experiments showed CNP's anabolic effect in osteoblastic activity.

6. CNP's role in vascular homeostasis

One of the most important roles of CNP is in the venous system. CNP via its NPR2 a d NPR3 receptor signaling in the vascular wall regulates vasodilatation particularly on the venous wall. Enhanced osteoblastic and osteoclastic activities. In addition, serum levels of osteocalcin and tartrate-resistant acid phosphatase-5b, were elevated in the Tg mice. The same study showed that open and Vascular endothelial cells express and secrete CNP. CNP is suppressed by the VEGF secretion and is known to act as a vasodilator [64]. Also, CNP has been suggested to have a major role in angiogenesis [47, 65]. Once the growth plate is closed after puberty, the chondrogenic CNP will no longer available. Then CNP needed for trabecular bone remodeling will then have to be secreted partially by osteoblasts as a paracrine/autocrine factor and/or by vascular endothelium. Steady serum levels of NT-proCNP may also be regulating the cartilage and bone homeostasis and the main source of NT-proCNP might only be the vascular endothelium. Due to the vascular wall expression of CNP and its vasodilator effect, CNP's role in hypertension, vasculitis and myocardial infarction has been studied.

7. Lack of CNP signaling in growth plate causes short stature and dwarfism

Heterozygous carriers of a mutation in NPR-B, the receptor for CNP, have idiopathic short stature suggesting a quantitative effect of the CNP pathway on skeletal growth [66]. Serum levels of CNP's N-terminal pro-peptide (NT-proCNP), the inactive form of CNP, were found to be highest at birth, gradually decreased by puberty, and plateau after 18 years of age [67]. The levels of NT-proCNP correlate with levels of alkaline phosphatase (bone formation markers) in humans [67, 68]. More importantly, serum NT-proCNP levels are maintained at a level in adults.

Individuals with acromesomelic dysplasia-type Maroteaux (AMDM), a type of human dwarfism, develop periarticular osteopenia, loss of trabecular bone structure. AMDM is caused by loss of function mutations in the CNP's receptor, natriuretic peptide-B (Npr2 gene). AMDM patients have disproportional growth retardation and abnormal development of bone tissue and appear to have (juxta-articular) metaphyseal flaring and osteopenia but do not have any other health problems [58, 69]. The trabecular bone loss is more significant in the juxta-articular area resembling osteopenia of inflammatory arthritis.

8. CNP in skeletal overgrowth

Before CNP and it effectors can be used as a remedy for short stature and growth delay, its effects in humans need to be studied well. Evidence for complications of excess systemic CNP came after the description of two novel mutations that resulted in gain of function in humans. The C-type natriuretic peptide (CNP), encoded by NPPC gene, is located on chromosome 2q37.1. Two independent studies have described three patients with a Marfan-like phenotype presenting a de novo balanced translocation involving the same chromosomal region 2q37.1 and overexpression of NPPC [70]. One study reported on two partially overlapping interstitial 2q37 deletions. These two patients showed opposite phenotypes characterized by short stature and skeletal overgrowth, respectively. The patient with short stature presented a 2q37 deletion causing the loss of one copy of the NPPC gene with normal CNP plasma concentration. The deletion identified in the patient with a Marfan-like phenotype interrupted the DIS3L2 gene without involving the NPPC gene. In addition, a strongly elevated CNP plasma concentration was found in this patient with Marfanoid features and a tall stature [71, 72].

9. CNP roles in energy metabolism

CNP was first isolated from porcine brain and was expected to be a neuropeptide [73], but the physiological significance of the CNP/GC-B system has been established in the vascular and skeletal systems [53, 58, 71, 72, 74–78]. It was reported that CNP and GC-B are expressed in the central [79–83] and peripheral nervous systems [84, 85]. It has been shown that the hypothalamus is an important center to control food intake and energy expenditure [86]. CNP mRNA was detected in the rat hypothalamus indicating this peptide's role in numerous

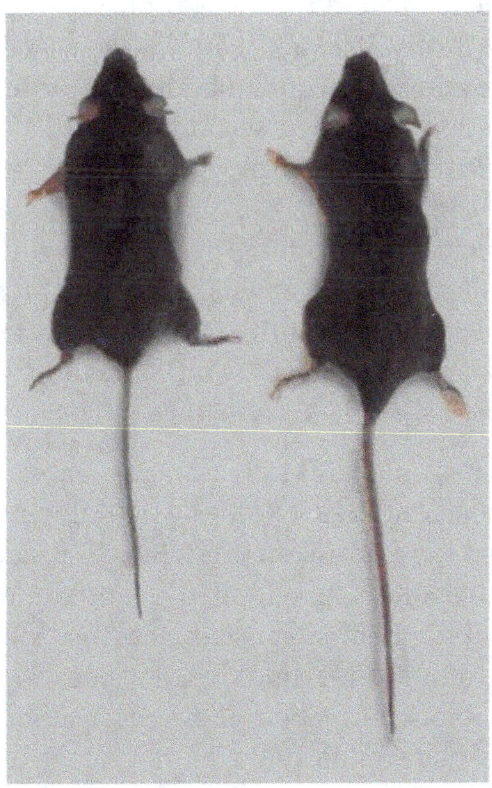

Figure 3. CNPcol2a1TG mice (on the right) are tall and slender as compared to the wild type littermates (on the left).

neuroendocrine regulation [87]. CNP is suggested to play important roles in central energy expenditure and food intake via its effects on the central nervous system (**Figure 3**).

10. CNP during inflammatory disease activity

Initial reports about CNP's effect on inflammatory disease activity came from osteoarthritis disease models. Since both nitric oxide and CNP are the two main activators of cGMP in cartilage they were checked for their role in development of osteoarthritis. The production of nitric oxide (NO) regulates host defense and inflammation. Nitric oxide has vasodilation, cytotoxicity, and it has a role in cytokine-dependent tissue injury. NO effects have been blamed in the tissue injury of a variety of rheumatologic conditions including systemic lupus erythematosus, rheumatoid arthritis, and osteoarthritis. Pro-inflammatory effects of nitric oxide include vasodilation, edema, cytotoxicity, and the mediation of cytokine-dependent processes that can lead to tissue destruction. In contrast to NO effect in the cartilage, NO secretion from vascular wall is protective against neutrophil adhesion and related vascular injury. Thus, nitric oxide has been found as a clear role player in osteoarthritis pathogenesis but not in microvasculature injury [88, 89]. Although CNP is known to induce articular chondrocyte hypertrophy, it was never blamed to be involved in osteoarthritis pathogenesis, while it was considered to contribute to the disease progression. On the other hand, we were able to show in an inflammatory arthritis murine model that cartilage overexpression of CNP increased the chondrocyte number, matrix synthesis, and maintained a thicker hypertrophic cartilage in the growth plate and in the joints and thus was protective against the cartilage degenerative effects of inflammatory arthritis. The mouse model we used was for a K/BxN rheumatoid arthritis mouse model that developed severe inflammatory arthritis which was evident from first synovitis, pannus formation, and then secondary cartilage deterioration [28, 90]. Our transgenic mouse under Col2a1 promoter overexpressed CNP in the cartilage tissue mainly in the growth plate and in the joint cartilage. CNP transgenic mice developed thick growth plates with enlarged chondrocytes and wider growth plates with proliferating chondrocytes that produced a rich matrix. Furthermore, when CNP overexpressing mice was crossed with K/BxN mouse and developed systemic arthritis, we observed that cartilage matrix integrity and cartilage structure was protected against the inflammation. CNP transgenic mice did not develop severe complications of arthritis (**Figure 4**) [27, 91].

Another evidence for CNP's systemic anti-inflammatory effect was reported in a rat model of hemorrhagic shock and resuscitation. CNP infusion to this model lowered the myeloperoxidase activity and decreased the expression of TNF-α, IL-6, and IL-1β in the kidneys. CNP treatment suppressed oxidative stress, ameliorated the inflammatory response, and caused acute kidney injury [92]. Investigators suggested that they demonstrated CNP infusion's inhibitory effect on the generation of reactive oxygen species (ROS) and pro-inflammatory cytokines after hemorrhagic shock induction and subsequently suppressed the activation, recruitment, and adherence of neutrophils in the kidney. Neutrophil recruitment is one of the fundamental pathways in hemorrhagic shock. It is suggested that neutrophil recruitment is also delayed after CNP treatment. In an earlier study, Chen et al. showed that CNP treatment

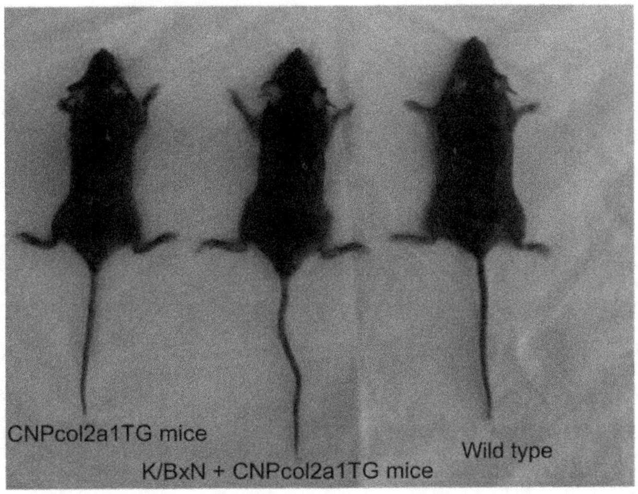

Figure 4. K/BxN+CNPcol2a1TG double transgenic mice do not develop growth retardation or severe complications of arthritis.

effectively attenuates lipopolysaccharide (LPS)-induced endothelial activation by eliminating intracellular ROS production, inhibiting the NF-κB and MAPK p38 signaling pathways and activating the PI3 K/Akt/HO-1 pathway in human umbilical vein endothelial cells (HUVECs), [93] suggesting an anti-inflammatory effect for CNP.

Another study that showed CNP's effect in reducing the LPS-induced lung injury suggested that mechanism of action might involve downregulation of inflammatory cytokine expression in lung parenchyma and again downregulation of neutrophil migration in the lungs [94].

Finally, evidence for CNP and its derivate anti-inflammatory treatment potential were shown in a wounded cartilage explant model in steers. In this study, wounded explants were cultured with 0 or 10 ng/mL IL-1β and/or microcapsules loaded with or without CNP for a period of 48 h. The presence of CNP microcapsules had a concentration-dependent effect with significant inhibition of NO release in response to IL-1β at 2000 ($p < 0.01$), 10,000 ($p < 0.01$), and 50,000 microcapsules/well ($p < 0.001$) [45]. Others suggested that the effect of CNP on preventing the inflammatory effects of IL-1β in chondrocytes depends on local protein concentration. While low concentrations (pM) were shown to promote a proliferative response, high concentrations (μM) lead to anabolic effects such as matrix synthesis in chondrocytes [95, 96].

Acute inflammation and the inflammatory mediators seems to suppress the activity of CNP in growing organisms [97]. It is possible that in chronic inflammatory diseases, serum NT-proCNP levels are also low and contribute to the growth arrest during active disease in children.

11. Other conditions in which circulating CNP levels are affected

CNP regulates fat metabolism in adipogenic tissue, and adipogenic CNP transgenic mice is resistant to obesity when fed by high fat content. Natriuretic peptides regulate intracellular cGMP and phosphorylated vasodilator-stimulated phosphoprotein (VASP). Adipogenic CNP transgenic mice showed a decrease in fat weight and adipocyte hypertrophy and increases in fatty acid β-oxidation, lipolysis-related gene expression, and energy expenditure during high fat diet (HFD)-induced obesity. Furthermore it seems like CNP overexpression diminished the inflammatory activity in adipogenic tissue. Adipogenic cell CNP transgenic mice were reported to have significantly decreased gene expression of TNF-α, interleukin-6 (IL-6), monocyte chemoattractant protein-1 (MCP-1), and F4/80 in mature adipocytes [98]. Adipogenic CNP transgenic mice also developed better glucose tolerance and insulin sensitivity, which were found to be associated with enhanced insulin-stimulated Akt phosphorylation. It was suggested that CNP overexpression in adipocytes protects against adipocyte hypertrophy, excess lipid metabolism, inflammation, and decreased insulin sensitivity during HFD-induced obesity. An earlier report also suggested that overexpression of endothelial-specific CNP overexpression protects against visceral adipose tissue hypertrophy, systemic inflammation, and insulin resistance during the development of obesity due to the feeding of a high-fat diet (HFD) [99]. Overall current knowledge suggests that natriuretic peptides are new pathways controlling human adipose tissue lipolysis operating via a cGMP-dependent pathway.

One of the intriguing studies is one that examined serum levels of 53 patients with Behçet's disease and showed that all patients with active disease had lower levels of CNP indicating its suppression by inflammatory disease activity [100]. Thus, there is evidence that during chronic inflammatory diseases CNP serum levels might be suppressed which can impact the skeletal growth if the individuals affected have open growth plates and ongoing longitudinal growth process.

12. Current clinical use of CNP

Use of CNP and its analogues in achondroplasias: gain-of-function mutations in the FGFR3 gene result in achondroplasia. Achondroplasia is known as the most common form of dwarfism. In patients with achondroplasia there is impaired proliferation and differentiation of the chondrocytes in the growth plate cartilage that causes stunted longitudinal growth due to endochondral growth suppression and skull abnormalities due to membranous ossification disruption. In achondroplasia, FGFR3 mutations induce increased phosphorylation of the tyrosine kinase receptor FGFR3 and increase the mitogen-activated protein kinase (MAPK). It is known that C-type natriuretic peptide (CNP) suppresses FGFR3 downstream signaling by inhibiting the pathway of mitogen-activated protein kinase (MAPK) in vivo and in vitro. Mice overexpressing CNP rescues FGFR3 gain of mutation-related dwarfism. Exogenous administration of CNP has been challenging since it is rapidly cleared and degraded in vivo through receptor-mediated and proteolytic pathways such as proteolytic-neutral endopeptidase degradation. Therefore, multiple variants of CNP molecules have been tested for their efficacy. Recently, a variant of CNP called BMN111, neutral endopeptidase-resistant CNP analog, showed significant ability to stimulate signaling downstream of the CNP receptor, natriuretic peptide receptor B. Initial trial of continuous delivery of CNP through intravenous (IV) infusion in the form of BMN111 in 2014 showed normalization of dwarfism [101].

Since subcutaneous (SC) route of administration is preferred over continuous infusion in pediatric individuals, it is expected that BMN 111, a 39 amino acid CNP pharmacological analog, would be very effective in diseases where CNP signaling pathway is impaired. BMN 111 can be applied once daily via SC administration at physiological concentrations [101].

In the near future, CNP analogues might be used in other diseases where CNP signaling is impaired or blocked by chronic inflammation affecting cartilage and bone. Use of CNP analogues can be applicable to both adult and pediatric diseases.

Author details

Hulya Bukulmez

Address all correspondence to: hxb38@case.edu

Department of Pediatrics, Division of Pediatric Rheumatology, MetroHealth Medical Center, Case Western Reserve University, Cleveland, Ohio, United States

References

[1] Olsen BR, Reginato AM, Wang W. Bone development. Annual Review of Cell and Developmental Biology. 2000;**16**:191-220

[2] Wagner EF, Karsenty G. Genetic control of skeletal development. Current Opinion in Genetics & Development. 2001;**11**(5):527-532

[3] Karsenty G, Wagner EF. Reaching a genetic and molecular understanding of skeletal development. Developmental Cell. 2002;**2**(4):389-406

[4] Provot S, Schipani E. Molecular mechanisms of endochondral bone development. Biochemical and Biophysical Research Communications. 2005;**328**(3):658-665

[5] DeLise AM, Fischer L, Tuan RS. Cellular interactions and signaling in cartilage development. Osteoarthritis and Cartilage. 2000;**8**(5):309-334

[6] Kronenberg HM. Developmental regulation of the growth plate. Nature. 2003;**423**(6937): 332-336

[7] van der Eerden BC, Karperien M, Wit JM. Systemic and local regulation of the growth plate. Endocrine Reviews. 2003;**24**(6):782-801

[8] Beier F et al. Cell cycle genes in chondrocyte proliferation and differentiation. Matrix Biology. 1999;**18**(2):109-120

[9] Lefebvre V, Smits P. Transcriptional control of chondrocyte fate and differentiation. Birth Defects Research. Part C, Embryo Today. 2005;**75**(3):200-212

[10] Kronenberg HM. PTHrP and skeletal development. Annals of the New York Academy of Sciences. 2006;**1068**:1-13

[11] Alvarez-Nava F, Lanes R. GH/IGF-1 Signaling and current knowledge of epigenetics; a review and considerations on possible therapeutic options. International Journal of Molecular Sciences. 2017;**18**(10)

[12] Savino W et al. The thymus gland: A target organ for growth hormone. Scandinavian Journal of Immunology. 2002;**55**(5):442-452

[13] Ying H et al. Dual functions of the steroid hormone receptor coactivator 3 in modulating resistance to thyroid hormone. Molecular and Cellular Biology. 2005;**25**(17):7687-7695

[14] Welbourne TC, Milford L, Carter P. The role of growth hormone in substrate utilization. Baillière's Clinical Endocrinology and Metabolism. 1997;**11**(4):699-707

[15] Cittadini A et al. Growth hormone and the heart. Mineral and Electrolyte Metabolism. 1999;**25**(1-2):51-55

[16] Hochberg Z. Mechanisms of steroid impairment of growth. Hormone Research. 2002;**58** (Suppl 1):33-38

[17] Gevers EF et al. Single cell enzyme activity and proliferation in the growth plate: Effects of growth hormone. Journal of Bone and Mineral Research. 1996;**11**(8):1103-1111

[18] Claramunt D et al. Effects of growth hormone treatment on growth plate, bone, and mineral metabolism of young rats with uremia induced by adenine. Pediatric Research. 2017;**82**(1):148-154

[19] Teixeira CC, Agoston H, Beier F. Nitric oxide, C-type natriuretic peptide and cGMP as regulators of endochondral ossification. Developmental Biology. 2008;**319**(2):171-178

[20] Barnes PJ, Karin M. Nuclear factor-kappaB: A pivotal transcription factor in chronic inflammatory diseases. The New England Journal of Medicine. 1997;**336**(15):1066-1071

[21] Cirillo F et al. Inflammatory diseases and growth: Effects on the GH-IGF axis and on growth plate. International Journal of Molecular Sciences. 2017;**18**(9)

[22] Kim H et al. Extracellular S100A4 negatively regulates osteoblast function by activating the NF-kappaB pathway. BMB Reports. 2017;**50**(2):97-102

[23] Soysa NS, Alles N. NF-kappaB functions in osteoclasts. Biochemical and Biophysical Research Communications. 2009;**378**(1):1-5

[24] Iotsova V et al. Osteopetrosis in mice lacking NF-kappaB1 and NF-kappaB2. Nature Medicine. 1997;**3**(11):1285-1289

[25] De Benedetti F et al. Interleukin 6 causes growth impairment in transgenic mice through a decrease in insulin-like growth factor-I. A model for stunted growth in children with chronic inflammation. The Journal of Clinical Investigation. 1997;**99**(4):643-650

[26] Liu Z et al. SOCS3 promotes inflammation and apoptosis via inhibiting JAK2/STAT3 signaling pathway in 3T3-L1 adipocyte. Immunobiology. 2015;**220**(8):947-953

[27] Bukulmez H et al. C-type natriuretic peptide (CNP) over expression in chondrocytes prevents growth delay in murine model of inflammatory arthritis. Arthritis and Rheumatism. 2008;**58**(9):S645-S645

[28] Kyburz D, Corr M. The KRN mouse model of inflammatory arthritis. Springer Seminars in Immunopathology. 2003;**25**(1):79-90

[29] Wit, J.M. and F. de Luca, Atypical defects resulting in growth hormone insensitivity. Growth Hormone & IGF Research. 2016;**28**:57-61

[30] Wolters TLC et al. IGF1 potentiates the pro-inflammatory response in human peripheral blood mononuclear cells via MAPK. Journal of Molecular Endocrinology. 2017;**59**(2):129-139

[31] Cirillo F et al. MicroRNAs link chronic inflammation in childhood to growth impairment and insulin-resistance. Cytokine & Growth Factor Reviews; 2018

[32] Liem JJ, Rosenberg AM. Growth patterns in juvenile rheumatoid arthritis. Clinical and Experimental Rheumatology. 2003;**21**(5):663-668

[33] Bozzola E et al. Changes in growth hormone receptor gene expression during therapy in children with juvenile idiopathic arthritis. Hormone Research in Pædiatrics. 2012;**77**(1):52-58

[34] Uettwiller F et al. Effect of biologic treatments on growth in children with juvenile idiopathic arthritis. The Journal of Rheumatology. 2014;**41**(1):128-135

[35] De Benedetti F et al. Catch-up growth during tocilizumab therapy for systemic juvenile idiopathic arthritis: Results from a phase III trial. Arthritis & Rhematology. 2015;**67**(3):840-848

[36] Svantesson H. Treatment of growth failure with human growth hormone in patients with juvenile chronic arthritis. A pilot study. Clinical and Experimental Rheumatology. 1991;**9**(Suppl 6):47-50

[37] Simon D. Management of growth retardation in juvenile idiopathic arthritis. Hormone Research. 2007;**68**(Suppl 5):122-125

[38] Simon D. rhGH treatment in corticosteroid-treated patients. Hormone Research. 2007;**68**(1):38-45

[39] Simon D. Safety of growth hormone treatment in children with juvenile idiopathic arthritis. Hormone Research. 2009;**72**(Suppl 1):65-68

[40] Simon D, Bechtold S. Effects of growth hormone treatment on growth in children with juvenile idiopathic arthritis. Hormone Research. 2009;**72**(Suppl 1):55-59

[41] Simon D, Prieur A, Czernichow P. Treatment of juvenile rheumatoid arthritis with growth hormone. Hormone Research. 2000;**53**(Suppl 1):82-86

[42] Shamir R. Nutrition and growth in inflammatory bowel disease. World Review of Nutrition and Dietetics. 2013;**106**:156-161

[43] Sanderson IR. Growth problems in children with IBD. Nature Reviews. Gastroenterology & Hepatology. 2014;**11**(10):601-610

[44] Bukulmez H et al. Role of C-type natriuretic peptide (CNP) in osteogenesis and treatment of osteoporosis. OAC. 2010;**18**(S2):185

[45] Peake NJ et al. Controlled release of C-type natriuretic peptide by microencapsulation dampens proinflammatory effects induced by IL-1beta in cartilage explants. Biomacromolecules. 2015;**16**(2):524-531

[46] Del Ry S et al. High concentration of C-type natriuretic peptide promotes VEGF-dependent vasculogenesis in the remodeled region of infarcted swine heart with preserved left ventricular ejection fraction. International Journal of Cardiology. 2013;**168**(3):2426-2434

[47] Doi K et al. Expression of natriuretic peptide system during embryonic stem cell vasculogenesis. Heart Vessels. 1997;(Suppl 12):18-22

[48] Potter LR, Abbey-Hosch S, Dickey DM. Natriuretic peptides, their receptors, and cyclic guanosine monophosphate-dependent signaling functions. Endocrine Reviews. 2006;**27**(1):47-72

[49] Baxter GF. The natriuretic peptides. Basic Research in Cardiology. 2004;**99**(2):71-75

[50] Cea LB. Natriuretic peptide family: New aspects. Current Medicinal Chemistry. Cardiovascular and Hematological Agents. 2005;**3**(2):87-98

[51] Chusho H et al. Dwarfism and early death in mice lacking C-type natriuretic peptide. Proceedings of the National Academy of Sciences of the United States of America. 2001;**98**(7):4016-4021

[52] Jaubert J et al. Three new allelic mouse mutations that cause skeletal overgrowth involve the natriuretic peptide receptor C gene (Npr3). Proceedings of the National Academy of Sciences of the United States of America. 1999;**96**(18):10278-10283

[53] Matsukawa N et al. The natriuretic peptide clearance receptor locally modulates the physiological effects of the natriuretic peptide system. Proceedings of the National Academy of Sciences of the United States of America. 1999;**96**(13):7403-7408

[54] John SW et al. Genetic decreases in atrial natriuretic peptide and salt-sensitive hypertension. Science. 1995;**267**(5198):679-681

[55] John SW et al. Blood pressure and fluid-electrolyte balance in mice with reduced or absent ANP. The American Journal of Physiology. 1996;**271**(1 Pt 2):R109-R114

[56] Suda M et al. Skeletal overgrowth in transgenic mice that overexpress brain natriuretic peptide. Proceedings of the National Academy of Sciences of the United States of America. 1998;**95**(5):2337-2342

[57] Yasoda A et al. Natriuretic peptide regulation of endochondral ossification. Evidence for possible roles of the C-type natriuretic peptide/guanylyl cyclase-B pathway. The Journal of Biological Chemistry. 1998;**273**(19):11695-11700

[58] Bartels CF et al. Mutations in the transmembrane natriuretic peptide receptor NPR-B impair skeletal growth and cause acromesomelic dysplasia, type Maroteaux. American Journal of Human Genetics. 2004;**75**(1):27-34

[59] Bukulmez H et al. Role of C-type natriuretic peptide (Cnp) in osteogenesis and treatment of osteoporosis. Osteoarthritis and Cartilage. 2010;**18**:S89-S89

[60] Hagiwara H et al. cGMP produced in response to ANP and CNP regulates proliferation and differentiation of osteoblastic cells. The American Journal of Physiology. 1996;**270**(5 Pt 1):C1311-C1318

[61] Suda M et al. C-type natriuretic peptide as an autocrine/paracrine regulator of osteoblast. Evidence for possible presence of bone natriuretic peptide system. Biochemical and Biophysical Research Communications. 1996;**223**(1):1-6

[62] Bukulmez H et al. Protective effects of C-type natriuretic peptide on linear growth and articular cartilage integrity in a mouse model of inflammatory arthritis. Arthritis & Rhematology. 2014;**66**(1):78-89

[63] Kondo E et al. Increased bone turnover and possible accelerated fracture healing in a murine model with an increased circulating C-type natriuretic peptide. Endocrinology. 2015;**156**(7):2518-2529

[64] Doi K et al. Vascular endothelial growth factor suppresses C-type natriuretic peptide secretion. Hypertension. 1996;**27**(3 Pt 2):811-815

[65] Pedram A, Razandi M, Levin ER. Natriuretic peptides suppress vascular endothelial cell growth factor signaling to angiogenesis. Endocrinology. 2001;**142**(4):1578-1586

[66] Olney RC. C-type natriuretic peptide in growth: A new paradigm. Growth Hormone & IGF Research. 2006;**16**(Suppl A)S6-14

[67] Olney RC et al. Heterozygous mutations in natriuretic peptide receptor-B (NPR2) are associated with short stature. The Journal of Clinical Endocrinology and Metabolism. 2006;**91**(4):1229-1232

[68] Prickett TC et al. Identification of amino-terminal pro-C-type natriuretic peptide in human plasma. Biochemical and Biophysical Research Communications. 2001;**286**(3):513-517

[69] Kant SG et al. Acromesomelic dysplasia Maroteaux type maps to human chromosome 9. American Journal of Human Genetics. 1998;**63**(1):155-162

[70] Ko JM et al. Skeletal overgrowth syndrome caused by overexpression of C-type natriuretic peptide in a girl with balanced chromosomal translocation, t(1;2)(q41;q37.1). American Journal of Medical Genetics. Part A. 2015;**167A**(5):1033-1038

[71] Bocciardi R, Ravazzolo R. C-type natriuretic peptide and overgrowth. Endocrine Development. 2009;**14**:61-66

[72] Bocciardi R et al. Overexpression of the C-type natriuretic peptide (CNP) is associated with overgrowth and bone anomalies in an individual with balanced t(2;7) translocation. Human Mutation. 2007;**28**(7):724-731

[73] Hama N et al. Detection of C-type natriuretic peptide in human circulation and marked increase of plasma CNP level in septic shock patients. Biochemical and Biophysical Research Communications. 1994;**198**(3):1177-1182

[74] Kake T et al. Chronically elevated plasma C-type natriuretic peptide level stimulates skeletal growth in transgenic mice. American Journal of Physiology. Endocrinology and Metabolism. 2009;**297**(6):E1339-E1348

[75] Waschek JA. Developmental actions of natriuretic peptides in the brain and skeleton. Cellular and Molecular Life Sciences. 2004;**61**(18):2332-2342

[76] Chusho H et al. Dwarfism and early death in mice lacking C-type natriuretic peptide. USA: Proc Natl Acad Sci; 2001;**98**(7):4016-21

[77] Damgaard P et al. Evidence of physiotherapy interventions for patients with chronic neck pain: A systematic review of randomised controlled trials. ISRN Pain. 2013;**2013**:567175

[78] Fujii T et al. Circulating C-type natriuretic peptide (CNP) rescues chondrodysplastic CNP knockout mice from their impaired skeletal growth and early death. Endocrinology. 2010;**151**(9):4381-4388

[79] Wiedemann K, Jahn H, Kellner M. Effects of natriuretic peptides upon hypothalamo-pituitary-adrenocortical system activity and anxiety behaviour. Experimental and Clinical Endocrinology & Diabetes. 2000;**108**(1):5-13

[80] Vatta MS et al. B and C types natriuretic peptides modulate norepinephrine uptake and release in the rat hypothalamus. Regulatory Peptides. 1996;**65**(3):175-184

[81] Imura H, Nakao K, Itoh H. The natriuretic peptide system in the brain: Implications in the central control of cardiovascular and neuroendocrine functions. Frontiers in Neuroendocrinology. 1992;**13**(3):217-249

[82] Shimekake Y, Ohta S, Nagata K. C-type natriuretic peptide stimulates secretion of growth hormone from rat-pituitary-derived GH3 cells via a cyclic-GMP-mediated pathway. European Journal of Biochemistry. 1994;**222**(2):645-650

[83] Totsune K et al. C-type natriuretic peptide in the human central nervous system: Distribution and molecular form. Peptides. 1994;**15**(1):37-40

[84] Kishimoto I et al. C-type natriuretic peptide is a Schwann cell-derived factor for development and function of sensory neurones. Journal of Neuroendocrinology. 2008; **20**(11):1213-1223

[85] Ter-Avetisyan G, Rathjen FG, Schmidt H. Bifurcation of axons from cranial sensory neurons is disabled in the absence of Npr2-induced cGMP signaling. The Journal of Neuroscience. 2014;**34**(3):737-747

[86] Gardi J et al. The effects of brain and C-type natriuretic peptides on corticotropin-releasing factor in brain of rats. Life Sciences. 1997;**60**(23):2111-2117

[87] Herman JP, Langub MC Jr, Watson RE Jr. Localization of C-type natriuretic peptide mRNA in rat hypothalamus. Endocrinology. 1993;**133**(4):1903-1906

[88] Abramson SB et al. The role of nitric oxide in tissue destruction. Best Practice & Research. Clinical Rheumatology. 2001;**15**(5):831-845

[89] Abramson SB et al. Nitric oxide and inflammatory mediators in the perpetuation of osteoarthritis. Current Rheumatology Reports. 2001;**3**(6):535-541

[90] Kouskoff V et al. Organ-specific disease provoked by systemic autoimmunity. Cell. 1996;**87**(5):811-822

[91] Bukulmez H et al. C-type Natriuretic Peptide Over Expression in Chondrocytes Prevents Growth Delay in Murine Model of Inflammatory Arthritis. Arthritis and Rheumatism. 2008;**58**:S645

[92] Chen G et al. C-type natriuretic peptide prevents kidney injury and attenuates oxidative and inflammatory responses in hemorrhagic shock. Amino Acids. 2017;**49**(2):347-354

[93] Chen G et al. C-type natriuretic peptide attenuates LPS-induced endothelial activation: Involvement of p38, Akt, and NF-kappaB pathways. Amino Acids. 2014;**46**(12):2653-2663

[94] Kimura T et al. C-type natriuretic peptide attenuates lipopolysaccharide-induced acute lung injury in mice. The Journal of Surgical Research. 2015;**194**(2):631-637

[95] Waldman SD et al. Differential effects of natriuretic peptide stimulation on tissue-engineered cartilage. Tissue Engineering. Part A. 2008;**14**(3):441-448

[96] Ramachandran M et al. Biomechanical signals and the C-type natriuretic peptide counteract catabolic activities induced by IL-1beta in chondrocyte/agarose constructs. Arthritis Research & Therapy. 2011;**13**(5):R145

[97] Prickett TC et al. Acute inflammation in young children inhibits C-type natriuretic peptide. Pediatric Research. 2013;**74**(2):191-195

[98] Bae CR et al. Adipocyte-specific expression of C-type natriuretic peptide suppresses lipid metabolism and adipocyte hypertrophy in adipose tissues in mice fed high-fat diet. Scientific Reports. 2018;**8**(1):2093

[99] Bae CR et al. Overexpression of C-type natriuretic peptide in endothelial cells protects against insulin resistance and inflammation during diet-induced obesity. Scientific Reports. 2017;**7**(1):9807

[100] Yagci R et al. Serum levels of natriuretic peptides in patients with Behcet's disease. Clinical Rheumatology. 2008;**27**(9):1153-1158

[101] Legeai-Mallet L. C-type natriuretic peptide analog as therapy for achondroplasia. Endocrine Development. 2016;**30**:98-105

6

Osteonecrosis of the Jaws

Vladimira Schwartzova, Marcel Riznic,
Branislav Borza and Peter Kizek

Abstract

Osteonecrosis of the jaw is a very severe complication in patients using antiresorptive drugs, which have been widely applied for the last 10 years. It has prompted an increase in number of negative complications such as significantly restricted food intake, reduced quality of life with a negative impact on the general health status of the patient as a whole. The negative influence of antiresorptive drugs on jaw bones is still not precisely known and is the subject of research. More than 30% of patients with rheumatic diseases develop osteonecrotic lesions in the jaws due to a relation with bisphosphonates, corticosteroids or other antiangiogenic treatment administered orally or parenterally. The treatment is often protracted, variable and very complicated. The clinical symptoms and treatment possibilities are presented, and, based on the clinical results, compared with many investigative researches and multicenter studies all over the world. Preventive measures are often consistent with other studies, where precautions such as radical dental treatment were observed, especially before antiresorptive treatment initiation. Despite the clinical results, which widely differ, the best way to prevent the osteonecrosis of the jaw is a necessary interdisciplinary approach and further research.

Keywords: osteonecrosis of the jaw, antiresorptive drugs, interdisciplinary approach, quality of life, rheumatic diseases

1. Introduction

Medication-related osteonecrosis of the jaw (MRONJ) was first described in patients with multiple myeloma treated with intravenously administered bisphosphonates in 2003. At the time, the disease was classified as bisphosphonate-related osteonecrosis of the jaw (BRONJ). However, 15 years of development in diagnosing, treating and monitoring the course of the disease revealed the correlation with drugs other than the bisphosphonates. The American Association of Maxillofacial Surgeons (AAOMS) standardized the diagnostic criteria for BRONJ in 2009, and updated the disease to MRONJ, eventually merging both diseases in 2014 [1].

Recently, there have been a growing number of cases with osteonecrosis of the jaw diagnosed in patients treated with cytostatics, hormonal preparations combined with corticosteroids and human monoclonal antibodies. This group of drugs is known as antiresorptive medicaments (ARM), with proven cytotoxic effect on mucous membrane of the oral cavity. Most often, however, following an invasive procedure in oral cavity that breaches its integrity and exposes the alveolar bone, while simultaneously failing to implement measures that promote wound healing, they lead to a necrosis. Osteonecrosis of the jaw is confirmed by the clinical picture of non-healing post-extraction wound (or dental trauma), which has not healed in 8 months without medical history of radiation therapy in head and neck region, edema, loose teeth, foetor ex ore, fistulas and, in advanced stages, pain.

It is possible to locate the affected area by employing the modern methods such as MRI, CBCT or through bone resorption biomarker findings. These diagnostic methods aid in determining the stage of the disease and subsequent method of treatment. The treatment is difficult and often ineffective, with recurrent complications. When the preventive measures are observed and the disease is diagnosed early, followed up by an adequate treatment, the disease can be cured, or at least in certain cases, the symptoms in the oral cavity can be alleviated. In the majority of cases, however, MRONJ patients who have been treated with antiresorptive drugs tend to also suffer from breast cancer, prostate cancer or multiple myeloma (**Figures 1** and **2**). We also encounter increasing number of patients with osteoporosis and rheumatoid arthritis [2]. Most cases of MRONJ arise after prolonged intravenous use of nitrogen-containing bisphosphonates. Orally administered nitrogen-containing bisphosphonates cause MRONJ less often [3].

The scope and course of the disease depends on the correlation between other drugs and the patient's overall health status. Antiresorptive treatment is a common treatment method, only excluding patients with cancer, rheumatoid arthritis, osteoporosis or the so-called skeletal-related

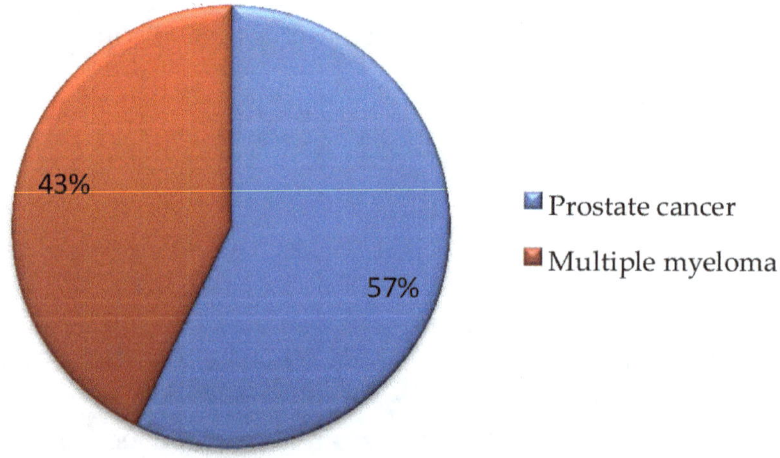

Figure 1. The basis of disease in men.

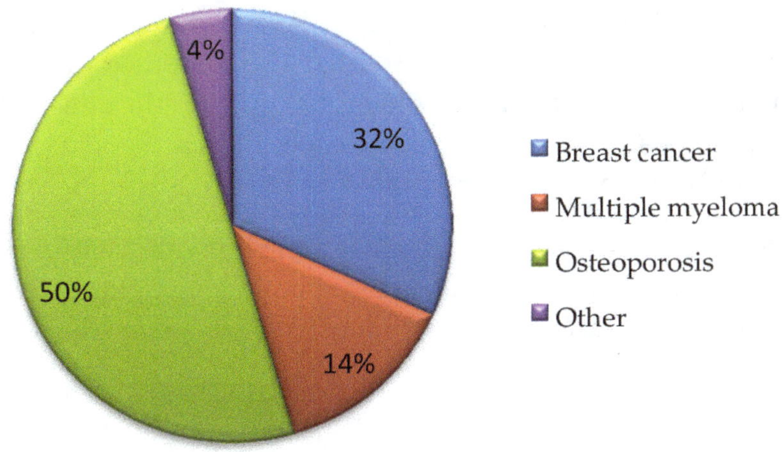

Figure 2. The basis of disease in women.

events (SREs). This term refers collectively to specific serious complications relating to the metastatic bone disease. SREs include pathological fractures of vertebrae and long bones, malignant spinal cord compression, hypercalcemia and cases requiring orthopedic and analgesic radiotherapy. This treatment improves the quality of life for such patients, and provides them with longer lifespan, with minimal undesirable effects.

2. Etiopathogenesis

There are a number of theories concerning the cause of this complication. They are mostly related to the formation of necrotic bone caused by the inhibition of bone remodeling with bisphosphonates and an antiangiogenic therapy. However, several studies on the development of the disease indicate that the bone remodeling inhibition itself cannot cause bone exposure. It is necessary for local risk factors to also be present.

The most significant theories about the possible cause are based on the following arguments:

1. The only barrier between the bone and the mouth is a thin mucosa that is easily damaged by mechanical irritation (chewing, prosthesis-related trauma).
2. Oral cavity contains a diverse microbial flora that may induce pulpo-periodontal diseases, when the area becomes pathologic.
3. A surgical procedure in the area exposes the alveolar bone to a high concentration of bacteria.
4. Bone remodeling rate of the jaw and mandible is very high, which leads to a greater accumulation of bisphosphonates in the mineralized bone tissue [4].

According to a theory, keratinocytes undergo bisphosphonate-induced apoptosis resulting in diminished mucous barrier in the oral cavity, which plays a role in the development of MRONJ. If an infection in the oral cavity is caused by the naturally occurring post-surgery bacteria (*Actinomyces israelii, Escherichia coli*), they will cause the drop in the wound area pH, and will release bisphosphonates and calcium salts. The hypothesis is that high concentrations of bisphosphonates increase apoptosis of keratinocytes in the attached gingiva and consequently, allow the penetration of bacteria into deeper tissues. This hypothesis may explain why MRONJ occurs only in maxilla and mandible, but not in other bones of the skeleton.

Another theory considers the unique role of bone remodeling rate. Both maxilla and mandible are examples of a bone that is subject to an increased bone remodeling, mainly in the alveolar socket area and periodontal area, as a result of intensive mechanical stress acting on teeth during chewing and other movements of the teeth. It turns out that the bone turnover is constant during the life of an individual, regardless of their age [5].

The suppression of remodeling and decrease of bone turnover results from bisphosphonates directly affect osteoclasts and their function. Studies examining osteogenesis imperfecta in kids reveal that bisphosphonates do not always reduce the level of osteoclasts, but contrary to that, under certain conditions, they tend to increase their levels [6, 7]. Suppression of bone remodeling could therefore occur through other mechanisms such as intravenous bisphosphonate application.

Longitudinal animal studies with long-term application of bisphosphonates revealed increased number of multilocular phosphatase-positive cells in jaw and long bones. On the surface of the bone, however, the number of osteoclasts is decreased, while the number of osteoclasts in the woven bone is increased [8]. A traumatized alveolar compact bone with damaged periosteal and endosteal covering and diminished osteoprogenitor cells will activate osteoclasts and start the bone remodeling process. However, osteoclasts are unable to bind themselves to the bone surface and resorp the bone matrix as a result of incorporated bisphosphonates. Traumatized bone can hold the attempted osteoclast activation signal, and the osteoclasts then accumulate near the bone surface. The purpose of these accumulated unconnected osteoclasts in bone tissue is currently unclear [9].

2.1. Infectious agents

The oral cavity is colonized by a number of microorganisms that may become pathogenic even after the slightest superficial trauma to the oral mucosa, which then acts as a gateway for jaw bone infection. An organism treated with ARM has altered immune response and is unable to react efficiently against infectious agents and curb the spread of infection to surrounding tissues of the oral cavity and alveolar processes.

Various in vivo studies on rats describe a link between the periodontal infection and the osteonecrosis development. Young adult rats have been administered bisphosphonates for 15 weeks and had a circumdental wire applied to the first molar for 3 weTeks to induce an aggressive periodontitis. Osteonecrosis of the jaw diagnosed in this study had the identical course and histological finding to the human manifestations of the disease, with bone sequestration, numerous empty osteocyte lacunas and an expression of inflammation. Culture results proved that Fusobacterium nucleatum were present. After the subsequent ATB application, the signs of osteonecrosis have subsided; however, the healing ad integrum did not happen.

Numerous similar longitudinal studies confirm the significant role of infectious agents in the oral cavity with expressed osteonecrosis [10]. Surgical procedures conducted during a bisphosphonate therapy or a periodontal pathology indicating bone remodeling of the alveolar bone make it easier for bisphosphonates to accumulate in maxilla or mandible. After bisphosphonates in a bone reach the critical concentration, a trigger (tooth extraction) activates the bone remodeling, simultaneously releasing local deposits of bisphosphonates that inhibit the bone healing process. Necrotic osteomyelitis is induced by the slowed-down repair process, accompanied by a bone wound contamination by the Actinomyces bacteria.

Hence, efficient debridement, application of antimicrobial mouthwash and application of ATB directly on the bone defect and the wound play a very important role in the treatment of ONJ.

3. Clinical picture

In the past, osteonecrosis of the jaw proved to be a serious problem not only in the view of possible treatments, but also in the view of the diagnosis itself. Such lesions and conditions were usually considered to be osteitis, osteomyelitis or alveolitis, which were thought to have been the result of a preceding extraction.

Complications in the oral cavity in patients with MRONJ are usually diverse. The complications may emerge due to the progression of the disease, or as a result of medical procedures, which produce functional problems such as diminished chewing function, loss of teeth and limited rehabilitation of the chewing function. In addition, aesthetic obstructions may also emerge due to the loss of teeth, facial contour defects (owing to partial bone resections) or due to enduring oroantral fistulas. Patients experience sore mouth, impaired wound healing and drug-induced mucositis.

The most common clinical sign of MRONJ (up to 93.9%) is an exposed necrotic bone. The scope of bone exposure may vary greatly and is directly connected neither with the scope of the necrosis nor with the severity of the disease. Signs of infection such as swelling of soft tissues, intra/extra oral purulent discharge or abscesses may also be present. Patients may suffer from severe pain if the infection breaks out of the necrotic tissue, although this symptom is not a requirement—many patients do not report any pain. In severe cases, local infection may develop into abscesses in the deeper areas of the head and neck, resulting in life-threatening conditions. It may even lead to an abscess in brain tissues. Some rare cases of septic systemic infection have been documented.

Rare, although typical, symptom of MRONJ is the paresis of alveolar nerve, also known as the Vincent's symptom. It is interesting that it manifests itself in the earlier and in the advanced stages of MRONJ. Reduced sensitivity of nervus alveolaris inferior can also be a sign of metastatic infiltration. Histologic examination is recommended. Other symptoms associated with MRONJ include loss of teeth due to structural changes within the necrotic bone and bad breath due to bacterial inflammation.

Loss of teeth is the result of a progress of the necrotic damage to the alveolar bone. Bad breath as a symptom commonly occurs in patients suffering from MRONJ based on previous changes within the necrotic bone and the surrounding soft tissues. This can also be the result of a bacterial colonization of the affected area, usually combined with a non-sterile infection of the bone and the surrounding soft tissue. This symptom occurs in 71–84% of MRONJ patients with periodontitis which form an inflammatory periodontal disease. Polymicrobial biofilm swab samples from oral cavity reveal specific bacteria such as Porphyromonas gingivalis, Treponema denticola, Tannerella forsythia or Aggregatibacter actinomycetemcomitans.

Thanks to the adequate and effective management of these diseases and their various possible stages, it is now possible to correctly diagnose the patient and consequently, try and treat them. Though, the treatment itself usually does not bring neither adequate nor successful results, which is the reason why such an amount of studies and in vivo and in vitro experiments exist. The status of oral cavity in patients undergoing intravenous bisphosphonate therapy after primary prevention can be maintained to such an extent that the cancer treatment may continue without any negative impact on the quality of life of the patient, even when osteonecrotic defects and lesions are present. **Figures 3** and **4** describe the clinical picture of ONJ.

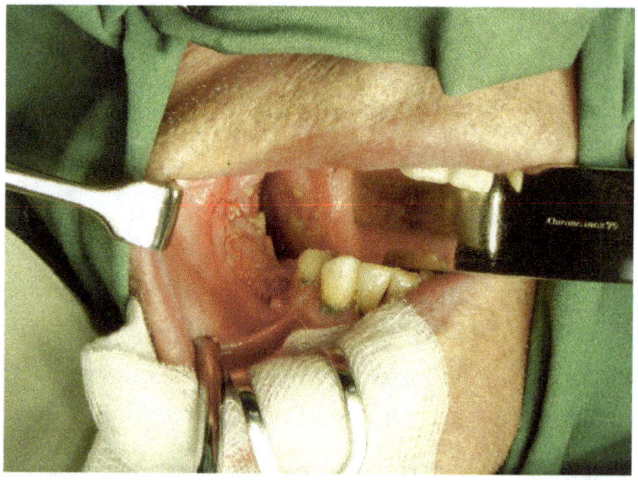

Figure 3. Osteonecrosis of the right mandible.

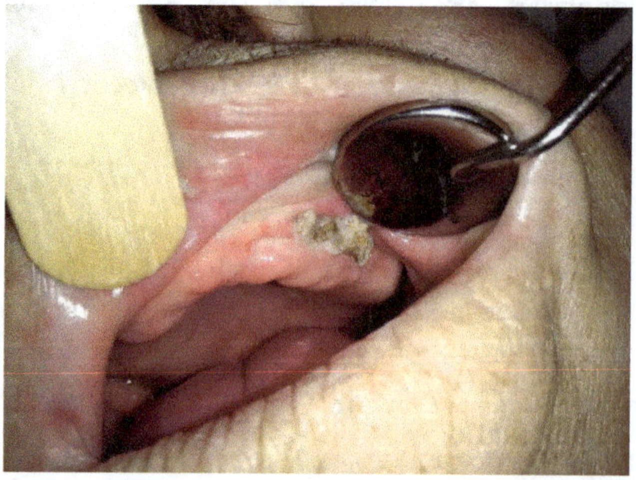

Figure 4. Osteonecrosis of the left maxilla.

4. Prevention

Considering how complex the bisphosphonate-related osteonecrosis of the jaw therapy is, primary prevention may be the most important strategic approach to this complication.

Preventive measures are able to reduce, albeit not eliminate, the risk of formation of lesions. The rationale behind the primary prevention is the elimination of all focuses of infection in the jaw and total denture restoration lege artis.

The radical form of the therapy is comparable to denture restoration in patients before a radiation therapy in the head and neck region. All dentists should be familiar with the form of the therapy. Every patient should be subject to dental examination and panoramic dental X-ray before their planned antiresorptive therapy (**Figure 5**). In case surgical procedures in oral cavity (usually teeth extractions) are necessary as a part of the denture restoration procedure, it is recommended, if possible, to postpone the launch of ARM treatment by 2–3 weeks, or, preferably, until clear signs of bone healing show up on the skiagram. Other dental examinations and good oral hygiene are, of course, essential in the course of the ARM treatment.

In cancer patients taking intravenous bisphosphonates, the most conservative therapy possible is indicated for dental diseases. All invasive procedures involving jaw bones are strictly contraindicated (tooth extractions, periodontal-dentoalveolar surgery, implantology). It is recommended to refer the patients for whom these procedures are necessary to a specialized department of maxillofacial surgery. Such preventive measures are recommended to be followed not only in cancer patients who are subject to bisphosphonate treatment, but also in patients who use other drugs affecting bone metabolism or osteoclast function inhibitors.

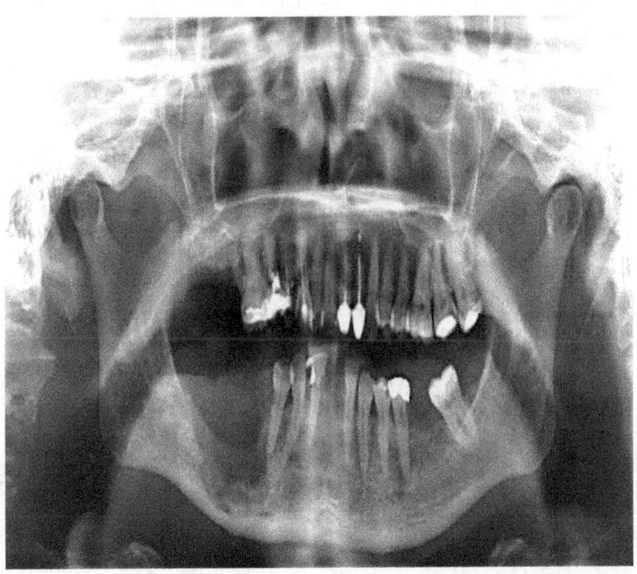

Figure 5. Panoramic X-ray with osteonecrosis of the right mandible.

The secondary prevention, in terms of ARM treatment interruption—the so-called drug holiday—is bit problematic. So far, there is no scientific evidence that the interruption of a therapy prior to surgery in the oral cavity reduced the risk of developing osteonecrosis of the jaw. According to AAOMS, suspending intravenous bisphosphonates has no significant short-term benefit in case the lesions are already present. Long-term treatment suspension, however, may stabilize the affected area, alleviate the clinical signs and also reduce the risk of new sites being affected. The priority still lies in the treatment of malignant diseases, and therefore, the suspension of bisphosphonates has to be thoroughly assessed.

The situation with monoclonal antibodies is different. Based on current knowledge about the effect of denosumab on bone remodeling, it is recommended to suspend the drug prior to any planned surgery in the oral cavity, in order to reduce the risk of developing osteonecrosis of the jaw. Suspending denosumab treatment seems to be appropriate, even in cases of an already developed osteonecrosis of the jaw, which can lead to heightened healing of the lesion. Some authors recommend suspending bevacizumab 6–8 weeks before surgery and resuming the medication 4 weeks after the procedure to prevent complications with wound healing.

5. Treatment

The primary goal of the treatment is to minimize the occurrence of MRONJ. Even though cases of spontaneous formation of MRONJ do exist, the majority of cases develop after a surgery.

In the first place, it is necessary to carry out a preservation treatment and consequent prosthetic and surgical treatment lege artis. This includes restorations of carious teeth, repairing of overhanging fillings, or extracting devitalized or destroyed teeth with extensive periapical findings. ARM treatment should initiate or resume only after the extraction wound in the socket has healed thoroughly. Prevention is important in terms of maintaining the functionality of healthy teeth.

Examination of the affected mucosa is necessary in patients with prosthetic replacement, since decubiti, traumatic lesions or fissural granuloma may emerge in the area. For these reasons, temporary restoration is contraindicated in many cases. Dentoalveolar procedure must be carried out in the gentlest manner, preferably at a maxillofacial surgery facility. It is necessary to inform the patient about the possible risks. Chlorhexidine mouth washes are indicated both before and after the dentoalveolar procedure. The surgery is performed under the influence of antibiotics, which continue to be employed after the procedure.

MRONJ treatment is very demanding in terms of time; therefore, AAOMS recommends a conservative approach, in an attempt to delay the surgical resection treatment, which is indicated in the advanced stages of the disease. Palliative conservative treatment is usually applied, since only a small percentage of patients will experience complete healing ad integrum. The conservative approach consists of equalization of sharp bone edges, sequestrectomy, necrotic area teeth extractions, and incisions and drainages under total antibiotic and topical treatment.

Surgical treatment consists of complete removal of the necrotic foci, which serve as a fertile ground for infection, followed by wound closure with soft tissue that is finely vascularized, using layered suture. During the radical surgical resection, there are still concerns about the resulting wounds, difficulty in healing and progression of osteonecrotic foci.

Several studies point to the possibility of employing new treatment methods such as PRP, ozone or hyperbaric oxygen therapies. The benefit for cancer patients who are undergoing intravenous bisphosphonate treatment is bone pain relief and retreat of other bone complications. The basic rule is to preserve the quality of life for these patients, which includes a thorough oral health care, patient education, regular visits to the dentist, pain management and reports on health status, edemas, pain or bone exposure. It is also important to prevent the spread of new necrotic sockets by observing the proper prevention. Staging and management is described in **Table 1**.

Patients with aforementioned drugs in their medical history need to be treated as risk patients in view of invasive procedures in the oral cavity. Currently, the majority of osteonecrosis are of iatrogenic nature, caused by the incorrect choice of treatment for risk patients by the medical

Staging and Management of The ARM-Induced Osteonecrosis of The Jaw	
Stage	**Clinical Stages and Management**
Risk	**No evidence of necrotic bone. Patients who were, and still are treated with oral or intravenous antiresorptive drugs.** • Asymptomatic • Not requiring treatment • Patient education
0.	**No clinical records of necrotic bone, with non-specific finding and symptoms** • Systematic management • Analgesia
I.	**Asymptomatic patient with an exposed bone, without pain and infection of the surrounding tissues** • Daily use of an antibacterial mouthwash (chlorhexidine 0.12%) • Follow-up • X-RAY checks, analgesia
II.	**Osteonecrosis with signs of pain, inflammation and erythema** • Daily use of an antibacterial mouthwash (chlorhexidine 0.12%) • Analgesia, ATB p.o. based on the cultivation and sensitivity identification • Supportive treatment, polyvitaminosis (Tocopherol, Calcium)
III.	**Extensive osteonecrosis accompanied by pain, infection, fistula, osteolysis, extraoral fistula and pathological fracture. Exposed necrotic bone, or fistula that probes to bone in patients with pain and infection and at least one associated complication: exposed and necrotic bone extended beyond the area of the alveolar bone (i.e., the lower border of the ramus in mandible, or sinus and zygomatic bone area in maxilla), which leads to pathological fractures, extra and intra oral fistulas, oronasal and oroantral communication, or osteolysis extended to the lower border of the mandible** • Daily use of an antibacterial mouthwash (chlorhexidine 0.12%) • Surgical debridement/necrectomy • Analgesia, ATB p.o./i.v. based on the cultivation and sensitivity identification • Supportive treatment, polyvitaminosis (Tocopherol, Calcium)

Table 1. Staging and management.

staff. The cause of this unfavorable situation lies in the lack of communication between the specialist prescribing the high-risk drug and the treating dentist. The lack of awareness of the issue, both in patients and treating dentists, also plays its role. Medical specialist prescribing a high-risk drug is obligated to inform the patient about the risks and adverse effects of the planned treatment and to remind them to specifically inform their dentist about this fact. By disregarding this obligation on the part of the specialist (clinical oncologist, internist, rheumatologist, urologist, gynecologist, endocrinologist, orthopedist, etc.), the patient usually has no idea about the risk involved; however, the development of iatrogenic osteonecrosis may be prevented by the right approach by the treating dentist. They should not underestimate drug anamnesis prior to any invasive procedure in the oral cavity. Precise and targeted medical history can help identify at-risk patients and to choose the right treatment plan.

The incidence of MRONJ can be divided into two groups: patients with non-oncological disease (osteoporosis, rheumatoid arthritis) and patients with cancer who take high doses of intravenous bisphosphonates.

In the second group, the incidence after 36 months of treatment ranges from 1 to 12%. The majority of cases described are connected with the use of zoledronate and pamidronate in treatment of multiple myeloma and bone metastases. So far, the results and recommendations on potential treatment for these conditions refer to the multicenter studies conducted in the last 15 years.

The study named DEFEND (Denosumab Evaluation for Preserving Bone Density) was a double-blind, multicenter, placebo-controlled, third phase study on 332 postmenopausal women with osteopenia and respective T-scores in the range of 1.5–2.5 SD. Denosumab was applied in 6-month intervals at a dose of 60 mg subcut, in contrast to placebo. Both groups of patients took a calcium supplement (100 mg a day) and vitamin D. The primary objective was to observe the lumbar spine bone mineral density after 24 months of treatment.

The results of the study showed that, compared with placebo, denosumab significantly increased the value of BMD in lumbar spine (by 6.5%). Denosumab also increased the density in the proximal part of femur (3.4%) and in the distal end of radius (by 1.4%). In the placebo group, the BMD decreased in these areas.

In another study, titled DECIDE (Determining Efficacy: Comparison of Initiating Denosumab vs. Alendronate), the effectiveness of denosumab with the same dosage as in the study DEFEND was compared to alendronic acid with a dosage of 70 mg, once a week, in order to reduce the risk of osteoporotic fractures. The yearlong study enrolled 1189 postmenopausal, relatively older women with more serious osteopenia than in the DEFEND, with half the women having a fracture in their medical history. Calcium and vitamin D supplementation has been the norm throughout the study. The primary measured indicator was the change in the density of proximal femur. Moreover, bone densities of lumbar spine, femoral neck, trochanter and distal radius were also monitored.

The results showed that denosumab improved bone density in all the monitored areas markedly better than alendronic acid, as early as at the end of the first month. At the same time, resorption markers significantly decreased in the group treated with denosumab, compared to the alendronic acid group.

Large, randomized, placebo-controlled study called FREEDOM (Fracture Reduction Evaluation of Denosumab in Osteoporosis Every 6 Months) studied the reduction of incidence of osteoporotic fractures. The authors monitored 7868 women aged 60–90, with an average BMD T-score of −2.5, but not lower than −4.0.

After 3 years, the incidence of new vertebral fractures identified on X-rays in women treated with denosumab was 2.3%, while the incidence in the control group was 7.2%. The treatment reduced the relative risk of vertebral fractures by 68%. The cumulative incidence of hip fractures was 0.7% in the treatment group and 1.2% in the control group (40% reduction in the risk of fractures). There were no recorded significant differences in incidence of side effects such as cardiovascular complications, infections, fracture healing time and hypercalcemia between the treated and the control group [11].

An important outcome of these studies was the discovery that denosumab significantly increases bone density, even in areas with prevalence of cortical bones. From these results, it can be concluded that alendronate has the longest half-life decay (10 years), while denosumab has a reversible effect because it does not deposit into bone tissue.

5.1. Combining antiresorptive drugs and hormonal therapy

Several studies refer to clinical cases of patients with antiresorptive drug-related osteonecrosis of the jaw that describe improvement in local findings and bone remodeling and an increase in patient's quality of life after switching bisphosphonates for hormonal therapy with recombinant parathyroid hormone teriparatide [12, 13].

Teriparatide was approved for the treatment of postmenopausal osteoporosis. Unlike the antiresorptive treatment, teriparatide has anabolic effect in bone which stimulates bone remodeling and bone tissue density. Intermittent administration (once a day) leads to a temporary increase of serum concentrations and preferential stimulation of the osteoblast activity, which leads to bone formation stimulation. The effect lies in the increase of bone mass and the number of osteoblasts, and the consequent strength of bones.

Some clinical trials document a positive effect of teriparatide and parathyroid hormone which reduces the risk of vertebral fractures while increasing the bone mineral density (BMD). The preparation is administered subcutaneously, one injection a day. Recommended treatment duration is 18 months. Side effects include cephalalgia, nausea and hypercalcemia. After its administration, osteal healing in mouth cavity was documented.

According to the trial results, hormonal preparations used after stimulating the activity of osteoblast and osteoclasts could be employed in the treatment of non-oncological osteonecrosis. However, current trials are very small, and there is no sufficient evidence, which calls for more studies. Treatment is difficult, and it is therefore available only for some patients.

Teriparatide should not be used in cancer patients due to an increased risk of osteosarcomas, which were found in preclinical trials on rats. The teriparatide therapy should not be indicated in patients who inject their bisphosphonates, zoledronic acid or pamidronic acid because of the increased incidence of necrosis and associated severe complications, in contrast to orally administered bisphosphonates.

6. Conclusion

The aforementioned clinical recommendations are based on relevant data, scientific evidence, available literature and the empirical experience of the authors. Despite the effort, neither standard nor recommended procedure may still be defined.

Clinical recommendation and subsequent treatment should be assessed by the treating physician based on the patient's status and their needs and preferences, which should alleviate their difficulties and improve the quality of life of the patient suffering from the osteonecrosis of the jaw. Compliance with preventive measures before and during the antiresorptive treatment seems beneficial; however, it is also considerably complicated.

The ARM-induced osteonecrosis of the jaw poses a current problem with a number of yet unanswered questions. In general, it is believed that the cause of the osteonecrosis is multifactorial, dependent not only on administered preparations, but also on the underlying oncological disease, type of chemotherapy, hormonal treatment, associated illnesses, age and addiction case history. It is therefore necessary to correctly set up and indicate the pharmacological and surgical treatment, monitor the bone antiresorptive therapy, with focus on prevention and complications.

Author details

Vladimira Schwartzova[1], Marcel Riznic[2*], Branislav Borza[1] and Peter Kizek[1]

*Address all correspondence to: dr.riznic@gmail.com

1 Dental Clinic, Kosice, Slovakia

2 Department of Stomatology and Maxillofacial Surgery, Kosice, Slovakia

References

[1] Ruggiero l et al. American association of oral and maxillofacial surgeons special committee position paper on medication-related osteonecrosis of the jaw. Journal of Oral and Maxillofacial Surgery. 2014;**72**(10):1938-1956

[2] Abdu-id MH et al. "Bis-Phossy jaws"—High and low risk factors for bisphosphonate-induced osteonecrosis of the jaw. Journal of Cranio-Maxillo-Facial Surgery. 2008;**36**(2): 95-103

[3] Otto S et al. Osteoporosis and bisphosphonates-related osteonecrosis of the jaw: Not just a sporadic coincidence—A multi-centre study. Journal of Cranio-Maxillo-Facial Surgery. 2011;**39**(4):272-277

[4] Ruggiero LS et al. American association of oral and maxillofacial surgeons positions paper on bisphosphonate-related osteonecrosis of the jaws—2009 Update. Journal of Oral and Maxillofacial Surgery. 2009;**67**(Suppl 1):2-12

[5] Yamashita J, McCauley LK, Van Poznak C. Updates on osteonecrosis of the jaw. Current Opinion in Supportive and Palliative Care. 2010;**4**:200-206

[6] Weinstein RS, Roberson PK, Manolagas SC. Giant osteoclast formation and long-term oral bisphosphonate therapy. The New England Journal of Medicine. 2009;**360**:53-62

[7] Cheung MS, Glorieux FH, Rauch F. Large osteoclasts in pediatric osteogenesis imperfecta patients receiving intravenous pamidronate. Journal of Bone and Mineral Research. 2009;**24**:669-674

[8] Allen MR, Kubek DJ, Burr DB. Cancer treatment dosing regimens of zoledronic acid result in near-complete suppression of mandible intracortical bone remodeling in Beagle dogs. Journal of Bone and Mineral Research. 2010;**25**:98-105

[9] Bertoldo F et al. Bisphosphonates and osteomyelitis of the jaw: A pathogenic puzzle. Nature Clinical Practice Oncology. 2007;**4**(12):711-721

[10] Aghaloo TL, Kang B, Sung EC, et al. Periodontal disease and bisphosphonates induce osteonecrosis of the jaws in the rat. Journal of Bone and Mineral Research. 2011;**26**: 1871-1882

[11] Zaheer S, LeBoff M, Lewiecki EM. Denosumab for the treatment of osteoporosis. Expert Opinion on Drug Metabolism & Toxicology. 2015 Mar;**11**(3):461-470

[12] Harper RP, Fung E. Resolution of bisphosphonate-associated osteonecrosis of the mandible: Possible application for intermittent low-dose parathyroid hormone [Rhpth (1-34)]. Journal of Oral and Maxillofacial Surgery. 2007;**65**:573-580

[13] Kwon YD, Lee DW, Choi BJ, et al. Short-term teriparatide therapy as an adjunctive modality for bisphosphonate-related osteonecrosis of the jaws. Osteoporosis International. 2012;**23**(11):2721-2725

7

The Gut Microbiota and Inflammation in Rheumatoid Arthritis

Reem Hamdy A. Mohammed and
Hesham Ibrahim I. Elmakhzangy

Abstract

"Mutualism" is a well-defined relationship that describes a form of cooperation between two living organisms of different species that ends up with a beneficial outcome for each one. Any disruption to such a relationship by an external trigger or a potential intruder puts at risk the well-being of both. In humans, oral and gut microbiota provide a noteworthy model of beneficial mutualism. Multiple recent evidences point to the possible pathologic consequences of a disruption to this ecosystem (altered microbiota profile or dysbiosis) on human well-being. The gut-joint axis found its clear way "Proof of Principle" in the pathogenesis of autoimmune rheumatic diseases including rheumatoid arthritis (RA), seronegative spondyloarthropathies, and Behcet's disease in a number of studies. Current therapeutic trends are directed towards the diverse biologic and immune-pathogenic factors involved in the disease process. Addressing dysbiosis in RA features an attractive future therapeutic target. In this chapter, authors aim to explore the recent evidences regarding the pathogenic role of "gut dysbiosis" in rheumatoid arthritis (RA), highlighting the spectrum of immune-pathogenic events that might contribute to disease evolution and inspecting future directives of research.

Keywords: Mutualism, microbiota, dysbiosis, pathogenesis, autoimmune rheumatic diseases, rheumatoid arthritis

1. Rheumatoid Arthritis and The Microbiome Theory "The Revival of an Old Hypothesis"

Rheumatoid arthritis (RA) is a systemic immune-mediated chronic inflammatory disease that predominantly targets diarthrodial joints contributing to synovial inflammation, joint destruction, and deformity. The disease has been initially recognized as a complex genetically based inflammatory joint disease, a concept that was redefined toward a multifactorial immune-mediated etiology. The etiopathogenesis of rheumatoid arthritis is typically a challenge incorporating complex network of genetic factors (HLA genes), environmental and biological factors (infections, a dominant pro-inflammatory profile, dysbiosis), as well as individual habits (smoking) interacting to shape up disease phenotype [1, 2].

An infectious etiology of RA has been proposed for decades, Banntyne and Wohlmann in 1896 were the first to suggest a mycobacterial etiology behind the development of rheumatoid arthritis, a theory that awaited solid scientific evidence. The hypothesis of "molecular mimicry" and cross-reactivity between epitopes of microbial origin with a self-protein was among the proposed mechanisms to explain the role of infectious agents in the breakdown of immune tolerance in RA. Certain viral infections like Epstein-Barr virus (EBV), cytomegalovirus (CMV), and Parvovirus B19 have been additionally claimed as potential etiopathogenic agents in RA [3–9].

1.1. The oral sepsis hypothesis

In the 1900s, the oral sepsis hypothesis and its relation to arthritis led to the use of teeth extraction as a prevalent treatment of disease for several decades. The impact of polymicrobial phylotypes and the pro-inflammatory burden in periodontitis proved its contribution to the pro-inflammatory drive in RA. The *Porphyromonas gingivalis,* a Gram-negative anaerobe bacterium and part of periodontopathic microbiome, contributes to protein citrullination, which leads to anticitrullinated autoantibody (ACPA) formation and joint inflammation in RA [6–13].

The infectious profile further extended to include other pathogenic bacterial species as wells as cell membrane proteins of mycoplasma in RA like *Proteus mirabilis* (*sharing sequence similarities to peptide sequences at amino acid position 67–74 of the HLA-shared epitope in RA and bacterial-specific antibodies detected in sera of RA patients*) [14, 15]. The presence of specific *Escherichia coli, Mycoplasma fermentans,* and *Klebsiella pneumonia* in the gut has been associated with RF positivity and has been linked to inflammatory arthritis in many ethnic populations [16].

1.2. The infectious hypothesis and therapeutic evidences

The relationship between infections and arthritis was indirectly reinforced by the time antimicrobials showed an observable beneficial effect in the amelioration of arthritis. In the 1940s, sulfasalazine was the first rationally designed drug in the field of rheumatology, where RA was thought to be caused by Streptococci found in milk. Sulfasalazine was designed as a deliberate attempt to combine a sulfonamide antibiotic with a salicylate anti-inflammatory agent through an azo bond. Such "combination therapy" brought up good initial responses in RA as well as enteropathies. The triple DMARD therapy (a combination of methotrexate, sulfasalazine and hydroxychloroquine) currently stands among the first few recommendations in RA patients with poor prognostic features and moderate to high levels of disease activity [17–21].

Certain antibiotics like tetracycline have proven efficacy in the treatment of early seropositive RA which led to the approval of minocycline, as a DMARD [22, 23]. Clarithromycin is another example that gave observable beneficial effects in some refractory cases [24]. Treatment with probiotics, particularly *Bifidobacterium, Lactobacillus,* and *Faecalibacterium prausnitzii,* showed protective effects in NSAID-treated animal models of arthritis. Theories regarding supplementations of microbiome-derived molecules with immune-modulating properties (e.g., Polysaccharide A, short-chain fatty acids) provide promising novel immune regulatory effects by possibly downregulating pro-inflammatory cytokines with upregulation of the anti-inflammatory profile [25–27].

2. The human gut ecosystem

Mutualism is a well-defined relationship between living organisms. The term describes a form of cooperation between two living organisms of different species that ends up with a beneficial outcome for each one. Partners in a mutualistic relationship make headway together with each forming a part of the other's environment and maintaining its homeostasis in a typically harmless yet useful way. A disruption to such a relationship by an external trigger or a potential intruder puts at risk the well-being of both. In humans, oral and gut microbiota provide a noteworthy model of beneficial mutualism. Multiple recent evidences point to the possible pathologic consequences of a disruption to this ecosystem (altered microbiota profile or dysbiosis) on human well-being. The gut-joint axis found its clear way "Proof of Principle" in the pathogenesis of autoimmune rheumatic diseases including RA, seronegative spondyloarthropathies, and Behcet's disease in a number of studies.

The term "microbiota" is defined as the ecological community of symbiotic, commensal, and pathogenic microorganisms that literally inhabit the human body and effectively contribute to human health and might contribute to disease. According to their contributions to human health, they can be classified to symbiomes and pathobiomes. The symbiome microbiota are groups of microorganisms predominantly bacterial as well as fungal (previously recognized as normal flora) that get acquired at birth and inhabit every part of the human body from the skin to mucosa (mouth, eyes, gut, and genital tracts). The alimentary tract represents an established microbial habitat for almost 29–30% of the overall commensal/symbiome population in the human body. They involve over 500 bacterial species encoding around three million different genes constituting a complex challenging ecosystem, difficult to differentially analyze or understand [28, 29].

2.1. The development of the human microbiota profile

The general composition of gut microbiota is much similar in most healthy individuals; however, the individuals' microbiota profile retains a highly personalized pattern (fingerprint). This pattern helps to keep in situ homeostasis in healthy individuals; therefore triggers of dysbiosis are expected to offer a threat to the humans' well-being in a variety of forms.

At birth: The initial shape up of the different microbial colonies of the gut begins as early as childbirth by the time the newborn gets exposed to microorganisms that inhabit the maternal genital tract during normal vaginal delivery (first encounter), maternal fecal bacteria, or the skin in the case of caesarian section. The fetal fingerprint of microbiota gets additionally shaped up by the skin as well as breast milk microbiota that add their signature to this microbial network [30].

Adulthood: The typical adult microbiota profile emerges by the end of the first year with more than 1000 different species from a dozen different divisions colonizing the gastrointestinal tract (4×10^{13} colonizing bacteria). The profile becomes increasingly stable with age. The acquired bacterial species pass through a series of modifications with colonies competing for survival, alternating their dominance aiming to establish phylogenetic richness and species diversity at the same time. Serial microbial evolutions are proven to be largely dependent on a multiplicity of host as well as environmental factors (the host genetics, the maternal microbiota, and mode of delivery as major determinants). Breast milk composition is another proven shaping factor of individuals' microbiota profile (*Bifidobacterium* is among the dominant gut microbiota in breast-fed infants compared to artificially fed ones and is deficient in patients with RA). Aging; lifestyle patterns including diet, smoking, and obesity; and infections also contribute [31–34].

2.2. The identification and characterization of gut microbiota

The human microbiome project served as a major contributor toward better understanding of the human microbiome. For a sufficient period of time, the conventional culture-based methods were the only methods available and routinely used for identification of gut microbiota, with over 500 bacterial species successfully isolated, cultured, and characterized from the human GI tract [35].

The majority of gut microbiota (over 80%) could not be technically cultivated ranking the culture-based methods as an investigative technique of limited value in determining the actual microbial diversity. The revolutionary era of the human microbiome project announced in 2007 and the utilization of novel culture-independent molecular techniques have successfully contributed to the in-depth understanding of such complex human microbiome network. Such culture-independent techniques target the highly conserved 16S ribosomal RNA (rRNA) gene sequence (a component the 30S subunit of prokaryotic ribosomes) of bacterial and archaeal microorganisms. Universal PCR primers targeting these conserved regions can be used for gene amplification to provide the complete nucleotide sequence of the 16S rRNA without prior knowledge of which bacterial species are present. Concomitantly, the 16S rRNA gene also contains hypervariable regions that provide species-specific signature sequences and enable unbiased bacterial identification utilizing next-generation sequencing platforms. Examples of these molecular techniques include quantitative polymerase chain reaction (qPCR), temperature or denaturing gradient gel electrophoresis (TGGE or DGGE), terminal-restriction fragment length polymorphism (T-RFLP), and fluorescent in situ hybridization (FISH). The next-generation sequencing and phylogenetic microarrays promote the in-depth analysis of the complete phylogenetic diversity of the intestinal microbiota, whereas the whole-genome shotgun sequencing is a technique currently applied for identification of the metabolic and enzymatic pathways present in these microbial communities. Such techniques were able to identify a portion of predominant species in the human gut [36–38].

Genomic culture-independent techniques disclosed that the human intestine is dominated by two divisions of bacteria, Bacteroidetes and Firmicutes, and both contribute to more than two-thirds of the total gut microbiota including anaerobes such as *Bacteroides, Porphyromonas, Bifidobacterium, Lactobacillus*, and *Clostridium* [13, 34, 39, 40].

2.3. The human-microbiota interdependence

Microbiota are involved in a number of structural, biological, protective, and metabolic processes including angiogenesis, postnatal intestinal maturation, and xenobiotic metabolism. They are additionally involved in the synthesis of vitamins, the digestion, and uptake of nutrients. Microbiota are capable of metabolically simplifying nutritional components through the process of fermentation; an important example is the indigestible carbohydrates (complex starch and dietary fibers) as well as short-chain fatty acids (SCFA, e.g., acetate, butyrate, and propionate) which constitute a critical prerequisite in a number of host physiological functions [41].

2.3.1. Microbiota and immunity

A unique harmonious and complex interplay exists between gut microbiota and the local as well as the systemic immune response in humans. Colonizing microbiota and their products have a profound effect on the development and maintenance of the immune system integrity [42–45].

2.3.1.1. The microbiota and T-cell differentiation, proliferation, and functions

Evidences support the existence of immune cross talks between the microbiota-derived products and the gut epithelium that involves molecular exchange of bacterial signals recognized by host receptors to mediate beneficial outcomes for both the microbiome and human beings [42–47]. The gut microbiota have the potential to effectively stimulate and direct the host innate and adaptive immune responses in humans by triggering instructional signals to the immune cells, particularly regulatory T (Treg)-cell and T-helper (Th) cell differentiation.

2.3.1.2. Short-chain fatty acids and Treg cells

SCFAs are actively produced by anaerobic microbiota in the colon as fermentation products of digestion-resistant dietary fibers [46, 47]. SCFAs produced locally in the colon are either absorbed and metabolized within the colonocytes or transported into the circulation to reach other organs, such as the liver and muscles. SCFAs exert direct and indirect regulatory effects on epithelial cells, antigen-presenting cells, and T cells via multiple mechanisms including metabolic regulation, histone deacetylase inhibition (HDAC inhibition), and G-protein–coupled receptor (GPCR) activation.

SCFAs can be converted to Acetyl-CoA and integrated into the citric acid cycle (Krebs cycle). Acetyl-CoA is a central molecule that stores energy and is eventually oxidized to CO_2 for energy production (the cellular energy [ATP/ADP] level increases). This boosts a homeostatic T-cell sensor mammalian target of rapamycin (mTOR) to be activated in T cells which skews T-cell differentiation into effector T cells such as Th1 and Th17 cells at the expense of FoxP3$^+$ T cells. mTOR activation also promotes the generation of IL-10$^+$ cells. Thus, the SCFA regulation of cell metabolism and mTOR accounts for the increased generation of Th1 cells, Th17 cells, and IL-10^{+} cells.

The activation of SCFA-binding G-protein–coupled receptors (GPCRs) such as GPR41, GPR43, GPR109A, and Olfr78 initiates T-cell differentiation.

All major SCFAs such as C2, C3, C4, and C5 have HDAC inhibitor activity. Class I/II HDACs are major targets of SCFA inhibition in a concentration-dependent pattern. Treg generation was increased as a result of HDAC inhibition by SCFAs and histone H3 acetylation in key regulatory regions of the Foxp3 locus.

SCFAs can indirectly affect T cells through their effects on DCs. They suppress the development of bone marrow progenitors into myeloid DCs and inhibit functional maturation of DCs in vitro. For example, C4 suppressed the maturation of bone marrow-derived DCs and production of IL-12 but increased the expression of IL-23p19. Valproic acid, a branched short-chain fatty acid and potent HDAC inhibitor that suppressed the maturation of human DCs in vitro, inhibits the upregulation of T-cell–activating molecules such as MHC II, CD80, CD86, and IL-12.

These effects are combined to create the overall tolerogenic gut environment with a strong barrier function.

2.3.1.3. Microbiota and cytokine production

Microbiota produce stimulatory signals to gut macrophages to produce interleukin-1 (IL-1). IL-1 acts on type 3 innate lymphoid cells in the intestine, producing colony-stimulating factor 2 (CSF-2). CSF-2 induces myeloid cells (including dendritic cells and macrophages) to produce immune regulatory cytokines (retinoic acid and IL-10) which support the conversion and expansion of regulatory T cells (Treg) critical for maintaining immune tolerance in the gut.

Microbiota have the capacity to produce a certain set of microbial products—gut microbiota–derived butyrate and polysaccharide A PSA (e.g., *Bacteroides fragilis*) that mediates the conversion of CD4+ T cells into Interleukin (IL)-10 producing Foxp3+ Treg cells offering immune protection. Such microbiome-derived molecule further promotes immunologic tolerance via TLR2 signaling pathway directly on Foxp3(+) Treg cells [47, 48].

The "segmented filamentous bacterium (SFB)" is another symbiotic gut commensal that is capable of inducing the appearance and activation of Th17 cells in the lamina propria, which secrete the pro-inflammatory cytokine (IL-17) and thereby enhance mucosal immune responses of the host [49].

2.3.1.4. Experimental evidences illustrated the impact of dysbiosis on the immune system and T-cell function

Multiple experimental evidences revealed that a germ-free environment is associated with a decline in neutrophil count and function [42–45]. Recognition of peptidoglycans from gut microbiota by the cytosolic recognition receptor nucleotide oligomerization domain 1 (NOD1) is capable of enhancing the killing activity of marrow-derived neutrophils contributing to immune integrity. A germ-free environment was associated with impaired neutrophil phagocytic function, superoxide function, and nitric oxide generation, which could not be restored upon pathogen exposure. Germ-free rats lack the microbe-derived ATP capable of stimulating dendritic cells (CD70 and CX3CR1) involved in the subsequent differentiation of Th17 cells. Additionally, in germ-free rats, systemic, not gut macrophages, were reduced, and gut macrophages lack macrophage-activation markers, such as MHC class II.

Early-life microbial exposures alter sex hormone levels and modify the progression to autoimmunity in the nonobese diabetic (NOD) mouse model of type 1 diabetes (T1D). Colonization by commensal microbes elevated serum testosterone and protected NOD males from T1D. Furthermore, transfer of gut microbiota from adult males to immature females altered the recipient's microbiota, resulting in elevated testosterone and metabolomic changes, reduced islet inflammation and autoantibody production, and T1D protection [45].

3. The gut-microbiome checkpoints

Under normal conditions the human body has established a number of locally protective mechanisms and checkpoints to maintain immune integrity. These checkpoints include:

3.1. Mucosal buffer zone: "first-line defense"

Mucosal buffer zone represents an effective physicochemical barrier which is composed of the thick mucus layer, a number of antimicrobial proteins, and secretory IgA antibodies. The components of this barrier coalesce to minimize the contact and dilute any possible pathological microbial trigger between the commensal microbes in the gut lumen and intestinal epithelial cells that line the gut wall [50, 51].

3.2. Intestinal epithelial cells: "second-line defense"

Microbiota that escape the initial "buffer zone" encounter a second defense strategy represented by the tight junctions formed between the intestinal epithelial cells featuring a physical barrier.

Epithelial cells produce a variety of antimicrobial/bactericidal proteins, such as defensins, cathelicidins, and C-type lectins and express Toll-like receptors (TLRs) in their cell membrane. Toll-like receptors (TLRs) present on the surface of cells of innate immunity recognize pathogen-associated molecular patterns (PAMPs) with activation of the signaling adaptor molecule MyD88 (myeloid differentiation primary-response protein 88) provoking a downstream inflammatory responses. Lipopolysaccharides (LPS) are important components of the outer membrane of all Gram-negative bacteria. TLR4 is a natural ligand for LPS and upon binding to LPS leads to activation of cell and secretion of inflammatory cytokines. Cytokines in turn activate cells of the adaptive immune system that generates antigen-specific response [52].

3.3. The Innate and Adaptive Immune responses of the Lamina Propria "Third-Line Defense"

The composition and function of the gut microbiota play a critical role in regulating the Th17/Treg cell balance in the lamina propria. The innate cells in lamina propria constitute an important local line of immune defense that constantly surveys the gut lumen tracing undesirable antigens. The first is the intestinal macrophage system that phagocytoses microorganisms bypassing the first- and second-line barriers. The second is the lamina propria dendritic cells (DCs, antigen-presenting cells) that present foreign peptides complexed with MHC class II molecules for priming of antigen-specific B- or T-cell receptors to initiate an adaptive immune response.

T helper cells feature another key player when primed via a complex network of receptors, cytokines, and transcription factors enabling their differentiation into several pro-inflammatory or anti-inflammatory subsets. The type 1 T helper (Th1) response develops in response to intracellular pathogens, while type 2 T helper (Th2) and type 17 T helper (Th17) cells are predominantly stimulated after identification of extracellular organisms [53, 54].

4. Dysbiosis and autoimmune inflammatory arthritis

Multiple animal models of human autoimmune diseases (AD) suggest the direct involvement of commensal microbiota in disease development. A change to a single bacterial species and/or the entire community leads to an imbalance between the pathobiome and the symbiome immune responses with breakdown of self-immune tolerance provoking a number of ADs [47]. Mono-colonization with *Lactobacillus bifidus* in IL-1 receptor antagonist knockout mice resulted in rapid onset of arthritis which was dependent on Toll-like receptor activation by *L. bifidus*. The arthritis onset was preventable by promoting a germ-free environment [52]. Mono-colonization of germ-free mouse with single gut-microbiome "segmented filamentous bacterium (SFB)" is sufficient to induce fully functional TH17 cells that produce pro-inflammatory cytokines IL-17 and drive the onset of arthritis. The SFB upregulates the production of acute-phase isoforms of serum amyloid A (SAA) in the ileum, which can act on dendritic cells (DCs) from the small intestinal lamina propria to induce Th17 differentiation [49, 55]. Also, colonization of the mice gut with *Prevotella copri* (*P. copri*) can enhance experimental dextran sulfate sodium-induced colitis which is capable of initiating a pro-inflammatory drive in human arthritis. The *P. copri* genome encodes phosphoadenosine phosphosulfate reductase, an oxidoreductase that participates in the production of thioredoxin. Thioredoxin (TRX) is a cellular reducing catalyst induced by oxidative stress and is involved in the redox regulation of transcription factors such as NF-kappa B. TRX has been widely implicated in the pathogenesis of RA with significantly increased concentrations observed in both RA serum and synovial fluid [56–58].

Finally, commensal bacteria can produce and secrete large amounts of adenosine 51-triphosphate (ATP) that can activate a unique subset of lamina propria cells, CD70highCD11clow cells. The CD70highCD11clow subset cells could express Th17-inducing molecules, such as IL-6, IL-23p19, and transforming-growth-factor-_-activating integrin AV, and induce Th17 differentiation [59].

The metabolome theory: The analysis of bacterial metabolites and their association with specific taxa unveiled significant scientific data on potential mechanistic link in RA. The abundance of the *Collinsella* genus correlated strongly with high levels of three metabolites (beta-alanine, alpha-aminoadipic acid, and asparagine) in RA. The immune-stimulatory role of the *Collinsella* in RA was confirmed using a human epithelial cell line and a humanized mouse model of collagen-induced arthritis (CIA). *Collinsella* increased gut permeability by reducing the expression of tight junction protein in the human intestinal epithelial cell line CACO-2, induced production of the pro-inflammatory cytokine interleukin IL-17A. In humanized CIA, *Collinsella* enhanced disease severity. All together, these data suggest that it seems to have an essential role in altering gut permeability and disease severity as confirmed in experimental arthritis [60].

5. Altered Gut Microbiota and Inflammation in Rheumatoid Arthritis.

The Th17 pathway is one of the main inflammatory pathways. Th17 cells and its signature cytokine IL-17 have been involved in mediating pannus growth, osteoclastogenesis, and synovial neo-angiogenesis. Circulating Th17 cells as well as the IL-17 are significantly elevated in patients with RA. IL-17 induces RANKL expression in human synovial fibroblasts, leading to the loss of the RANKL/OPG balance with subsequent enhancement of osteoclastogenesis and bone erosion. IL-17 also increases the production of vascular endothelial growth factor (VEGF) in rheumatoid fibroblast-like synoviocytes (FLS), contributing to the angiogenesis in rheumatoid synovium. Finally, IL-17 stimulates the expression of various pro-inflammatory cytokines (e.g., IL-1β, TNF-α, and IL-6) and matrix-degrading enzymes (e.g., matrix metalloproteinase (MMP)-1, matrix metalloproteinase-2, matrix metalloproteinase-9, and matrix metalloproteinase-13) in whole synovial tissue, synovial fibroblasts, and cartilage, thus promoting inflammation, extracellular matrix breakdown, and cartilage destruction during RA development [61–65].

The gut mucosa represents a strategic landscape promoting a variety of interactions between the environment and the human host. They possess the potential to trigger autoimmunity in diverse ways. When genetic and/or environmental factors alter the balance in the microbiota composition, dysbiosis ensues. The metagenomics shotgun sequencing technique has revealed significant alterations in the microbiota profile in patients with RA. Evidences illustrated that changes in the symbiotic relationship between intestinal microflora and opportunistic bacteria as well as bacterial translocation from the gut to nasal mucosa or urinary tract may additionally enhance the risk of developing RA as well as disease-related comorbid conditions. Partial depletion of natural gut flora by antibiotic in experimental animals aggravates CIA [53].

Potentially harmful microorganisms/pathobiomes (such as SFB or *Lactobacillus*) dominate and create a local pro-inflammatory profile with local expansion of autoreactive Th1 and Th17-cell compartments, via secretion of stimulatory molecules as ATP adenosine-5′-triphosphate, SAA serum amyloid A, or CCL5 CC-chemokine ligand 5 signaling. The autoreactive T cells migrate to peripheral immune compartments and activate B cells to differentiate into autoantibody-producing plasma cells. These cells and antibodies then migrate to synovial tissue where the inflammatory cascade is amplified through the activation of effector components, including macrophages, fibroblasts, osteoclasts, cytokines, and proteinases provoking arthritis and pannus formation. Dysbiosis in RA is associated with clinical indices of immune-mediated inflammation, such as the titers of immunoglobulin, autoantibodies, anti-cyclic citrullinated peptide (anti-CCP), and rheumatoid factor (RF) [17, 52, 55, 66].

5.1. Microbial colonies overpresented in RA

5.1.1. The Lactobacillus species

Lactobacillus fecal microbiome communities were found to be significantly increased in patients with early RA with those from healthy individuals [25] (**Table 1**). The abundance of *Lactobacillus salivarius* was associated with an increase in disease severity associating the increase in bacterial load.

Study	Patients vs. controls (number)	Sample	Technique	Microbiota profile Increased (++), decreased (--)
Vaahtovuo et al. [67]	Early RA (n= 51) vs. fibromyalgia (n= 50)	Stool	16S rRNA hybridization and DNA staining	Bifidobacteria --, *Bacteroides* --, Porphyromonas --, *Prevotella* --, *Bacteroides fragilis* --, *Clostridium coccoides* --
Gul'neva et al. [68]	Treatment-naïve RA (n= 94) vs. healthy (n= 97)	Stool, dental, saliva	Metagenomic shotgun sequencing	*Lactobacillus salivarius* ++, *Gordonibacter pamelaeae* ++, *Clostridium asparagiforme* ++, *Haemophilus* spp. --
Liu et al. [69]	Early RA (n= 15) vs. healthy (n= 15)	Stool	Quantitative real-time PCR	*Lactobacillus* ++
Scher et al. [57]	New-onset RA (n= 44) vs. healthy (n= 28)	Stool	16S rRNA gene and WGS sequencing	Prevotella copri ++, Bacteroidetes --
Zhang et al. [70]	RA (n= 30) vs. healthy (n= 30)	Stool	16S rRNA gene and WGS sequencing	Enterococci ++, Clostridia ++, Colibacteria ++, Lactobacteria --

Table 1. Microbiota profile in RA [57, 67–70].

5.1.2. The Prevotella copri species

A strong positive correlation was illustrated between the *Prevotella copri* (*P. copri*) and new-onset untreated RA (NORA). *Prevotella* was found to be overrepresented in NORA patients, and the relative abundance of *P. copri* in RA patients negatively correlates with the presence of HLA-DRB1-shared epitope. The relation between this specific microbiome and RA was further confirmed by the observation that the expansion of *P. copri* in RA patients could be suppressed to a similar state that was observed in healthy subjects after treatment with DMARDs that control of RA disease activity.

5.1.3. Other forms of gut microbiota

RA patients showed a dysbiotic gut microbiota characterized by a decrease in *Faecalibacterium* and an increase in *Collinsella* and *Eggerthella*. Large microbiota clusters including *Gordonibacter pamelaeae, Clostridium asparagiforme, Eggerthella lenta,* and Lachnospiraceae bacterium as well as small clusters of *Bifidobacterium dentium* and *Ruminococcus lactaris* were enriched in the gut of RA patients.

On the other hand, RA patients have significantly less bifidobacteria and microbiome of the *Bacteroides-Porphyromonas-Prevotella* group, *Bacteroides fragilis* subgroup, and *Eubacterium rectale-Clostridium coccoides* group and *Haemophilus* spp. in comparison to patients with non-inflammatory rheumatic diseases.

5.1.4. Protective microbiota species: Prevotella histicola "P. histicola"

Oral feeding of *P. histicola* in mouse models of RA led to decreased symptom frequency and severity and fewer signs of inflammation in diseased vs. controls. *P. histicola* administration is associated with an upregulation of the anti-inflammatory cytokine IL-10 and Treg cells in the lamina propria and spleen of mice with CIA with subsequent amelioration of immune inflammatory responses. *P. histicola* preserves gut epithelium integrity by lowering gut permeability and increased expression of tight junction proteins (zonulin and occludin) in treated mice compared to control. Treatment with *P. histicola* had fewer side effects (such as weight gain, villous atrophy, and increased gut permeability) that are linked with nonsteroidal anti-inflammatory drugs and other traditional medications used for treating RA. This microbiome is currently considered as potential future novel therapy in RA [71].

6. Future perspectives

Multiple lines of evidence support the potential pathogenic role of gut dysbiosis in RA which makes gut microbiota a possibly promising new territory for drug targeting [72]. Restoring balance of gut microbiota might contribute to the improvement of disease symptoms in RA. Experimental models demonstrated the ability of certain microbial colonies to drive inflammation such as *P. copri* and SFB.

Thus, it is plausible to hypothesize that targeting the postulated pathobiomes might contribute to clinical improvement in RA. Despite the successful use of antimicrobials in RA, they lack microbial specificity in most studies.

"Mapping of the individual's microbiota profile and tracking their metabolic signatures might serve in the future design of a predictive profile of the potential to develop inflammatory arthritis, anticipate disease course, severity and specify more therapeutic strategies."

"Restoring balance in dysbiosis represents an advent toward novel treat to target therapeutic strategies in RA, a promising step toward an effective personalized medical approach."

Author details

Reem Hamdy A. Mohammed[1,*] and Hesham Ibrahim I. Elmakhzangy[2]

*Address all correspondence to: rmhamdy@yahoo.com

1 Department of Rheumatology/Clinical Immunology and Rehabilitation, School of Medicine, Cairo University-FRCP, Egypt

2 Department of Gastroenterology/Hepatology and Tropical Medicine, School of Medicine, Cairo University, Egypt

References

[1] Gregersen PK, Silver J, Winchester RJ. The shared epitope hypothesis. An approach to understanding the molecular genetics of susceptibility to rheumatoid arthritis. Arthritis Rheum. 1987;30:1205–13.

[2] Wellcome Trust Case Control Consortium. Genome-wide association study of 14,000 cases of seven common diseases and 3,000 shared controls. Nature. 2007;447:661–78.

[3] Taneja V. Arthritis susceptibility and the Gut Microbiome. FEBS Lett. 2014;588(22): 4244-4249.

[4] Alauzet C, Mory F, Carlier JP, Marchandin H, Jumas-Bilak E, Lozniewski A. *Prevotella nanceiensis* sp. nov., isolated from human clinical samples. Int. J. Syst. Evolut. Microbiol. 2007;57:2216–2220.

[5] de Pablo P, Dietrich T, McAlindon TE. Association of periodontal disease and tooth loss with rheumatoid arthritis in the US population. J. Rheumatol. 2008;35:70–76.

[6] Bannatyne G, Wohlmann A. Rheumatoid arthritis: its clinical history, etiology, and pathology. Lancet. 1896; 147 (3791):1120–5.

[7] Human Microbiome Project Consortium, Huttenhower C, Gevers D, Knight R, Abubucker S, Badger JH, et al. Structure, function and diversity of the healthy human microbiome. Nature. 2012; 486 (7402):207–14.

[8] Pineda MLA, Thompson SF, Summers K, de Leon F, Pope J, Reid G. A randomized, double-blinded, placebo-controlled pilot study of probiotics in active rheumatoid arthritis. Med. Sci. Monitor. 2011;17(6):CR347–5.

[9] Moen K, Brun JG, Valen M, Skartveit L, Eribe EK, Olsen I, et al. Synovial inflammation in active rheumatoid arthritis and psoriatic arthritis facilitates trapping of a variety of oral bacterial DNAs. Clin. Exp. Rheumatol. 2006; 24:656–63.

[10] Hunter W. Oral sepsis as a cause of disease. Br. Med. J. 1900; 2: 215–216.

[11] Mikuls TR, et al. Antibody responses to *Porphyromonas gingivalis* (P. gingivalis) in subjects with rheumatoid arthritis and periodontitis. Int. Immunopharmacol. 2009; 9: 38–42.

[12] Hitchon CA, et al. Antibodies to *Porphyromonas gingivalis* are associated with anticitrullinated protein antibodies in patients with rheumatoid arthritis and their relatives. J. Rheumatol. 2010; 37: 1105–1112.

[13] Loyola-Rodriguez JP, Martinez-Martinez RE, Abud-Mendoza C, Patino-Marin N, Seymour GJ. Rheumatoid arthritis and the role of oral bacteria. J. Oral Microbiol. 2010; http://dx.doi.org/10.3402/jom.v2i0.5784.

[14] Rashid T, Jayakumar KS, Binder A, Ellis S, Cunningham P, Ebringer A. Rheumatoid arthritis patients have elevated antibodies to cross-reactive and non cross-reactive antigens from Proteus microbes. Clin. Exp. Rheumatol. 2007;25:259–267.

[15] Ebringer A, Rashid T, Wilson C. Rheumatoid arthritis, Proteus, anti-CCP antibodies and Karl Popper. Autoimmun. Rev. 2010; 9: 216–223.

[16] Newkirk MM, Zbar A, Baron M, Manges AR. Distinct bacterial colonization patterns of *Escherichia coli* subtypes associate with rheumatoid factor status in early inflammatory arthritis. Rheumatology (Oxford) 2010; 49:1311–1316.

[17] Scher JU, Abramson SB. The microbiome and rheumatoid arthritis. Nat. Rev. Rheumatol. 2011; 7: 569–578.

[18] Svartz, N. The primary cause of rheumatoid arthritis is an infection—the infectious agent exists in milk. Acta Med. Scand. 1972; 192, 231–239.

[19] Hannonen P, Mottonen T, Hakola M, Oka M. Sulfasalazine in early rheumatoid arthritis. A 48-week double-blind, prospective, placebo-controlled study. Arthritis Rheum. 1993; 36, 1501–1509.

[20] O'Dell JR, et al. Treatment of rheumatoid arthritis with methotrexate alone, sulfasalazine and hydroxychloroquine, or a combination of all three medications. N. Engl. J. Med. 1996; 334, 1287–1291.

[21] Saag KG, et al. American College of Rheumatology 2008 recommendations for the use of nonbiologic and biologic disease-modifying antirheumatic drugs in rheumatoid arthritis. Arthritis Rheum. 2008; 59, 762–784.

[22] Tilley BC, et al. Minocycline in rheumatoid arthritis. A 48-week, double-blind, placebo-controlled trial. MIRA Trial Group. Ann. Intern. Med. 1995; 122, 81–89.

[23] O'Dell JR, et al. Treatment of early seropositive rheumatoid arthritis: doxycycline plus methotrexate versus methotrexate alone. Arthritis Rheum. 2006; 54, 621–627.

[24] Saviola G, Abdi Ali L, Rossini P, Campostrini L, Coppini A, Gori M, Ianaro A, Bucci M, de Nucci G, Cirino G. Clarithromycin in rheumatoid arthritis patients not responsive to disease-modifying antirheumatic drugs: an open, uncontrolled pilot study. Clin. Exp. Rheumatol. 2002; 20: 373–378.

[25] Syer SD, Blackler RW, Martin R, de Palma G, Rossi L, Verdu E, Bercik P, Surette MG, Aucouturier A, Langella P, et al. NSAID enteropathy and bacteria: a complicated relationship. J. Gastroenterol. 2015; 50: 387–393.

[26] So JS, Kwon HK, Lee CG, Yi HJ, Park JA, Lim SY, Hwang KC, Jeon YH, Im SH. *Lactobacillus casei* suppresses experimental arthritis by down-regulating T helper 1 effector functions. Mol. Immunol. 2008; 45: 2690–2699.

[27] Smith PM, Howitt MR, Panikov N, Michaud M, Gallini CA, Bohlooly-Y M, Glickman JN, Garrett WS. The microbial metabolites, short-chain fatty acids, regulate colonic Treg cell homeostasis. Science 2013; 341: 569–573.

[28] Simon GL, Gorbach SL. Intestinal flora in health and disease. Gastroenterology. 1984;86(1):174–93.

[29] Savage DC. Microbial ecology of the gastrointestinal tract. Annu. Rev. Microbiol. 1977; 31:107–33.

[30] Yeoh N, Burton J P, Suppiah P, Reid G, Stebbings S. The role of the microbiome in rheumatic diseases. Curr. Rheumatol. Rep. 2013; 15:314.

[31] Isolauri E. Development of healthy gut microbiota early in life. J. Paediatr. Child Health. 2012; 48(3):1–6.

[32] Urbaniak C, Burton JP, Reid G. Breast, milk and microbes: a complex relationship that does not end with lactation. Women's Health (Lond Engl). 2012; 8(4):385–98.

[33] Qin J, et al. A human gut microbial gene catalogue established by metagenomic sequencing. Nature. 2010;464:59–65.

[34] Eckburg PB, et al. Diversity of the human intestinal microbial flora. Science. 2005; 308:1635–1638.

[35] Rajilić-Stojanović M, Smidt H, De Vos WM. Diversity of the human gastrointestinal tract microbiota revisited. Environ. Microbiol. 2007; 9(9):2125–2136.

[36] Van den Bogert B, De Vos WM, Zoetendal EG, Kleerebezem M. Microarray analysis and barcoded pyrosequencing provide consistent microbial profiles depending on the source of human intestinal samples. Appl. Environ. Microbiol. 2011;77(6):2071–2080.

[37] Zoetendal EG, Akkermans AD, De Vos WM. Temperature gradient gel electrophoresis analysis of 16S rRNA from human fecal samples reveals stable and host-specific communities of active bacteria. Appl. Environ. Microbiol. 1998; 64(10):3854–3859.

[38] Human Microbiome Jumpstart Reference Strains Consortium, Nelson KE, Weinstock GM, Highlander SK, Worley KC, Creasy HH, Wortman JR, Rusch DB, et al. A catalog of reference genomes from the human microbiome. Science. 2010; 328:994–999.

[39] Quigley EMM. Therapies aimed at the gut microbiota and inflammation: antibiotics, prebiotics, probiotics, synbiotics, anti-inflammatory therapies. Gastroenterol. Clin. North Am. 2011;40 (1):207–22.

[40] Dimmitt RA, Staley EM, Chuang G, Tanner SM, Soltau TD, Lorenz RG. Role of postnatal acquisition of the intestinal microbiome in the early development of immune function. J. Pediatr. Gastroenterol. Nutr. 2010; 51(3):262–73.

[41] Lerner A, Aminov R, Matthias T. Dysbiosis may trigger autoimmune diseases via inappropriate post-translational modification of host proteins. Front. Microbiol. 2016;7:84.

[42] Mortha A, Chudnovskiy A, Hashimoto D, Bogunovic M, Spencer SP, Belkaid Y, Merad M. Microbiota-dependent crosstalk between macrophages and ILC3 promotes intestinal homeostasis. Science 2014; 343: 1249-288.

[43] Aychek T and Jung S. The axis of tolerance. Science 2014; 343: 1439–1440.

[44] Furusawa Y, Obata Y, Fukuda S, Endo TA, Nakato G, Takahashi D, Nakanishi Y, Uetake C, Kato K, Kato T, et al. Commensal microbe-derived butyrate induces the differentiation of colonic regulatory T cells. Nature 2013; 504: 446–450.

[45] Markle JG, Frank DN, Mortin-Toth S, Robertson CE, Feazel LM, Rolle-Kampczyk U, von Bergen M, McCoy KD, Macpherson AJ, Danska JS. Sex differences in the gut microbiome drive hormone-dependent regulation of autoimmunity. Science 2013, 339: 1084–1088.

[46] Wu HJ, Wu E.. The role of gut microbiota in immune homeostasis and autoimmunity. Gut Microbes 2012; 3: 4–14.

[47] Kim CH, Park J, Kim M. Gut microbiota-derived short-chain fatty acids, T cells, and inflammation. Immune Network. 2014;14(6):277-288.

[48] Round JL, Lee SM, Li J, Tran G, Jabri B, Chatila TA, Mazmanian SK. The Toll-like receptor 2 pathway establishes colonization by a commensal of the human microbiota. Science 2011; 332: 974–977.

[49] Ivanov II, Atarashi K, Manel N, Brodie EL, Shima T, Karaoz U, Wei D, Goldfarb KC, Santee CA, Lynch SV, et al. Induction of intestinal Th17 cells by segmented filamentous bacteria. Cell 2009; 139: 485–498.

[50] Pullar T, Hunter JA, Capell HA. Which component of sulphasalazine is active in rheumatoid arthritis? Br. Med. J. 1985; 290: 1535–1538.

[51] Ogrendik M. Effects of clarithromycin in patients with active rheumatoid arthritis. Curr. Med. Res. Opin.2007; 23: 515–522.

[52] Abdollahi-Roodsaz S, Joosten LA, Koenders MI, Devesa I, Roelofs MF, Radstake TR, Heuvelmans-Jacobs M, Akira S, Nicklin MJ, Ribeiro-Dias F, et al. Stimulation of TLR2 and TLR4 differentially skews the balance of T cells in a mouse model of arthritis. J. Clin. Investig. 2008, 118: 205–216.

[53] Dorożyńska I, Majewska-Szczepanik M, Marcińska K, Szczepanik M. Partial depletion of natural gut flora by antibiotic aggravates collagen induced arthritis (CIA) in mice. Pharmacol. Rep. 2014; 66: 250–255.

[54] Xu J, Lian F, Zhao L, Zhao Y, Chen X, Zhang X, Guo Y, Zhang C, Zhou Q, Xue Z, et al. Structural modulation of gut microbiota during alleviation of type 2 diabetes with a Chinese herbal formula. ISME J. 2015; 9: 552–562.

[55] Wu HJ, Ivanov II, Darce J, Hattori K, Shima T, Umesaki Y, Littman DR, Benoist C, Mathis D. Gut-residing segmented filamentous bacteria drive autoimmune arthritis via T helper 17 cells. Immunity 2010; 32: 815–827.

[56] Yoshida S, Katoh T, Tetsuka T, Uno K, Matsui N, Okamoto T. Involvement of thioredoxin in rheumatoid arthritis: its costimulatory roles in the TNF-alpha-induced production of IL-6 and IL-8 from cultured synovial fibroblasts. J Immunol. 1999; 163(1):351-8

[57] Scher JU, Sczesnak A, Longman RS, Segata N, Ubeda C, Bielski C, Rostron T, Cerundolo V, Pamer EG, Abramson SB, et al. Expansion of intestinal Prevotella copri correlates with enhanced susceptibility to arthritis. Elife 2013; 2: e01202.

[58] Maurice, MM, Nakamura H, Gringhuis S, Okamoto T, Yoshida S, Kullmann F, Lechner S, van der Voort EA, Leow A, Versendaal J, et al. Expression of the thioredoxin-thioredoxin reductase system in the inflamed joints of patients with rheumatoid arthritis. Arthritis Rheum. 1999; 42: 2430–2439.

[59] Atarashi K, Nishimura J, Shima T, Umesaki Y, Yamamoto M, Onoue M, Yagita H, Ishii N, Evans R, Honda K, et al. ATP drives lamina propria T(H)17 cell differentiation. Nature 2008; 455: 808–812.

[60] Taneja V, Krco CJ, Behrens MD, Luthra HS, Griffiths MM, David CS. B cells are important as antigen presenting cells for induction of MHC-restricted arthritis in transgenic mice. Mol. Immunol. 2007; 44: 2988–2996.

[61] Lubberts E, van den Bersselaar L, Oppers-Walgreen B., Schwarzenberger P, Coenen-de Roo, CJ, Kolls JK, Joosten LA, van den Berg WB. IL-17 promotes bone erosion in murine collagen-induced arthritis through loss of the receptor activator of NF-_B ligand/osteoprotegerin balance. J. Immunol. 2003, 17, 2655–2662.

[62] Kim KW, Kim HR, Park JY, Park JS, Oh HJ, Woo YJ, Park MK, Cho ML, Lee SH. Interleukin-22 promotes osteoclastogenesis in rheumatoid arthritis through induction of RANKL in human synovial fibroblasts. Arthritis Rheum. 2012; 64: 1015–1023.

[63] Ryu S, Lee JH, Kim SI. IL-17 increased the production of vascular endothelial growth factor in rheumatoid arthritis synoviocytes. Clin. Rheumatol. 2006; 25: 16–20.

[64] Moran EM, Mullan R, McCormick J, Connolly M, Sullivan O, Fitzgerald O, Bresnihan B, Veale DJ, Fearon U. Human rheumatoid arthritis tissue production of IL-17A drives matrix and cartilage degradation: synergy with tumour necrosis factor-_Oncostatin M and response to biologic therapies. Arthritis Res. Ther. 2009; 11: R113.

[65] Jovanovic DV, Di Battista JA, Martel-Pelletier J, Jolicoeur FC, He Y, Zhang M, Mineau F, Pelletier JP. IL-17 stimulates the production and expression of proinflammatory cytokines, IL-_ and TNF-_, by human macrophages. J. Immunol. 1998; 160: 3513–3521.

[66] Catrina AI, Joshua V, Klareskog L, Malmström V. Mechanisms involved in triggering rheumatoid arthritis. Immunol. Rev. 2016; 269: 162–174.

[67] Vaahtovuo J, Munukka E, Korkeamäki M, Luukkainen R, Toivanen P. Fecal microbiota in early rheumatoid arthritis. J. Rheumatol. 2008, 35, 1500–1505.

[68] Gul'neva MIU, Noskov SM. Colonic microbial biocenosis in rheumatoid arthritis. Klin. Med. 2011; 89: 45–48.

[69] Liu X, Zou Q, Zeng B, Fang Y, Wei H. Analysis of fecal Lactobacillus community structure in patients with early rheumatoid arthritis. Curr. Microbiol. 2013; 67: 170–176.

[70] Zhang X, Zhang D, Jia H, Feng Q, Wang D, Liang D. The oral and gut microbiomes are perturbed in rheumatoid arthritis and partly normalized after treatment. Nat. Med. 2015; 21: 895–905.

[71] Jia W, Li H, Zhao L, Nicholson JK. Gut microbiota: a potential new territory for drug targeting. Nat. Rev. Drug Discov. 2008; 7: 123–129.

[72] Smith PM, Howitt MR, Panikov N, Michaud M, Gallini CA, Bohlooly-Y M, Glickman JN, Garrett WS. The microbial metabolites, short-chain fatty acids, regulate colonic Treg cell homeostasis. Science 2013; 341: 569–573.

8

BAFF System in Rheumatoid Arthritis: From Pathobiology to Therapeutic Targets

Codrina Ancuta, Cristina Pomirleanu,
Claudia Mihailov, Eugen Ancuta and Daniela Opris

Abstract

Recent advances in understanding the multifaceted pathobiology of rheumatoid arthritis have highlighted the pivotal role and continuing crosstalk between activated immune cells, pro-inflammatory cytokines, and matrix-degrading mediators, promoting chronic inflammation as well as irreversible tissue damage within an autoimmune background. B cells are widely recognized as leading players in immune mediated pathology based on their ability to produce not only different patterns of autoantibodies and driving cytokine synthesis but also as independent antigen-presenting cells and by modulating the specific activation of T cells. Overwhelming evidence emphasized the role of BAFF, a B-cell-activating factor, and BAFF receptors (TACI, BCMA, BAFF-R) in promoting B-cell homeostasis, proliferation, and survival under normal and autoimmune systemic disorders. We systematically reviewed data from literature focusing on BAFF, its homolog molecule APRIL, and BAFF-binding receptors biology, dysregulation of BAFF/BAFF receptor signaling in autoimmune settings, and current status of targeting BAFF/BAFF receptor pathway for rheumatoid arthritis.

Keywords: rheumatoid arthritis, autoimmunity, B-cell-activating factor (BAFF), BAFF-bounding receptors, BAFF antagonists

1. Introduction

Rheumatoid arthritis (RA) is a chronic immuno-inflammatory disease characterized by a multifaceted pathobiology, where a complex cytokine and cellular network contribute to excessive and extensive articular and systemic inflammatory events, accompanied by progressive tissue damage [1–4].

B cells are widely recognized as leading players in the mechanisms underlying the pathogenesis of RA based on their ability to produce not only different subsets of autoantibodies but also as independent antigen-presenting cells, cytokine synthesis, and modulators of T-cell activation. Moreover, their differentiation and survival are driven by positive feedback loops induced by cytokines, especially members belonging to the tumor necrosis factor (TNF) family [1–4].

Recent data highlighted the role of signaling crosstalk in B-lymphocytes, particularly of B-cell-activating factor (BAFF) and its receptors in early steps of the disease, advancing clinical development of BAFF antagonists for the treatment of RA [2–5]. Acting as an innate cytokine mediator, BAFF is known to modulate peripheral B- and T-cell homeostasis, promoting specific downstream signaling events through three different types of receptors [2, 4, 5].

Abnormal BAFF/BAFF receptor-signaling pathways were reported in several autoimmune disorders including systemic lupus erythematosus, Sjogren's syndrome, ANCA-associated vasculitis, and RA [2, 4, 5]. Of interest, elevated BAFF levels were detected in synovial fluid, serum, and saliva in very early stages of RA, suggesting its involvement in cell-cell interactions network in the synovial microenvironment, as well as B-cell activation and the development of autoreactive B cells [2–4]. Furthermore, the overexpression of BAFF receptors, as well as disturbed autocrine and paracrine BAFF network, seems to be related to inflammatory events and RA progression [1–6].

Although clinical development of BAFF antagonists as potential therapeutic target for systemic autoimmune conditions is promising, the benefit of specific agents such as belimumab, atacicept, or tabalumab in RA is controversial [2, 4, 6].

We systematically reviewed data from the literature focusing on the biology of BAFF, its homologue molecule APRIL and BAFF-binding receptors, dysregulation of BAFF/BAFF receptor signaling in RA and current status of targeting BAFF/BAFF receptor pathway.

2. BAFF and BAFF receptors physiology

2.1. BAF and APRIL

BAFF, also known as BLyS (B-lymphocyte stimulator), TALL-1 (TNF and apoptosis ligand-related leukocyte-expressed ligand 1), zTNF4, TNFSF13B (TNF ligand superfamily member 13B) or THANK, is a protein member of the TNF ligand family, critically involved in B-cell survival, maturation, and function [2–6]. As a vital cytokine for peripheral B-cell homeostasis, BAFF is acknowledged as a key regulator for both innate and adaptive immune responses [2–5].

Under normal conditions, BAFF is mainly expressed and secreted by a variety of cells including monocytes, dendritic cells, neutrophils, stromal cells, and activated T cells [2–14] and is typically upregulated by different cytokines, such as TNF-α, IFN-γ, and TGF-β [2–14].

BAFF is recognized under two isoforms, a biologically active full-length isoform and the alternatively spliced one, 4BAFF, meaning a protein with a small peptide deletion which does not bind to BAFF receptors, but has the ability to form heterotrimers with the original isoform [2–6]. Additionally, BAFF is expressed as a membrane-binding homotrimer and released as a soluble, biologically active molecule in peripheral blood after cleavage by a dedicated furinprotease [2, 4].

APRIL, a proliferation-inducing ligand known as the homolog molecule of BAFF or TNFSF13 (TNF ligand superfamily member 13), is also a key cytokine for B-cell activation and maturation; APRIL prompts B-cell proliferation, antibody class switching and survival, but is not required for the normal B-cell development [12–14].

Interestingly, BAFF and APRIL exhibit the ability to generate mixed molecules comprising BAFF/APRIL hetero-trimers [2–14] and TWE-PRIL (TNFSF12), an APRIL extracellular domain/TWEAK intracellular domain hybrid molecule [2, 4], as well as ΔBAFF, an alternatively spliced form of BAFF [4]. None of these molecules binds to BAFF receptors, but their co-expression with BAFF may have a deleterious impact on receptor signaling [2–14].

2.2. BAFF receptors signaling

Three distinct BAFF receptors typically expressed on B cells in different developmental stages are generally recognized: (i) BAFF receptor (BAFF-R, BR-3, TNFRSF13C or TNF receptor superfamily member 13C); (ii) transmembrane activator and calcium modulator ligand interactor (TACI, TNFRSF13B or TNF receptor superfamily member 13B); and (iii) B-cell maturation antigen (BCMA, TNFRSF17 or TNF receptor superfamily member 17) [2–14].

The expression of BAFF-binding receptors becomes evident only during the transitional stages of B-cells, varies according to the B-cell subset and is strictly dependent on various downstream mediators, further differentiation, maturation, and activation level as well [2–14]. Moreover, each receptor triggers its own set of signaling pathways [2, 4].

Thus, BAFF-R is essentially engaged in naïve and memory B-cell populations, with the highest expression in follicular and marginal zone B-lymphocytes, and is upregulated by B-cell receptor on mature B cells and enables most of the BAFF-dependent actions [2–14]. BAFF-R appears to be the most important receptor for mature B-cell survival and homeostasis in peripheral B cells [5].

TACI remains the predominant receptor on marginal zone B cells and short-lived plasma cells, while BCMA is typically expressed by long-lived plasma cells being essential for their optimal generation [2, 4]. The ability of TACI to act as a sink for BAFF, preventing the attachment of BAFF to its BAFF-R, may also reflect mixed regulatory functions on B cells [2, 4, 5, 10–14].

Although BAFF-R/BR3 stands as a specific receptor for both soluble and membrane-bound BAFF, TACI and BCMA can also bind to the homologous proliferation-inducing ligand APRIL [2, 4, 10–14].

Each of the three receptors has a different pattern of expression and mediates distinct functions [2, 4].

2.3. BAFF and BAFF receptors functioning

It is widely accepted that BAFF plays a crucial role in B-cell homeostasis, adjusting their maturation, proliferation, and survival under different backgrounds. BAFF may also indirectly interfere with T-cell functioning, providing several co-stimulatory signals in conjunction with T-cell receptor, mainly related to cellular proliferation and synthesis of mediators [2, 4].

Table 1 summarizes the BAFF/BAFF receptors functions in B and T cells (**Table 1**) [2–14].

Cell type	Function
B cells	Enhance B-cell and plasma cell survival Co-stimulate B-cell proliferation B-cell maturation Promote B-cell differentiation from transitional type 1 to type 2 cells Immunoglobulin synthesis T-cell-independent and T-cell-dependent antibody response
T cells	Enhance T-cell proliferation Enhance cytokine synthesis
Dendritic cells	Promote immune cell recruiting Promote cytokine synthesis

Source: Adapted from Ref. [2].

Table 1. Overview of main BAFF biological functions in immune cells.

2.3.1. BAFF and B-cell functioning

BAFF and APRIL mediate several important B-cell functions in normal settings, but dysregulated BAFF/BAFF receptors represent a significant event in different autoimmune conditions [2–14].

First, BAFF enhances long-term B-cell survival primarily through NF-kB pathway by upregulating anti-apoptotic Genes, particularly the expression of Bcl-2 gene family members [2–14]. While BAFF and APRIL typically improve the survival of plasmablasts, their role in promoting long-lived plasma cells persistence is still debatable [2, 4]. Moreover, either BAFF or APRIL accounts for the survival of plasma cells expressing TACI and/or BCMA [2, 4, 10–14]. By contrast, memory B cells do not require BAFF nor APRIL for their proliferation and survival [2, 4]. Thus, their survival and reactivation are both BAFF-independent [2, 4, 10–14]. Finally, BAFF-BAFF-R interface seems to be vital for the survival of B2 subpopulation from the transitional type 1 stage, with a minor input from TACI and without feedback from BCMA [2–14].

Second, BAFF enhances signaling through the B-cell receptor (BCR) by upregulating the expression of its co-receptors, namely CD21 and CD19, respectively [2–14]. The relation is bidirectional as BAFF-R expression is upregulated by B-cell receptor on mature B cells [2–14]. Additionally, there is a direct linkage between the intensity of BCR signaling and the extent of BAFF signal, particularly related to the non-classical NF-kB pathway which is operational for BAFF-R [2, 4–14]. Therefore, signaling through BAFF-R is able to promote B-lymphocytes survival in general, and individual late transitional and follicular B-cell survival [2–14].

Third, BAFF upregulates Toll-like receptor (TLR), endorses B-cell survival as well as Ig class switching and plasma cell differentiation [2–14]. The expression of BAFF-bound receptors on B cells, particularly TACI [2–14], is up-regulated via intracellular-activated TLR under the effect of specific immune complexes, with further relevance for augmented BCR-mediated signaling. Activated B cells by TLR-4 overexpress BAFF-R receptor types with subsequent susceptibility to apoptotic signals through Fas molecules [2–14].

Finally, the differentiation of peripheral autoreactive B cells depends on high BAFF levels [2–14].

2.3.2. BAFF and T-cell functioning: proliferation and cytokine production

While recent insights have extensively advanced our knowledge about BAFF/BAFF receptor intervention on B-cell activity in normal microenvironment and autoimmunity, the role of BAFF and APRIL in T-cell co-stimulation is still controversial [2, 4–14].

Classically, BAFF indirectly enhances T-cell proliferation [8] and arbitrates cytokine production, particularly during inflammation. Hence, the expansion of T-cell population may occur as a consequence of primary B-cell expansion/proliferation rather than a result of direct intervention of BAFF cytokine. Of interest, APRIL itself appears to mediate T-cell overflow [2–14]. T-cell-dependent immunoglobulin (Ig) responses strictly vary according to Ig subtype; IgM responses require BAFF intervention, whereas IgG responses are usually BAFF-independent [2–15]. Also, the intervention of BAFF receptors on T-cell function is debatable; while TACI might refashion T-cell functions, BAFF-R charge is unclear [2–14].

2.3.3. BAFF and dendritic cells functioning

It is increasingly recognized that BAFF influences dendritic cells to be actively involved in many physiologic as well as pathologic processes. Dendritic cells not only overexpress BAFF under different mediators (e.g., type I interferons) but also express BAFF receptors, predominantly TACI required for cellular proliferation and function [2–14]. The interaction between BAFF and dendritic cells stimulates immune cell trafficking and recruitment to inflammatory sites, and delivery of different cytokines and chemokines, mainly IL-1 and IL-6 [2–14].

3. BAFF and BAFF receptors in rheumatoid arthritis

Dysregulated BAFF/BAFF receptor signaling is clearly a trigger for autoimmunity in particular settings as is the case of systemic lupus erythematosus and RA [1, 2, 4, 5, 15–24]. To better understand the relevance of BAFF/BAFF receptor system in the complex pathobiology of RA with direct involvement in both early stages and disease progression, we emphasized several aspects regarding cell networking and BAFF influences, BAFF levels, and BAFF receptor expression in RA [2, 4, 15–24].

3.1. BAFF and BAFF receptor influences on cell networking in rheumatoid arthritis

We already mentioned the effects of BAFF in B- and T-cell biological homeostasis in general, and we further provide information on how BAFF and APRIL influence immune cells and resident synovial cells in RA [2, 4, 15–24].

RA is thought to be the result of an interplay between multiple cells and their products (cytokines and mediators), from both innate and adaptive immunity that lead to systemic inflammatory and tissue-damaging events [1–4].

Persistent immune cell trafficking into the inflamed joints typically focuses on B- and T-lymphocytes, with special polarization for TCD4+ subpopulation, neutrophils, macrophages, and dendritic cells, which actively infiltrate the RA synovium and orchestrate inflammation and cartilage damage [1–4]. At least three different histological subtypes of immune infiltrates are actually recognized within the RA synovitis, meaning diffuse, nodular infiltrates, and lymphoid aggregates with germinal centers [2–4].

Excess of pro-inflammatory cytokines (mainly TNF-α, IL-1β, IL-6, IL-15, IL-17, and IL-23) and other inflammatory mediators (prostaglandin E2, reactive oxygen Species, nitric oxide) together with tissue-degrading enzymes (matrix metalloproteinases and other enzymes synthetized by activated neutrophils) are essential performers, maintaining local cellular networking in RA joints [1–3].

As innate cytokines, BAFF and APRIL are potentially involved in the dysregulated immuno-inflammatory synovial microenvironment, affecting both autocrine and paracrine feedback [1–6]. In addition, BAFF and APRILL are involved in an amplification loop which is locally activated by inflammation: B- and T-lymphocytes, together with plasmacytoid and myeloid dendritic cells, are interconnected through a continuing crosstalk [1–4]. Thus, B cells migrated to the inflamed tissues and activated produce pro-inflammatory and destructive cytokines and chemokines, but also exert their potent effector function by presenting self-antigens to and activating T cells [2–4]. Moreover, immune complexes as a result of aberrant functioning of B cells induce the activation of different subtypes of dendritic cells within the IFN direct supervision and further enhance B- and T-participation [4].

3.1.1. Neutrophils, macrophages, dendritic cells, and B-lymphocyte loop in rheumatoid arthritis

It is clear that activated neutrophils, macrophages, as well as dendritic cells represent fundamental sources of BAFF in the inflamed RA joints; however, these cells may have variable importance in different RA stages, with neutrophils releasing BAFF in early RA, while macrophages in established disease [1–4, 14–24].

Abundant BAFF levels further support a positive feedback from B-lymphocytes, the BAFF/BAFF-R signaling being an important stimulator of B-cell proliferation, survival, and activation, with subsequent dysregulated B-cell functioning, with synthesis of various cytokines, and autoantibodies [1–4, 14–24].

Neutrophils incoming in the inflamed synovial joint is able to produce high levels of soluble BAFF under the direct action of TNF-α and local G-CSF [1–4]. Additionally, through BAFF-R reverse signaling [2–4], macrophages are able to enhance MMP-9 and other matrix-degrading mediators [2–4]. Dendritic cells express BAFF molecule in early RA stages and turn into mature dendritic cells, mediating B-cell proliferation [2–4] with subsequent increase in antigen presentation, antibody production, immune complex formation, and cytokine secretion [1–4].

3.1.2. Neutrophils, macrophages, dendritic cells, and T-lymphocytes loop in rheumatoid

BAFF may also interfere with T cells-dendritic cells interaction. BAFF is obviously involved in T helper 1 (Th1)-related immune responses [1–4, 14–24] and facilitates significant in situ CD4+ T-cell proliferation and Th1 as well as Th17 polarization [1–4]. Interestingly, pro-inflammatory cytokines such as IL-1, IL-6, and TNF-α are involved in upregulation of BAFF expression on various activated cells in the synovial microenvironment (macrophages, dendritic cells, neutrophils) enhancing Th17 polarization and subsequent synthesis of IL-17 cytokine [1–4].

3.1.3. Fibroblast-like macrophages, B- and T-cell loop in rheumatoid arthritis

Fibroblast-like macrophages are known to constitutively express BAFF in patients with RA, and BAFF expression is significantly upregulated under TNF-α and IFN-γ stimulation [2, 4]. Activated fibroblast-like macrophages are further able to secrete IL-6 and CXCL12, as well as adhesion molecules (VCAM-1) influencing the survival of mature B cells and synovial trafficking [2, 4]. Recent data suggest that CD4+ T cells under BAFF activation are able to induce the proliferation of fibroblast-like macrophages, with consequent overexpression of various pro-inflammatory cytokines, particularly TNF-α, IL-1β, and IL-6 [2–4, 14–24].

Overall, various residents as well as recruited cells in rheumatoid synovium are responsible for BAFF synthesis, especially dendritic cells, macrophages and fibroblast-like macrophages, neutrophils, and CD4+ T cells. Further, BAFF interventions on the effector cell network (dendritic cells, macrophages and fibroblast-like macrophages, neutrophils, TCD4+ lymphocytes, and B cells) are able to promote by positive feedback their differentiation, proliferation, activation with subsequent cytokine production, and survival [2, 4].

3.2. Abnormal BAFF levels in rheumatoid arthritis

Elevated levels of BAFF are found in several inflammatory diseases (lupus, Sjogren's, RA), and are related to disease activity [2–4]; RA exhibits a positive correlation between BAFF and disease activity, so that BAFF was recommended as a new index of RA activity [2, 4, 14–24].

Interestingly, a recent study designates BAFF as a predictor of RA prognosis and outcomes as serum level of BAFF parallels radiographic progression and higher plasma BAFF correlates with advanced radiographic joint damage [2, 4, 14–24].

Elevated levels of both BAFF and APRIL along with their receptors in patients with RA, particularly in rheumatoid factor (RF) positive, anti-cyclic citrullinated peptide antibodies (ACPA)-positive subtype, active, erosive disease, support their role in the pathobiology of the disease [2, 4, 14–24]. Although abnormal BAFF was typically found in both serum and synovial fluid in RA, significantly higher synovial levels suggest local BAFF production, driving the maturation as well as preserving autoreactive B cells within the inflamed tissue, with subsequent amplification of inflammatory processes and generation of autoantibodies [2, 4, 14–24]. Furthermore, seropositive RA status is clearly associated with higher concentrations of BAFF than seronegative disease [2–4, 14–24], and there is a statistically significant correlation Between RF titer and BAFF level [2–4, 14–24].

Finally, it seems that BAFF levels depend on RA stage, and disease duration as well [2, 4, 14–24]; thereby, patients with very early RA (disease duration less than 6 weeks) have highest BAFF levels, followed by those with established (lasting more than 12 months) and long-standing disease [2, 4, 14–24]. Undifferentiated early arthritis also has lower BAFF levels as compared to very early RA supporting a role for BAFF in the initial steps of disease development [2, 4, 14–24].

However, local BAFF overexpression in RA joints is independent of the histologic subtype of RA synovitis (diffuse, nodular, and germinal center) [2, 4, 14–24]. BAFF also contributes to local B-lymphocyte function and survival, their activation and differentiation with subsequent production of autoantibodies [2, 4, 14–24]. Moreover, BAFF induces an autoreactive B-cell polarization as stressed by several studies in experimental arthritis models [2, 4, 14–24]. Thus, there is an interrelation between BAFF levels and humoral immune response [2, 4, 14–24], particularly RF, ACPA, as well as circulating immune complexes [2, 4, 14–24].

3.3. Abnormal expression of BAFF receptors in rheumatoid arthritis

BAFF receptors are also altered in RA [2, 4, 14–24]. The three receptor subtypes are expressed as follows: TACI-excessive levels are detected during first steps of RA development (early RA), BAFF-R has an obvious increase with disease progression, while BCMA expression has the same pattern as healthy population [2, 4, 14–24]. Furthermore, TACI receptor distribution and expression are typically lower than BAFF-R/BR3, without any relation with the histological subtype of synovitis [2, 4, 14–24]. On the other hand, it seems that only BCMA and its gene expression correlate with different patterns of B- and T-cell distribution among the synovial tissue [2, 4, 14–24]. Thereby, BCMA is significantly enhanced in synovial tissue presenting with follicular lymphocyte aggregation with or without germinal centers formation than in diffuse lymphoid infiltration synovitis [2, 4, 14–24]. Finally, aberrant expression of BCMA in resident synovial cells, Fibroblast-like synoviocytes, was reported in RA [2, 4, 14–24].

4. Targeting BAFF and BAFF receptors for rheumatoid arthritis

Accumulating data on the importance of B cells in various autoimmune diseases have reshaped the therapeutic armamentarium, specifically directed toward B-lymphocytes [2, 4, 25, 26].

While playing a pivotal role in B-cell survival and functioning, BAFF/BAFF receptor system recently emerged as a reasonable target for different autoimmune conditions [2, 4, 25, 26]; furthermore, several BAFF antagonists are already under development exploring the appropriate therapeutic intervention based on BAFF blockade in RA [2, 4, 25, 26].

Generally, therapeutic BAFF antagonism accounts not only for direct B-cell depletion and indirect impairment of B-cell-mediated processes such as antigen presentation, cytokine synthesis, and humoral immune response, but may also influence T-cell biology based on co-stimulatory signals [2, 4, 25, 26].

Several mechanisms were proposed to explain potential efficacy of BAFF/BAFF receptors antagonists in autoimmune conditions [2, 4, 25, 26]: (i) substantial B-cell depletion, particularly for bone-marrow-derived B2 subpopulation, known to undergo BAFF-mediated differentiation into follicular cells or marginal zone B cells [2, 4, 25, 26]; (ii) impaired immunoglobulin synthesis, especially in newly emerging B cells, while established memory B cells are spared; decreased transitional B-cell survival along with disturbed B-cell receptor co-signaling may further support altered immunoglobulin repertoire [2, 4, 25, 26]; (iii) indirect effect on other cells belonging to the BAFF amplification loop (T cells, dendritic cells, and macrophages) and their inflammatory mediators promoting decreased antigen presentation, decreased epitope spreading, immune complexes formation, and cytokine synthesis [2, 4, 25, 26]; (iv) selective depletion of plasmablasts expressing different BAFF-binding receptors [2, 4, 25, 26].

At least two classes of BAFF antagonists are currently recognized including (i) BAFF-blockers or monoclonal anti-BAFF antibodies (e.g., belimumab and tabalumab) and (ii) receptor fusion proteins (e.g., atacicept), specifically binding soluble BAFF, membrane BAFF, or APRIL [2, 4, 25, 26].

A simplified view of BAFF/APRIL/BAFF-binding receptor pathway and their targeted therapy in immune mediated is presented (**Figure 1**).

We reviewed the current status of targeting BAFF/BLyS, APRIL and their receptors in RA.

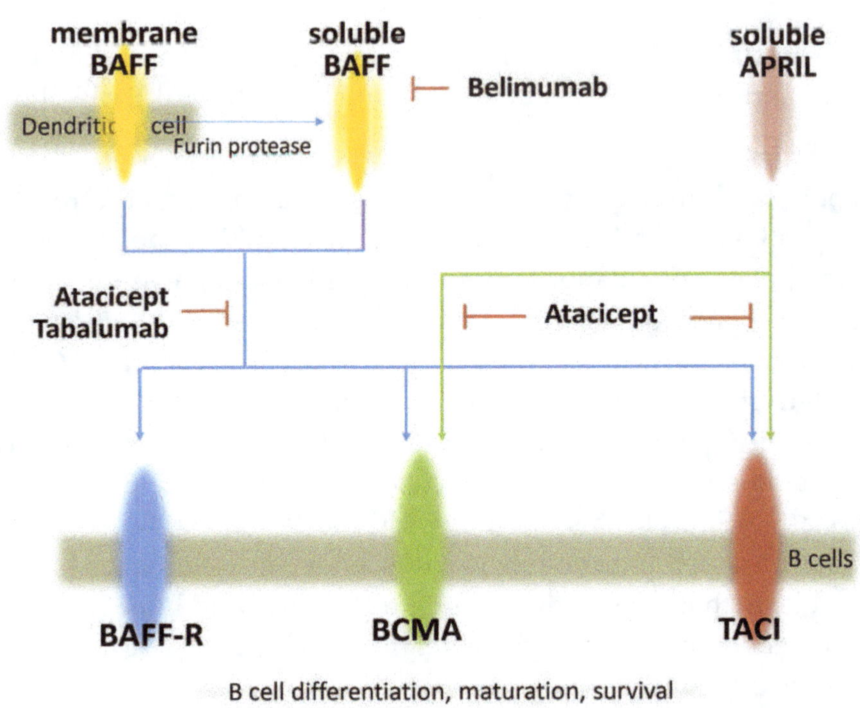

Figure 1. BAFF/APRIL/BAFF-binding receptor pathway and targeted therapy. Source: Adapted from Vincent F. et al., Nat Rev Rheum. 2014; Ref. [43].

4.1. Belimumab

Belimumab, the first targeted biological therapy for systemic lupus erythematosus, is a recombinant fully human immunoglobulin G subclass 1 (IgG1k) anti-BAFF monoclonal antibody recently approved for antinuclear antibody-positive lupus, selectively targeting soluble BAFF, but not membrane-bound BAFF or other members of the TNF ligand family. Moreover, belimumab demonstrates inhibitory activity on all three BAFF receptors (TACI, BCMA, BR3) with equivalent potency [2, 4, 26–30].

BAFF overexpression in RA theoretically induces local (synovial) autoreactive B-cell proliferation and survival. Preventing BAFF from binding to B cells is able to impair B-cell-mediated autoimmune response and could be an attractive target for RA patients [2, 4, 26–30].

The efficacy and tolerability of a novel, fully human variant of anti-BLyS monoclonal antibody was further evaluated in patients with active RA non-responsive to standard therapy in different clinical trials [2, 4, 26–30]. While safety data are convincing across all the studies and belimumab seems to be a promising agent for a specific RA population, optimal clinical efficacy needs further evaluation [2, 4, 26–30]. The majority of trials have demonstrated positive outcomes under belimumab BAFF-blockade, meaning significant response rates according to American College of Rheumatology (ACR) improvement ≥20% criteria but not ACR50 or ACR70, specifically for RA patients classified as having high disease activity (disease activity score DAS28>5.1), RF and ACPA-positive status, naïve to other biologics including TNF antagonists, previous methotrexate failure or low baseline BAFF levels [2, 4, 26–30].

4.2. Tabalumab

Tabalumab, formerly LY2127399, is another fully human IgG4 anti-BAFF monoclonal antibody that binds to and neutralizes soluble and membrane-bound BAFF, but not to APRIL [2, 4, 25, 31–35].

Efficacy and safety of tabalumab in active RA despite ongoing methotrexate was assessed in several phase 2 and 3 randomized-controlled studies and their open-label extensions performed on diverse patient populations comprising either bio-naive or bio-experienced RA with an inadequate response to TNF inhibitors (non-responders or intolerant) [2, 4, 25, 31–35]. Clinical efficacy parameters included standardized measures such as ACR20, ACR50, and ACR70 improvement criteria, DAS28-C-reactive protein (DAS28-CRP), and Health Assessment Questionnaire-Disability Index (HAQ-DI), while total B-cell counts or CD3-CD20 B cells and serum immunoglobulins were used for biological impact [2, 4, 25, 31–35]. Of interest, each one of the four phase 2 clinical trials (identifier NCT00308282, NCT00689728, NCT00785928, and NCT00837811) provided encouraging results under flexible doses of anti-BAFF and a background of stable methotrexate, with meaningful clinical and biological RA improvement as compared to placebo, regardless of prior treatment [2, 4, 25, 31–35]. However, tabalumab received no further validation following two phase 3 randomized, double-blind, placebo-controlled studies aiming to demonstrate drug efficacy and safety in patients with moderate-to-severe RA with inadequate response to one or more TNF inhibitors [25, 30, 34–36]. The interim analyses prompted the withdrawal of tabalumab due to lack of efficacy, not to safety concerns [2, 4, 25, 31–35].

To summarize, although tabalumab showed clinical and biological efficacy in phase 2 clinical trials irrespective of prior exposure to synthetic remissive drugs (methotrexate) or biologics, phase 3 trials fail to promote clinical benefit in patients with moderate-to-severe RA with prior inadequate response to TNF antagonists. Despite demonstrating biological improvement as supported by substantial change in B-cell count and decline in serum immunoglobulin levels, it is obvious that targeting the BAFF pathway alone is not a feasible strategy in RA [2, 4, 25, 31–35].

4.3. Atacicept

Atacicept is a recombinant fusion protein between the extracellular domain of one of the BAFF receptors (TACI) and the Fc portion of human IgG1, able to inhibit B-cell maturation, differentiation, and survival, as well as immunoglobulin synthesis by disconnecting B cells from standardized growth and development signals [2, 4, 25, 36–41]. In contrast to BAFF monoclonal antibodies, atacicept not only binds to and neutralizes BAFF but also targets APRIL molecule [2, 4, 25, 36–41] and could be an efficient target for RA treatment by inhibiting activation of TACI-mediated signaling [2, 4, 25, 36–42].

Preclinical and phase 1 clinical studies showed promising results as atacicept was well tolerated, with no increased incidence of infections, and displayed a meaningful biological activity with impaired levels of immunoglobulin, RF and ACPA, and a biphasic response in B-cell count [2, 4, 25, 36–41]. Moreover, atacicept induced substantial clinical improvement, despite the nonlinear pharmacokinetic profile [2, 4, 25, 36–41].

Nevertheless, AUGUST I (Clinical Trials.gov: NCT00430495) and AUGUST II (Clinical Trials.gov: NCT00595413), two phase 2 clinical trials, failed to demonstrate the efficacy of atacicept in moderate-to-severe RA patients. Both studies were specifically designed to assess efficacy, safety, and biological activity of atacicept in RA with an inadequate response to TNF inhibitors (AUGUST I) [2, 4, 25, 36–41] or biologically naive patients suboptimally controlled or intolerant to classic remissive agents (methotrexate) [2, 4, 25, 36–41].

Although the primary efficacy end point (ACR20 response) was not achieved in none of phase 2 studies, atacicept significantly reduced the immunoglobulin (IgM, IgG, and IgA) and rheumatoid factor levels in a dose-dependent manner. The safety profile was acceptable as atacicept did not show an increased susceptibility to infections, although the overall rate of adverse events was somewhat higher than placebo and lupus [2, 4, 25, 36–41].

To summarize, despite clinical and biological efficacy expressed in preclinical arthritis models and phase 1 clinical trial, phase 2 studies with atacicept fail to promote clinical benefit in patients with moderate-to-severe RA with inadequate response to either prior TNF antagonists or methotrexate [2, 4, 25, 36–41].

4.4. Other BAFF antagonists (AMG-623 and BR3-Fc)

Other BAFF-blockade agents are under development, targeting different BAFF receptor-binding molecules. A good example is A-623, previously known as AMG-623, a polypeptide fusion protein containing both IgG and the ligand-binding section of the BAFF-R, able to block both membrane and soluble BAFF and, therefore, to impair normal B-cell functioning

[43]. Briobacept or BR3-Fc is another distinct BAFF-blocking molecule acting as a homodimeric fusion glycoprotein including the extracellular ligand-binding portion of BAFF-R and the Fc portion of an IgG. This new drug was typically designed to induce further B-cell apoptosis interfering with BAFF/BAFF-R signaling [2, 4, 43].

5. Conclusions

Abnormal BAFF signaling (throughout either overexpression of B-cell-related activation and survival genes, or BAFF receptors) represents an important step in the pathobiology of rheumatoid arthritis, particularly by promoting the development of autoreactive B cells in early disease, but also by supporting disease progression.

Although BAFF/APRIL/BAFF receptors targeting therapy seems to be an attractive option for systemic autoimmune conditions, particularly systemic lupus erythematosus, considerable response heterogeneity and safety concerns are reported in rheumatoid arthritis.

Author details

Codrina Ancuta[1*], Cristina Pomirleanu[1], Claudia Mihailov[2], Eugen Ancuta[3] and Daniela Opris[4]

*Address all correspondence to: codrina_ancuta@yahoo.com

1 Rheumatology Department, Clinical Rehabilitation Hospital, Rheumatology 2 Department, 'Grigore T. Popa' University of Medicine and Pharmacy, Iasi, Romania

2 Clinical Port Hospital of Constanta, Faculty of Medicine, 'Ovidius' University of Constanta, Constanta, Romania

3 'Elena Doamna' Cinical Hospital, Research Department, Iasi, Romania

4 Internal Medicine and Rheumatology Department, 'Sfanta Maria' University Hospital, 'Carol Davila' University of Medicine and Pharmacy, Bucuresti, Romania

References

[1] Bugatti S, Vitolo B, Caporali R, et al. Cells in rheumatoid arthritis: from pathogenic players to disease biomarkers. BioMed Res Int. 2014;**2014**:681678 (1–14).

[2] Wei F, Chang Y, Wei W. The role of BAFF in the progression of rheumatoid arthritis. Cytokine. 2015;**76**(2):537–544.

[3] Moura RA, Graca L, Fonseca JE. To B or not to B conductor of rheumatoid arthritis orchestra. Clinic Rev Allerg Immunol. 2012;**43**(3):281–291.

[4] Ramanujam M, Davidson A. The current status of targeting BAFF/BLyS for autoimmune. Arthritis Res Ther. 2004;**6**:197–202.

[5] Woo YJ, Yoon BY, Jhun JY, et al. Regulation of B cell activating factor (BAFF) receptor expression by NF-κB signaling arthritis B cells. Exp Mol Med. 2011;**43**(6):350–357.

[6] Striz I, Brabcova E, Kolesar L, et al. Cytokine networking of innate immunity cells: a potential target of therapy. Clin Sci. 2014;**126**(9):593–612.

[7] Davidson A. Targeting BAFF in autoimmunity. Curr Opin Immunol. 2010;**22**:732–739.

[8] Lin Z, Davidson A. BAFF and selection of autoreactive B cells. Trends Immunol. 2011;**32**(8):388–394.

[9] Pillai S, Mattoo H, Cariappa A. B cells and autoimmunity. Curr Opin Immunol. 2011;**23**(6):721–731.

[10] Liu Z, Davidson A. BAFF inhibition: a new class of drugs for the treatment of autoimmunity. Exp Cell Res. 2011;**317**(9):1270–1277.

[11] Mackay F, Schneider P, Rennert P, et al. BAFF and APRIL: a tutorial on B cell. Ann Rev Immunol. 2003;**21**:231–264.

[12] Martin F, Kearney JF. B-cell subsets and the mature preimmune repertoire. Marginal zone and B1 B cells as part of a 'natural immune memory'. Immunol Rev. 2000;**175**:70–79.

[13] Marckay F, Mackay CR. The role of BAFF in B-cell maturation. T-cell activation and autoimmunity. Trends Immunol. 2002;**23**(3):1113–1125.

[14] Moisini L, Davidson A. BAFF: a local and systemic target in autoimmune diseases. Clin Exp Immunol. 2009;**1582**(2):155–163.

[15] De la Torre I, Moura RA, Leandro MJ, et al. B-cell-activating factor expression on naïve and memory B cells: relationship with relapse in patients with rheumatoid arthritis following B-cell depletion therapy. Ann Rheum Dis. 2010;**69**:2181–2188.

[16] Dong W, Li X, Liu Zhu P. Infiltrations of plasma cells in synovium are highly associated with synovial fluid levels of APRIL in inflamed peripheral joints of rheumatoid arthritis. Rheumatol Int. 2009;**29**:801–806.

[17] Geng Y, Zhang ZL. Comparative study on the level of B lymphocyte stimulator (BlyS) and frequency of lymphocytes between sero-negative and sero-positive rheumatoid arthritis patients. Int J Rheuma. 2012;**15**(5):478–485.

[18] Tan SM, Xu D, Roschke V, et al. Local production of B lymphocyte stimulator protein and APRIL in arthritic joints of patients with inflammatory arthritis. Arthritis Rheum. 2003;**48**(4):982–992.

[19] Seyler TM, Park YW, Takemura S, et al. BLyS and APRIL in rheumatoid arthritis. J Clin Invest. 2005;**115**(11):3083–3092.

[20] Nakajima K, Itoh K, Nagatani K, et al. Expression of BAFF and BAFF-R in the synovial tissue of patients with rheumatoid arthritis. Scand J Rheumatol. 2007;**36**:365–372.

[21] Leandro MJ, Cambridge G. Expression of B cell activating factor (BAFF) and BAFF-binding receptors in rheumatoid arthritis. J Rheumatol. 2013;**8**:1247–1250.

[22] Moura RA, Canhäo H, Polido-Pereira J, et al. BAFF and TACI gene expression are increased in patients with untreated very early rheumatoid arthritis. J Rheumatol. 2013;**40**(8):1293–1302.

[23] Moura RA, Cascäo R, Perpétuo I, et al. Cytokine pattern in very early rheumatoid arthritis favours B-cell activation and survival. Rheumatology. 2011;**50**(2):278–282.

[24] Moura RA, Weinmann P, Pereira PA, et al. Alternations on peripheral blood B-cell subpopulations in very early arthritis. Rheumatology. 2010;**49**:1082–1092.

[25] Blüml S, McKeever K, Ettinger R, et al. B-cell targeted therapeutics in clinical development. Arthritis Res Ther. 2013;15(1):54.

[26] Stohl W, Scholz JL, Cancro MP. Targeting BLyS in rheumatic disease: the sometimes – bumpy road from bench to bedside. Curr Opin Rheumatol. 2011;23(305-310)

[27] Jin X, Ding C. Belimumab –an anti-BLyS human monoclonal antibody for Rheumatoid Arthritis. Expert Opin Biol Ther. 2013;13(2):315-322.

[28] Eli Lilly and Company. ttps://newsroom.lilly.com/releasedetail.cfm?ReleaselD=738769. Press Release 2013 [Internet]. 2013 [Updated: 2013]. [Accessed: 26.08.2016]

[29] Genovese M, Filipowicz-Sosnowska A, Merrill J, et al. Differential responsiveness to belimumab in combination with standard of care therapy in RF+, TNF-inhibitors and methotrexate partial responder of subjects with moderate-severe rheumatoid arthritis. Arthritis Rheum. 2005;52:s1989.

[30] Stohl W, Merrill JT, McKay JD, et al. Efficacy and safety of belimumab in patients with rheumatoid arthritis: a phase II, randomized, double-blind, placebo-controlled, dose-ranging Study. J Rheumatol. 2013;40(5):579-589.

[31] Combe B, van Vollenhoven. Novel targeted therapies: the future of rheumatoid arthritis? Mavrilumab and tabalumab as examples. Ann Rheum Dis. 2013; 72 (9):1433-1435.

[32] Genovese MC, Fleischmann RM, Greenwald M, et al . Tabalumab, an anti-BAFF monoclonal antibody, in patients with active rheumatoid arthritis with an inadequate response to TNF inhibitors. Ann Rheum Diss. 2013;72(9):1461-1468.

[33] Greenwald M, Szczepanski L, Kennedy A, et al. A 52-week, open-label study evaluating the safety and efficacy of tabalumab, an anti-B-cell activating factor monoclonal antibody, for rheumatoid arthritis. Arthritis Res Ther. 2014;**16**(4):415–425.

[34] Smolen JS, Weinblatt ME, van der Heijde D, et al. Efficacy and safety of tabalumab, an anti-B-cell-activating factor monoclonal antibody, in patients with rheumatoid arthritis who had an inadequate response to methotrexate therapy: results from a phase III multicenter, randomized, double-blind study. Ann Rheum Dis. 2015; 74:1567-1570.

[35] Genovese MC, Lee E, Satterwhite J, et al. A phase 2 dose-ranging study of subcutaneous tabalumab for the treatment of patients with active rheumatoid arthritis and an inadequate response to methotrexate. Ann Rheum Dis. 2013;**72**(9):1453–1460.

[36] Genovese MC, Kinnaman N, de La Bourdonnave G, et al. Atacicept in patients with rheumatoid arthritis and an inadequate response to tumor necrosis factor antagonist therapy: results of a phase II, randomized, placebo-controlled, dose- finding trial. Arthritis Rheum. 2011;**63**(7):1793–1803.

[37] Nanda S. Therapy: Atacicept lacks clinical efficacy in RA. Nat Rev Rheumatol. 2011;**7**(6):313.

[38] Richez C, Truchetet ME, Schaeverbeke T, et al. Atacicept as an investigated therapy for rheumatoid arthritis. Expert Opin Investig. 2014;**23**(9):1285–1294.

[39] Bracewell C, Isaacs JD, Emery P, et al. Atacicept, a novel B cell-targeting biological therapy for the treatment of rheumatoid arthritis. Expert Opin Biol Ther. 2009;**9**(7):909–919.

[40] Tak PP, Thurlings RM, Rossier C, et al. Atacicept on patients with rheumatoid arthritis: results of a multicenter, phase Ib, double-blind, placebo-controlled, dose-escalating, single- and repeated-dose study. Arthritis Rheum. 2008;**58**:61–72.

[41] Van Vollenhoven RF, Kinnman N, Vincent E, et al. Atacicept in patients with rheumatoid arthritis and an inadequate response to methotrexate: results of a phase II, randomized, placebo- controlled trial. Arthritis Rheum. 2011;**63**(7):1782–1792.

[42] Hsu H, Khare SD, Lee F, et al. A novel modality of BAFF-specific inhibitor AMG623 peptibody reduces B-cell number and improves outcomes in murine models of autoimmune disease. Clin Exp Rheumatol. 2012;**30**(2):197–201.

[43] Nakayamada S, Tanaka Y. BAFF- and APRIL-targeted therapy in systemic autoimmune diseases. Inflamm Regener. 2016;36:6.

9

Raynaud's Phenomenon

Sevdalina Nikolova Lambova

Abstract

Raynaud's phenomenon (RP) is a clinical consequence of recurrent vasospasm of the small arteries and arterioles of the fingers and toes provoked by cold and emotional stress. RP is classified into two categories, i.e., primary and secondary RP. Primary RP is an isolated finding in the absence of an underlying pathology, while secondary RP is a syndrome in the context of another disease. The patients with primary RP have a younger age at onset, sparing of the thumb, and benign course without development of digital ulcers. Contrarily, secondary RP is characterized with later age of onset above 30 years, thumb involvement, and more severe course with possible development of trophic changes. In these cases, a focused, complaint-directed history and physical examination aim to reveal clinical symptoms and findings that confirm the presence of an underlying disorder, e.g., connective tissue disease (CTD) or other pathology. Together with clinical examination, laboratory, immunological, and capillaroscopic assessments facilitate the internal differential diagnosis of secondary RP. The capillaroscopic examination should be performed in all patients with symptoms of RP even in those cases without signs of systemic rheumatic disease, because the abnormal capillaroscopic picture inherits a high positive predictive value for the development of CTD.

Keywords: Raynaud's phenomenon, primary, secondary, peripheral vascular syndromes, capillaroscopy

1. Definition

The term "Raynaud's phenomenon" (RP) originates from the name of the French physician Maurice Raynaud, who described transient digital ischemia provoked by cold exposure and hypothesized that the changes are associated with exaggerated response of the central nervous system. Currently, the term "RP" defines the clinical consequence of recurrent vasospasm of the small arteries, arterioles, and arteriovenous shunts of the fingers and toes provoked by cold and emotional stress [1]. Other acral parts, e.g., the nose, lips, and ears, may be also affected. It manifests usually in three phases, ischemia, asphyxia, and reactive hyperemia, during which skin color changes occur consecutively from white to blue and red. A characteristic feature of RP is the clear demarcation between the affected and unaffected area.

2. Diagnosis of Raynaud's phenomenon

The diagnosis of RP is clinical and is based on direct observation of the vasospastic attacks [1]. Photographs that document the vasospastic attacks could also be used to confirm the history [2]. In routine clinical practice, it is not necessary to perform a cold provocation test to make a definite diagnosis of RP [1].

Observation of at least biphasic color changes is necessary for the diagnosis, as pallor and cyanosis are considered to be the most important signs. In a recent international consensus for the diagnosis of RP (Maverakis et al. [3]), a three-step approach for the diagnosis of RP has been suggested. The first two steps include asking more general questions: (I) a question about unusual sensitivity of the fingers to cold and (II) a question about "occurrence of biphasic color changes during the vasospastic episodes (white and blue)." Finally, during step III, the physician calculates the disease score by asking seven questions to the patient ((1) episodes are triggered by factors other than cold, i.e., emotional stress; (2) episodes involve both hands even if they are asynchronous or asymmetric; (3) numbness and paresthesias accompany vasospastic attacks; (4) well-demarcated border between the affected and unaffected skin; (5) photographs provided by the patient; (6) vasospastic episodes that affect other body parts such as the nose, ears, feet, and areolas; (7) occurrence of triphasic color changes during vasospastic attacks, e.g., white, blue, and red). If the score from step III is ≥3, the patient is diagnosed with RP [3].

3. Classification of Raynaud's phenomenon

RP is classified into two categories, i.e., primary and RP [1, 4, 5, 6].

Primary RP is an isolated finding in the absence of an underlying pathology, while secondary RP is a syndrome in the context of another disease. The patients with primary RP have a younger age of onset (below 30 years), sparing of the thumb, and benign course without the development of digital ulcers [4, 6, 7].

On the contrary, secondary RP is characterized with later age of onset above 30 years, thumb involvement, and a more severe course with possible development of trophic changes in some cases (digital ulcerations, digital necrosis) [4, 6, 7]. In these cases, a focused, complaint directed history and physical examination aim to reveal clinical symptoms and findings that confirm the presence of an underlying disease, e.g., connective tissue disease (CTD) or other disorders. The secondary RP is a characteristic feature in a number of rheumatic diseases. In systemic sclerosis (SSc)/scleroderma, it is with the highest frequency of approximately 95% [8]. RP could also be a sign in a spectrum of nonrheumatic pathology that also should be recognized and properly differentiated by the rheumatologists in routine clinical practice (**Table 1**) [8–14].

Together with clinical examination, laboratory, immunological, and capillaroscopic assessments facilitate the internal differential diagnosis of secondary RP and reveal the definite final diagnosis.

Nailfold capillaroscopy is a noninvasive, easy-to-perform method for diagnosis and differential diagnosis of patients with primary and secondary RP in rheumatic diseases (particularly the scleroderma-spectrum disorders), which is of crucial importance because of the different severity, prognosis, and therapeutic approach. Normal capillaroscopic pattern is an established diagnostic criterion for the diagnosis of primary RP. In addition, it has been found that capillaroscopic pattern in healthy individuals is constant for long periods of time. During the follow-up of patients with RP, it has been found that the appearance of abnormal capillaroscopic findings inherits a positive predictive value of 47% for the development of CTD that is higher as compared with the predictive value of the positive antinuclear autoantibody (ANA) test (30%) [15]. The appearance of giant capillaries is the earliest capillaroscopic sign of microangiopathy and represents a local response to tissue hypoxia. In RP patients, nailfold capillaroscopic analysis should be performed every 6 months and more often if new alarming symptoms appear. The capillaroscopic examination should be performed in all patients with symptoms of RP even in those cases without clinical and laboratory signs of systemic rheumatic disease, because the abnormal capillaroscopic picture inherits a high positive predictive value for the development of CTD.

Systemic sclerosis
Mixed connective tissue disease
Undifferentiated connective tissue disease
Systemic lupus erythematosus
Dermatomyositis, polymyositis
Sjögren syndrome
Rheumatoid arthritis
Systemic vasculitides-Buerger disease, Takayasu arteritis, polyarteritis nodosa, granulomatosis with polyangiitis, etc.
Fibromyalgia
Cryoglobulinemia
Drug-induced Raynaud's phenomenon—beta-blockers, cytotoxic drugs, vinblastine, bleomycin, interferon, etc.
Paraneoplastic Raynaud's phenomenon—associated with solid tumors and hematological malignancies
Endocrine disorders—hypothyroidism
Neurologic disorders—carpal tunnel syndrome

Table 1. Differential diagnosis of secondary Raynaud's phenomenon in rheumatologic practice.

4. Pathogenesis of Raynaud's phenomenon

The vasospasm in primary RP is reversible, while the secondary Raynaud's phenomenon in systemic sclerosis is associated with endothelial injury and subsequent structural abnormalities that lead to tissue damage.

Adrenergic alpha-2 receptors that are more important than alpha-1 receptors in the control of vasoconstriction of digital arteries are suggested to be abnormal in RP. The receptor subtype alpha-2c is found to predominate in the vascular smooth muscle cells of distal cutaneous vessels [16, 17]. Alpha-2c adrenergic receptors are not active at room temperature. In response to cold exposure, they are activated as a result from translocation from the Golgi complex to the plasmatic membrane [18, 19]. Estrogens also activate alpha-2c adrenoreceptors that could explain the predominance of primary RP in females and the increased severity of symptoms between menarche and menopause [20]. An association between enhanced contractile response to alpha-2c agonists and increased protein tyrosine kinase activity and tyrosine phosphorylation has been found. Greater intracellular tyrosine phosphorylation in response to cooling (31°C) has been found in arterioles in both primary and secondary RP patients vs. controls using immunofluorescence and an antiphosphotyrosine antibody [21, 22].

The endothelium controls blood vessel tone via production of vasodilators (nitric oxide (NO), prostacyclin) and vasoconstrictors (endothelin-1, angiotensin). Endothelial damage in secondary RP in SSc leads to disbalance between vasodilators and vasoconstrictors [10, 23]. In SSc-related RP, increased level of asymmetric dimethylarginine (an endogenous NO synthesis inhibitor produced by endothelial cells) was observed. Elevated plasma level of endothelin-1 was found in SSc as compared with primary RP [24]. Increased expression of endothelin-1 in the skin of SSc patients was also detected [25]. Besides its properties of vasoconstrictor, it has been confirmed that endothelin-1 promotes fibrosis in scleroderma patients [26]. In SSc, endothelial injury represents a key pathogenic step that mediates the processes of inflammation, thrombus formation, and fibrosis [23]. The role of endothelin-1 in pathogenesis of primary RP has also been implicated in some studies, but the evidence is weaker in comparison with SSc [10, 27].

Calcitonin gene-related peptide (CGRP) is a neuropeptide and a potent vasodilator produced by peripheral sensory nerves. In RP (primary and secondary RP in SSc), especially the secondary forms in SSc, a reduction in the number of CGRP immunoreactive neurons in the skin was found [28].

5. Primary Raynaud's phenomenon

In a recent systematic literature review, the prevalence of primary RP is reported to vary from 1.6 to 7.2% (calculated pooled prevalence—4.85%) [29]. As mentioned above, the primary RP is characterized with early age of onset, mainly at puberty. This classic type of presentation predominates in female patients with family history. Despite the fact that the age of onset is considered to be a discriminating factor between primary and secondary RP, it should be interpreted individually as primary RP with late onset (above the age of 40) is also possible [30].

5.1. Diagnosis of primary Raynaud's phenomenon

Wide application in clinical practice have the diagnostic criteria of Le Roy and Medsger (1992) that encompass the following findings:

1. Vasospastic attacks precipitated by cold or emotional stress
2. Symmetric attacks
3. Absence of digital ulcerations or gangrenes
4. Normal erythrocyte sedimentation rate
5. Negative test for ANA
6. Normal capillaroscopic picture [31]

Maverakis et al. published an international consensus for diagnosis of primary RP, which includes the following criteria: (1) normal capillaroscopy; (2) negative physical examination for findings suggestive of secondary causes such as ulcerations, tissue necrosis or gangrene, sclerodactyly, calcinosis, or skin fibrosis; (3) no history of existing CTD; and (4) negative or low titer ANA as low titer is considered (1:40) by indirect immunofluorescence. In the newly accepted criteria of Maverakis et al., the presence of normal erythrocyte sedimentation rate is not included, and negative test for ANA is not required [3] (**Table 2**). Normal capillaroscopic pattern exists in both sets of criteria.

In primary RP, capillary morphology and capillary density are normal. Slightly enlarged capillary diameters could be found [32–34].

6. Secondary Raynaud's phenomenon

Older age of onset, thumb involvement, severe course with trophic alterations of the fingers (digital ulcers, digital necrotic lesions), clinical features suggestive of autoimmune disease, positive autoantibodies, and abnormal capillaroscopic findings are characteristic features of secondary RP in rheumatic diseases [4, 6, 7].

6.1. Raynaud's phenomenon in systemic sclerosis

RP is one of the most common symptoms in SSc with frequency of about 95% [8]. It is usually the initial clinical feature that appears years before other disease symptoms. SSc-related RP is severe and often complicates with development of digital ulcers. The capillaroscopic pattern in SSc is specific and is characterized with the presence of dilated and giant capillaries, hemorrhages, avascular areas, and neoangiogenic capillaries. It has been described by Maricq et al. and is termed "scleroderma" type capillaroscopic pattern, which is a reference capillaroscopic pattern in rheumatology. Maricq et al. also observed components of this pattern in diseases from the scope of scleroderma-spectrum disorders, e.g., mixed connective tissue disease (MCTD), undifferentiated connective tissue disease (UCTD), and dermatomyositis (DM)—the so-called "scleroderma-like" pattern [35–37].

Le Roy and Medsger [31]	Maverakis et al. [3]
1. Vasospastic attacks precipitated by cold or emotional stress	1. Normal capillaroscopy
2. Symmetric attacks	2. Negative physical examination for findings suggestive of secondary causes (e.g., ulcerations, tissue necrosis or gangrene, sclerodactyly, calcinosis, or skin fibrosis)
3. Absence of digital ulcerations or gangrenes	3. No history of existing CTD
4. Normal erythrocyte sedimentation rate	4. Negative or low titer ANA (e.g., 1:40 by indirect immunofluorescence)
5. Negative test for ANA	
6. Normal capillaroscopic picture	

Table 2. Diagnostic criteria for primary Raynaud's phenomenon (Le Roy and Medsger [31]; Maverakis et al. [3]).

Cutolo et al. [38] described three phases of capillaroscopic changes in SSc:

I. An "early" phase—appearance of few dilated and/or giant capillaries and few hemorrhages. In this phase, the distribution is relatively preserved without loss of capillaries.

II. An "active" phase—the changes in this phase include a higher number of giant capillaries and hemorrhages, a moderate loss of capillaries, slight derangement, and, in some cases, diffuse pericapillary edema (**Figure 1**).

III. A "late" phase—it is characterized with extensive avascular areas, severe capillary derangement, and bushy and ramified capillaries [38].

"Scleroderma" type capillaroscopic pattern is found in the majority of SSc patients (about 90%). Maricq et al. detected "scleroderma" pattern in 82–95% of SSc patients [36, 37]. In an own study, "scleroderma" pattern of the hands was detected in 97.2% (35/36) of SSc patients [34, 39, 40].

In addition, it has been found that a number of patients with a definite diagnosis of SSc (those with sclerodactyly, telangiectasia, subcutaneous calcinosis, esophageal dysmotility, etc.) do not fulfill the ACR (American College of Rheumatology) classification criteria for the disease (1980). An abnormal "scleroderma" type capillaroscopic pattern was found in these cases [41].

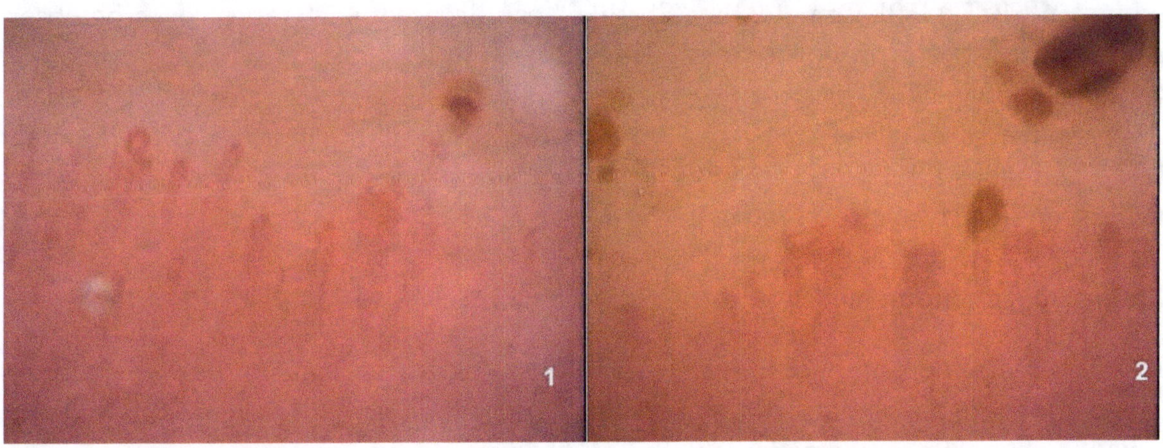

Figure 1. "Scleroderma type" capillaroscopic pattern in SSc (1) "early" phase, there is a single giant capillary loop and a single hemorrhage; (2) "active" phase, magnification 200×.

For establishing the diagnosis of SSc according to the ACR criteria (1980), the presence of the major criterion (skin thickening proximal to metacarpophalangeal joints of the hands) or two minor criteria ((1) sclerodactyly, (2) fingertip pitting scars, (3) bibasilar pulmonary fibrosis) is required [42]. These criteria have been proposed prior to the discovery of SSc-related autoantibodies and the characteristic capillaroscopic findings, which both had been found to improve the early diagnosis of SSc [43, 44]. Thus, Le Roy and Medsger suggested patients with RP and "scleroderma" type capillaroscopic changes or positive SSc-related autoantibodies to be diagnosed as "prescleroderma" *or limited SSc* even if other disease symptoms are absent [45]. The multicenter project VEDOSS (Very Early Diagnosis of Systemic Sclerosis) resulted in the new classification criteria for SSc (European League Against Rheumatism (EULAR)/ACR, 2013), which aim to detect SSc in early stages. In the new EULAR/ACR classification criteria, RP is scored with 3 points (1), the abnormal capillaroscopic pattern with 2 points (2), and presence of SSc-related autoantibodies (anticentromere, anti-topoisomerase I (anti-Scl-70), anti-RNA polymerase) with 3 points (maximum score for the immunologic criterion is 3) (3). The other criteria (overall 8 criteria) are as follows: telangiectasia (2 points) (4); fingertip lesions (digital tip ulcers - 2 points or fingertip pitting scars - 3 points), only the higher score is counted (5); pulmonary arterial hypertension and/or interstitial lung disease are scored with 2 points (6); skin thickening of the fingers (puffy fingers - score 2; sclerodactyly of the fingers - score 4), only the higher score is counted (7); skin thickening of both hands proximal to the metacarpophalangeal joints is scored with 9 points (8). A score ≥ 9 is necessary for a definite diagnosis of SSc [46, 47].

6.2. Raynaud's phenomenon in mixed connective tissue disease

MCTD combines symptoms of systemic lupus erythematosus (SLE), SSc, polymyositis (PM)/DM, arthritis, and the presence of a specific immunologic marker—anti-U1 RNP (an antibody against extractable nuclear antigen)—the latter being an obligatory classification criterion for the disease [48]. RP is met in 85% of patients with MCTD [8] and is the most common initial symptom [49]. Currently, the classification criteria for MCTD used in clinical practice are suggested by different author groups and not by professional organizations (criteria of Alarcon-Segovia, Kasukawa, Sharp, Kahn). RP is included in all of them because of its high frequency in MCTD [50]. Of note, the "SSc-like" capillaroscopic changes could be observed in a significantly lower proportion of MCTD patients in comparison with SSc. Maricq et al. have observed "SSc-like" pattern in 54% of cases in the examined group of 26 MCTD patients [36]. Bergman et al. detected "SSc-like" pattern in 50% (4/8) of the cases [51] and de Holanda Mafaldo Diógenes et al. in 65–71.5% [52]. Granier et al. observed a similar frequency of "scleroderma-like" capillaroscopic pattern—63.6% [53].

6.3. Raynaud's phenomenon in undifferentiated connective tissue disease

In UCTD patients, there are different symptoms of systemic rheumatic disease, but there is no full set of criteria of a well-defined rheumatic disorder. RP is a frequent symptom that may be observed in about 80% of the patients with UCTD. In evolution, a proportion of these patients (1/4–1/3) develop a distinct rheumatic disease, the most frequent being SSc, SLE, rheumatoid arthritis (RA), and Sjögren syndrome, but the majority of cases remain in a clinically and laboratory stable condition in the scope of the term "UCTD." In UCTD, the frequency of "scleroderma-like pattern" is lower as compared with SSc (13.8%, Nagy et al. [41]; 38%, Lambova et al.) [34, 54]. The presence of "scleroderma-like" capillaroscopic pattern in patients with UCTD is considered to be a reliable predictive factor for the development of SSc [41].

6.4. Raynaud's phenomenon in systemic lupus erythematosus

The prevalence of RP in SLE is between 10 and 45% [8]. Although in a proportion of cases with SLE peripheral vessel is affected by vasculitis, RP usually tends to have a benign course without the development of digital ulcers or necrosis [9]. Microvascular capillaroscopic changes in SLE are less specific vs. those in scleroderma-spectrum disorders. However, several capillaroscopic features have been noted in SLE that are termed "SLE" type capillaroscopic pattern [51, 53, 55], which includes the presence of elongated [53, 56] and dilated capillary loops, tortuous and meandering capillaries [55], and prominent subpapillary plexus [53, 56]. "Scleroderma-like" capillaroscopic pattern is a rare finding in SLE with frequency varying between 2 and 15% [36, 41, 51, 56, 57]. An association between "scleroderma-like" capillaroscopic pattern and the presence of RP and anti-U1 RNP antibody has been observed that is suggested to be in the context of a possible subclinical overlap syndrome with SSc [57]. In an own study of 30 SLE patients, RP was found in 73% of cases, and "scleroderma-like" capillaroscopic pattern in 13.3% of the patients (4/30). Such changes were observed in patients with high immunological activity, two of whom were with active vasculitis of peripheral vessels and two with secondary RP. They did not exhibit signs of overlap with SSc or other CTD. Anti-RNP antibody was positive in a single case in a patient with symptoms of secondary RP without peripheral vessel vasculitis, while in the other three cases with "scleroderma-like" pattern, this immunological marker was negative [34, 54]. Thus, it could be concluded that "scleroderma-like" capillaroscopic pattern could be found in SLE patients with high immunological activity, both in cases with active vasculitis of peripheral vessels and only with symptoms of secondary RP but without evidence for overlap with SSc or other CTD.

6.5. Raynaud's phenomenon in dermatomyositis and polymyositis

RP occurs in about 20% of DM/PM patients [8]. Digital gangrenes of the hands are usually not observed. When such changes are evident, the presence of neoplasm should be suspected. RP is characteristic for the antisynthetase syndrome, which is a subset of myositis characterized with positive anti-Jo-1 antibodies (against histidyl-tRNA synthetase), interstitial lung disease, nonerosive symmetric polyarthritis in small joints, and cracking and fissuring of the skin of the fingers ("mechanic's hands") [58]. In a part of the cases with DM, "scleroderma-like "capillaroscopic findings could be observed [35]. Although the capillaroscopic changes in DM and SSc are usually indistinguishable, it is suggested that bushy and branching capillaries could be found more frequently in DM [59]. The frequency of "SSc-like" pattern detected by Bergman et al. in 11 patients with DM was 63.6% [51].

6.6. Raynaud's phenomenon in rheumatoid arthritis

The prevalence of RP in RA varies between 3 and 17% (2.7%, Carrol et al., North Australia [60]; 4.6%, Grassi et al., Italy [61]; and 17.2%, Saraux et al., France) [62]. In 31 RA patients, Redisch et al. observed the following capillaroscopic changes: presence of elongated capillary loops, increased capillary tortuosity, and prominent subpapillary plexus. A "SSc-like" pattern was not detected in RA [55]. Nagy et al. also did not observe "SSc-like" pattern in a group of 14 patients with RA [41].

Of note, in an own study that included higher number of patients with RA (n = 62) with and without RP, a "SSc-like" pattern was observed in 14.5% (9/62; 2 males and 7 females). In one of the nine cases with such capillaroscopic changes, an overlap syndrome (RA overlap to SLE) with secondary RP and secondary vasculitis of peripheral vessels was evident. While in the rest eight out of nine patients, no overlap with other CTD was present. All RA patients with "SSc-like" capillaroscopic pattern (9/9) exhibited symptoms of secondary RP, and 2/9 a secondary vasculitis of peripheral vessels, respectively. Our results suggest that "SSc-like" capillaroscopic pattern could be observed in RA patients with secondary RP and with vasculitis of peripheral vessels although with low frequency. However, its presence is not mandatory in the context of overlap syndromes [34, 63].

6.7. Paraneoplastic Raynaud's phenomenon

RP may be a paraneoplastic symptom. When RP is newly appeared with late onset after the age of 60, it may also be an indicator for an underlying malignancy. Ischemia of the fingers has been reported in patients with carcinomas of the breast, the stomach, and the esophagus as well as in patients with oncohematologic disease (multiple myeloma, thrombocythemia, etc.). In a part of the cases, paraneoplastic RP is caused by secretion of vasoactive substances by the tumor cells and the respective immune response of the body, while in others like multiple myeloma and thrombocytopenia, it is associated with increased blood viscosity [64, 65]. We have not observed differences between microvascular changes in paraneoplastic rheumatic conditions in comparison with the respective idiopathic rheumatic diseases [66].

6.8. Raynaud's phenomenon in fibromyalgia

Fibromyalgia is an idiopathic, chronic, musculoskeletal, pain syndrome characterized with diffuse pain and presence of multiple tender points [67]. Primary fibromyalgia is an isolated disorder, while secondary fibromyalgia could be observed in different rheumatic diseases, e.g., RA, SLE, Sjögren syndrome, etc. [68]. RP is met in both primary and secondary fibromyalgia. The frequency of RP in fibromyalgia patients is about 17–30% [69, 70]. In an own study that included 26 patients with primary fibromyalgia, the most frequent capillaroscopic finding was the presence of dilated capillary loops analogous to primary RP. Capillaroscopic signs of microangiopathy were not detected [71].

7. Differential diagnosis of RP with other vascular acrosyndromes

Acrocyanosis represents painless bluish discoloration in the distal body parts, most commonly in the hands and feet and less frequently in the face that are affected symmetrically. In acrocyanosis, the bluish skin discoloration is a persistent finding that is aggravated by cold exposure and frequently is associated with local hyperhidrosis and edema of the hands and feet. In the absence of an accompanying cause, acrocyanosis is considered primary (idiopathic, essential) that is suggested to be a benign condition and typically does not require specific treatment. It does not evolve into CTD or other diseases and may spontaneously resolve. secondary acrocyanosis is a manifestation of other major diseases. Both acrocyanosis and RP are influenced by cold exposure and emotional stress, but in acrocyanosis, there is relative persistence of skin color changes, symmetry, and absence of paroxysmal pallor. Of note, RP may occur concomitantly with acrocyanosis. In addition, the persistence of acrocyanosis is also relative, and it may also demonstrate improvement in the summer as well as in horizontal and elevated position of the hand vs. dependent position [72].

Perniosis (chilblain) is a localized cutaneous inflammatory reaction in response to acute or repetitive exposure to damp cold above the freezing point. The skin lesions are edematous plaques that may be purple or red and are often painful or pruritic. In severe cases, ulceration, superinfection, and scarring may occur. Fingers and toes are most commonly affected although other areas, e.g., nose, ears, buttocks, or thighs, could also be involved. Primary and secondary forms are recognized. Secondary perniosis could be associated with a variety of underlying pathological conditions such as hepatitis, autoimmune disease, and cryopathies [73].

Erythromelalgia is characterized with episodic, symmetric, and painful hyperthermia and erythema of hands and feet. Contrary to RP, erythromelalgia is provoked by exposure to heat or physical exercise. Primary and secondary forms are also recognized, primary being a rare hereditary disease that manifests in children and young people, while secondary is met in the context of myeloproliferative disorders, diabetes, and SLE and during drug treatment with calcium channel blockers (CCBs) [74].

8. Treatment

8.1. Primary RP

The mild forms of primary RP are controlled by non-pharmacological measures, e.g., patient education in avoiding exposure to cold, use of warm clothes and gloves, smoking cessation, using protective devices in working with vibration. Caffeine consumption, administration of vasoconstrictors such as beta-blockers, and use of interferons should be avoided when possible [9].

Dihydropyridine-type CCBs have been the treatment of choice for patients with both primary and secondary RP for many years. They have proven efficacy for reduction of the severity and frequency of ischemic attacks in primary RP and secondary RP in SSc. Diltiazem (benzothiazepine class CCBs) could also be used in RP. It is administered at a dose of 30–120 mg three times daily orally. Verapamil (diphenylalkylamine class of CCBs) does not possess therapeutic effect in RP patients [75–77]. Nifedipine is the best studied and the most often used drug from dihydropyridine class CCBs. It is used at a dose of 10–40 mg twice daily orally. Other dihydropyridines commonly used in patients with RP are felodipine (2.5–10 mg twice daily orally) and amlodipine (5–10 mg daily orally) [1, 9]. Dihydropyridine class CCBs are vasodilators with direct effect on vascular smooth muscles. They are indicated for the treatment of arterial hypertension and stable angina, and some of them are also officially approved for vasospastic angina [78]. In RP patients, their use is off-label. Side effects of CCBs are common, e.g., flushing, hypotension, dizziness, headache, tachycardia, ankle edema, constipation, etc. Slow-release forms are better tolerated and preferred in clinical practice [1]. Pregnancy is a contraindication for administration of CCBs—a fact that deserves attention considering the high prevalence of primary RP in young women. This patient category requires specific instructions, and those women at childbearing age who plan conception or do not use effective contraception should not receive CCBs. Alternative, better-tolerated therapeutic options are often preferred in primary RP considering the milder clinical course and good prognosis of this condition as well as the side effects of CCBs.

Pentoxifylline inhibits phosphodiesterase and elevates cyclic adenosine monophosphate (cAMP) levels in polymorphonuclear leukocytes and other cells [79]. It exerts beneficial effects on microcirculation via improvement of blood fluidity, especially influencing erythrocyte flexibility [80]. Its maximal daily dose is 1200 mg (400 mg three times daily or 600 mg twice daily orally). It is not proven to be effective in severe forms of RP [1].

Therapeutic effect of *Ginkgo biloba* has been studied in patients with primary RP in double-blind, placebo-controlled trial. Significant reduction in the number of attacks has been observed in the group treated with high dose of *Ginkgo biloba* (360 mg daily) as compared with the placebo group (56 vs. 27%). It is suggested that *Ginkgo biloba* together with its vasodilator properties possesses also antiplatelet and radical scavenging effects [81].

8.2. Secondary RP in systemic sclerosis

EULAR recommends *dihydropyridine-type CCBs* as first-line therapy for RP in SSc [82]. A meta-analysis, including 8 randomized clinical trials (7 with nifedipine and 1 with nicardipine) with 109 SSc patients, indicates that dihydropyridine-type CCBs reduce the frequency and severity of ischemic attacks in SSc-related RP [77]. Apart from their effect to reduce the severity and frequency of vasospastic attacks, it has been demonstrated that CCBs lead to healing of digital ulcers [83]. In SSc with severe RP and/or those who do not respond satisfactorily to CCBs, *phosphodiesterase-5 enzyme inhibitors* are recommended (EULAR recommendation) [82]. NO is the main endothelium-derived vasodilator and an inhibitor of platelet activation and vascular smooth muscle proliferation. Its synthesis is regulated by the family of NO synthases, and its effect is mediated via cyclic guanosine monophosphate (cGMP). The intracellular concentration of cGMP is regulated by phosphodiesterases, which rapidly degrade cGMP in vivo [84]. A meta-analysis, including six randomized clinical trials (two with sildenafil, three with tadalafil, and one with vardenafil), demonstrated that phosphodiesterase-5 inhibitors have a significant effect on frequency and duration of RP attacks. Efficacy on healing of digital ulcers has been also reported. The therapeutic regimens used were as follows: sildenafil 50 mg twice daily or 200 mg once daily, tadalafil 20 mg daily or 20 mg on alternate days, and vardenafil 10 mg twice daily. The dosage regimens depend on half-lives of the different drugs that are 3–5 h for sildenafil and vardenafil (administered twice daily apart from modified-release sildenafil that is administered as a single dose) and about 18 h for tadalafil (administered once daily or on alternate days) [85]. Side effects during treatment with phosphodiesterase-5 inhibitors included different forms of vasomotor reactions, myalgias, allergic reaction, chest pain, dyspepsia, nasal stuffiness, and visual abnormalities. Considering long-term experience and good safety profile, EULAR experts recommend CCBs as first-line therapy for SSc-related RP and phosphodiesterase-5 inhibitors for SSc with severe RP and/or in cases with insufficient effect from the treatment with CCBs [82].

Intravenous iloprost possesses proven efficacy for reduction of the frequency and severity of SSc-related RP. Considering costs and feasibility, it is recommended after failure of oral therapies (CCBs and phosphodiesterase-5 inhibitors). Intravenous iloprost is also efficacious in the treatment of digital ulcers in SSc that is proved in randomized, placebo-controlled clinical trials [86, 87]. However, the need for hospitalization, the prolonged intravenous infusion (6 hours at the dose of 0.5–2 ng/kg/min), side effects, and high price are limiting factors for the administration of iloprost. Adverse effects include headache, nausea, vomiting, diarrhea, myalgia, arthralgia, chills, fever, arrhythmia, hypotension, chest pain (especially in patients with coronary heart disease), erythema, and pain at the infusion site. Thus, concomitant pathology should be assessed and hemodynamic parameters of the patients closely observed, e.g., blood pressure, heart rate, and pulse at the beginning and at every increase of the infusion rate. The risk for orthostatic hypotension should be also considered. Apart from its properties as a vasodilator, iloprost inhibits platelet aggregation, leukocyte chemotaxis, and adhesion to the endothelium. Iloprost also downregulates the expression of adhesion molecules on endothelial cells and phagocytes and enhances fibrinolytic activity [86–88].

In addition, in the most recent EULAR recommendation, *fluoxetine* (a serotonin-specific reuptake inhibitor and antidepressant) is suggested as an option in SSc-related RP despite the scarce published evidence [82]. In a small study that included 26 patients with primary RP and 27 with SSc-related RP, fluoxetine (20 mg daily) showed superior efficacy vs. nifedipine (40 mg daily). Observed side effects of fluoxetine were apathy, lethargy, and impaired concentration [89]. Despite the relatively low quality of published evidence, EULAR experts suggest fluoxetine as a useful alternative for treatment of SSc-related RP, especially in SSc patients who do not tolerate or fail to respond to vasodilators [82].

In SSc patients, in whom RP has complicated with digital ulcers, EULAR experts recommend *intravenous iloprost* and *phosphodiesterase-5 inhibitors* for treatment of digital ulcers and *bosentan (endothelin receptor antagonist)* for reduction of the number of new digital ulcers [82].

9. Prognosis

Being a first symptom in a number of CTD, the presence of RP requires regular follow-up that includes clinical, laboratory, immunological, and capillaroscopic assessment. The appearance of pathological capillaroscopic picture inherits a higher positive predictive value (47%) for the development of CTD vs. the predictive value of the positive ANA test (30%) [15]. Thus, nailfold capillaroscopy is the key investigation for monitoring RP patients. The interval of follow-up is 6 months, because a longer period of time is usually necessary for the development of morphological capillaroscopic changes, but this period may be shorter in cases with newly appeared alarming symptoms.

Author details

Sevdalina Nikolova Lambova

Address all correspondence to: sevdalina_n@abv.bg

Department of Propaedeutics of Internal Diseases, Faculty of Medicine, Medical University, Plovdiv, Bulgaria

References

[1] Wigley FM. Raynaud's phenomenon. The New England Journal of Medicine. 2002;**347**(13): 1001-1008

[2] Maricq HR, Weinrich MC. Diagnosis of Raynaud's phenomenon assisted by color charts. The Journal of Rheumatology. 1988;**15**:454-459

[3] Maverakis E, Patel F, Kronenberg DG, Chung L, Fiorentino D, Allanore Y, et al. International consensus criteria for the diagnosis of Raynaud's phenomenon. Journal of Autoimmunity. 2014;**48-49**:60-65

[4] Cortes S, Cutolo M. Capillaroscopic patterns in rheumatic diseases. Acta Reumatológica Portuguesa. 2007;**32**:29-36

[5] Ho M, Belch JJF. Raynaud's phenomenon: State of the art 1998. Scandinavian Journal of Rheumatology. 1998;**27**:319-322

[6] Wigley FM, Flavahan NA. Raynaud's phenomenon. The New England Journal of Medicine. 2016;**375**(6):556-565

[7] Chikura B, Moore T, Manning J, Vail A, Herrick AL. Thumb involvement in Raynaud's phenomenon as an indicator of underlying connective tissue disease. The Journal of Rheumatology. 2010;**37**:783-786

[8] Khan F. Vascular abnormalities in Raynaud's phenomenon. Scottish Medical Journal. 1999;**44**(1):4-6

[9] Block JA, Sequeira W. Raynaud's phenomenon. Seminar Lancet. 2001;**357**:2042-2048

[10] Herrick AL. The pathogenesis, diagnosis and treatment of Raynaud phenomenon. Nature Reviews Rheumatology. 2012;**8**(8):469-479

[11] Müller-Ladner U. Raynaud's Phenomenon and Peripheral Ischemic Syndromes. 1st ed. Bremen: UNI-MED Verlag AG; 2008. pp. 18-30

[12] Husein-Elahmed H et al. Severe Raynaud syndrome induced by adjuvant interferon alfa in metastatic melanoma. Current Oncology. 2010;**17**(4):122-123

[13] Lapossy E, Gasser P, Hrycaj P, et al. Cold-induced vasospasm in patients with fibromyalgia and chronic low back pain in comparison to healthy subjects. Clinical Rheumatology. 1994;**13**(3):442-445

[14] Steven AO. Raynaud's phenomenon. In: Sterling JB, editor. Secrets of Rheumatology. Moscow: Binom; 2001. pp. 614-619

[15] Spencer-Green G. Outcomes in primary Raynaud phenomenon: A meta-analysis of the frequency, rates, and predictors of transition to secondary diseases. Archives of Internal Medicine. 1998;**158**(6):595-600

[16] Coffman JD, Cohen RA. Role of alpha-adrenoceptor subtypes mediating sympathetic vasoconstriction in human digits. European Journal of Clinical Investigation. 1988;**18**: 309-313

[17] Flavahan NA, Cooke JP, Shepherd JT, Vanhoutte PM. Human postjunctional alpha-1 and alpha-2 adrenoceptors: Differential distribution in arteries of the limbs. The Journal of Pharmacology and Experimental Therapeutics. 1987;**241**(2):361-365

[18] Chotani MA, Flavahan S, Mitra S, et al. Silent alpha-2c-adrenergic receptors enable cold-induced vasoconstriction in cutaneous arteries. American Journal of Physiology. Heart and Circulatory Physiology. 2000;**278**(4):H1075-H1083

[19] Jeyaraj SC, Chotani MA, Mitra S, Gregg HE, Flavahan NA, Morrison KJ. Cooling evokes redistribution of α2c-adrenoceptors from golgi to plasma membrane in transfected human embryonic kidney 293 cells. Molecular Pharmacology. 2001;**60**:1195-1200

[20] Eid AH, Chotani MA, Mitra S, Miller TJ, Flavahan NA. Cyclic AMP acts through Rap1 and JNK signaling to increase expression of cutaneous smooth muscle alpha2C-adrenoceptors. American Journal of Physiology-Heart and Circulatory Physiology. 2008;**295**(1): H266-H272

[21] Furspan PB, Chatterjee S, Freedman RR. Increased tyrosine phosphorylation mediates the cooling-induced contraction and increased vascular reactivity of Raynaud's disease. Arthritis and Rheumatism. 2004;**1578-1585**(2004):50

[22] Furspan PB, Chatterjee S, Mayes MD, Freedman RR. Cooling-induced contraction and protein tyrosine kinase activity of isolated arterioles in secondary Raynaud's phenomenon. Rheumatology (Oxford). 2005;**44**:488-494

[23] Müller-Ladner U, Lambova S. Editorial: Vascular damage in systemic sclerosis. Current Rheumatology Reviews. 2013;**9**(4):233-236

[24] Rajagopalan S, Pfenninger D, Kehrer C, Chakrabarti A, Somers E, Pavlic R, et al. Increased asymmetric dimethylarginine and endothelin 1 levels in secondary Raynaud's phenomenon: Implications for vascular dysfunction and progression of disease. Arthritis Rheum. 2003;**48**(7):1992-2000

[25] Vancheeswaran R, Azam A, Black C, Dashwood MR. Localization of endothelin-1 and its binding sites in scleroderma skin. The Journal of Rheumatology. 1994;**21**:1268-1276

[26] Jing J, Dou TT, Yang JQ, Chen XB, Cao HL, Min M, et al. Role of endothelin-1 in the skin fibrosis of systemic sclerosis. European Cytokine Network. 2015;**26**(1):10-14

[27] Zamora MR, O'Brien RF, Rutherford RB, Weil JV. Serum endothelin-1 concentrations and cold provocation in primary Raynaud's phenomenon. Lancet. 1990;**336**:1144-1147

[28] Bunker CB, Terenghi G, Springall DR, Polak JM, Dowd PM. Deficiency of calcitonin gene-related peptide in Raynaud's phenomenon. Lancet. 1990;**336**:1530-1533

[29] Garner R, Kumari R, Lanyon P, Doherty M, Zhang W. Prevalence, risk factors and associations of primary Raynaud's phenomenon: systematic review and meta-analysis of observational studies. BMJ Open. 2015;**5**(3):e006389

[30] Planchon B, Pistorius M-A, Beurrier P, de Faucal P. Primary Raynaud's phenomenon: age of onset and pathogenesis in a prospective study of 424 patients. Angiology. 1994;**45**: 677-686

[31] Le Roy EC, Medsger TA Jr. Raynaud's phenomenon: a proposal for classification. Clinical and Experimental Rheumatology. 1992;**10**(5):485-488

[32] Anderson ME et al. Computerized nailfold videocapillaroscopy—A new tool for assessment of Raynaud's phenomenon. The Journal of Rheumatology. 2005;**32**:841-848

[33] Bukhari M et al. Quantitation of microcirculatory abnormalities in patients with primary Raynaud's phenomenon and systemic sclerosis by videocapillaroscopy. Rheumatology. 2000;**39**(5):506-512

[34] Lambova S. The role of capillaroscopy in rheumatology [dissertation]. Giessen, Germany: Justus Liebig University; 2011

[35] Maricq HR, Le Roy EC. Patterns of finger capillary abnormalities in connective tissue disease by "wide-field" microscopy. Arthritis & Rheumatism. 1973;**16**(5):619-628

[36] Maricq HR et al. Diagnostic potential of in vivo capillary microscopy in scleroderma and related disorders. Arthritis and Rheumatism. 1980;**23**(2):183-189

[37] Maricq HR et al. Microvascular abnormalities as possible predictors of disease subsets in Raynaud phenomenon and early connective tissue disease. Clinical and Experimental Rheumatology. 1983;**1**(3):195-205

[38] Cutolo M, Sulli A, Pizzorni C, Accardo S. Nailfold videocapillaroscopy assessment of microvascular damage in systemic sclerosis. The Journal of Rheumatology. 2000;**27**: 155-160

[39] Lambova S, Hermann W, Müller-Ladner U. Capillaroscopic pattern at the toes of systemic sclerosis patients: does it "tell" more than those of fingers? Journal of Clinical Rheumatology. 2011;**17**(6):311-314

[40] Lambova S, Müller-Ladner U. Capillaroscopic findings in systemic sclerosis--are they associated with disease duration and presence of digital ulcers? Discovery Medicine. 2011; **12**(66):413-418

[41] Nagy Z, Czirjac L. Nailfold digital capillaroscopy in 447 patients with connective tissue disease and Raynaud` disease. Journal of the European Academy of Dermatology and Venereology. 2004;**18**:62-68

[42] Subcommittee for scleroderma criteria of the American Rheumatism Association Diagnostic and Therapeutic Criteria Committee. Preliminary criteria for the classification of systemic sclerosis (scleroderma). Arthritis and Rheumatism. 1980;**23**(5):581-590

[43] Hudson M et al. Improving the sensitivity of the American College of Rheumatology classification criteria for systemic sclerosis. Clinical and Experimental Rheumatology. 2007;**25**(5):754-757

[44] Lonzetti LS et al. Updating the American College of Rheumatology preliminary classification criteria for systemic sclerosis: Addition of severe nailfold capillaroscopy abnormalities markedly increases the sensitivity for limited scleroderma. Arthritis and Rheumatism. 2001;**44**(3):735-736

[45] Le Roy EC, Medsger TA Jr. Criteria for the classification of early systemic sclerosis. The Journal of Rheumatology. 2001;**28**:573-576

[46] van den Hoogen F, Khanna D, Fransen J, et al. 2013 classification criteria for systemic sclerosis: An American college of rheumatology/European league against rheumatism collaborative initiative. Annals of the Rheumatic Diseases. 2013;**72**(11):1747-1755

[47] van den Hoogen F, Khanna D, Fransen J, et al. 2013 classification criteria for systemic sclerosis: An American college of rheumatology/European league against rheumatism collaborative initiative. Arthritis and Rheumatism. 2013;**65**(11):2737-2747

[48] Sharp GC, Irvin WS, Tan EM, Gould RG, Holman HR. Mixed connective tissue disease--an apparently distinct rheumatic disease syndrome associated with a specific antibody to an extractable nuclear antigen (ENA). The American Journal of Medicine. 1972;**52**(2):148-159

[49] Bennett RM, O'Connell DJ. The arthritis of mixed connective tissue disease. Annals of the Rheumatic Diseases. 1978;**37**(5):397-403

[50] Smolen JS, Steiner G. Mixed connective tissue disease: To be or not to be? Arthritis and Rheumatism. 1998;**41**(5):768-777

[51] Bergman R, Sharony L, Schapira D, et al. The handheld dermatoscope as a nail-fold capillaroscopic instrument. Archives of Dermatology. 2003;**139**:1027-1030

[52] de Holanda Mafaldo Diógenes A, Bonfá E, Fuller R, Correia Caleiro MT. Capillaroscopy is a dynamic process in mixed connective tissue disease. Lupus. 2007;**16**(4):254-258

[53] Granier F, Priollet P, Housset E. Nailfold capillary microscopy in mixed connective tissue disease. Comparison with systemic sclerosis and systemic lupus erythematosus. Arthritis and Rheumatism. 1986;**29**(2):189-195

[54] Lambova S, Müller-Ladner U. Capillaroscopic pattern in systemic lupus erythematosus and undifferentiated connective tissue disease—What we still have to learn? Rheumatology International. 2013;**33**(3):689-695

[55] Redisch W. Capillaroscopic observations in rheumatic diseases. Annals of the Rheumatic Diseases. 1970;**29**:244-253

[56] Kabasakal Y, Elvins DM, Ring EF, McHugh NJ. Quantitative nailfold capillaroscopy findings in a population with connective tissue disease and in normal healthy controls. Annals of the Rheumatic Diseases. 1996;**55**:507-512

[57] Furtado RNV, Pucinell MLC, Cristo VV, Andrade LEC, Sato EI. Scleroderma-like nailfold capillaroscopic abnormalities are associated with anti-U1-RNP antibodies and Raynaud's phenomenon in SLE patients. Lupus. 2002;**11**(1):35-41

[58] Seibold JR, Steen VD. Systemic sclerosis. In: Klippel JH, Dieppe PA, editors. Rheumatology. London: Mosby; 1994. pp. 6.8-6.11

[59] Kenik JG, Maricq HR, Bole GG. Blind evaluation of the diagnostic specificity of nailfold capillary microscopy in the connective tissue diseases. Arthritis and Rheumatism. 1981;**24**(7):885-891

[60] Carrol GJ, Withers K, Bayliss CE. The prevalence of Raynaud's syndrome in rheumatoid arthritis. Annals of the Rheumatic Diseases. 1981;**40**:567-570

[61] Grassi W, Blasetti P, Core P, Cervini C. Raynaud's phenomenon in rheumatoid arthritis. British Journal of Rheumatology. 1994;**33**:139-141

[62] Saraux A, Allain J, Guedes C, Baron D, Youinou P, Le Goff P. Raynaud's phenomenon in rheumatoid arthritis. British Journal of Rheumatology. 1996;**35**(8):752-754

[63] Lambova SN, Müller-Ladner U. Capillaroscopic pattern in inflammatory arthritis. Microvascular Research. 2012;**83**(3):318-322

[64] Ling SM, Wigley FM. Raynaud's phenomenon in older adults. Diagnostic considerations and management. Drugs & Aging. 1999;**15**(3):183-195

[65] Paw P, Dharan SM, Sackier JM. Digital ischemia and occult malignancy. International Journal of Colorectal Disease. 1996;**11**:196-197

[66] Lambova S, Müller-Ladner U. Capillaroscopic pattern in paraneoplastic Raynaud's phenomenon. Rheumatology International. 2013;**33**(6):1597-1599

[67] Di Franco M, Iannuccelli C, Valesini G. Neuroendocrine immunology of fibromyalgia. Annals of the New York Academy of Sciences. 2010;**1193**:84-90

[68] Wolfe F, Cathey MA, Kleinheksel SM. Fibrositis (Fibromyalgia) in rheumatoid arthritis. The Journal of Rheumatology. 1984;**11**(6):814-818

[69] Wolfe F, Smythe HA, Yunus MB, et al. The American College of rheumatology 1990 criteria for the classification of fibromyalgia. Report of the Multicenter Criteria Committee. Arthritis and Rheumatism. 1990;**33**(2):160-172

[70] Dinerman H, Goldenberg DL, Felson DT. A prospective evaluation of 118 patients with the fibromyalgia syndrome: Prevalence of Raynaud's phenomenon, sicca symptoms, ANA, low complement, and Ig deposition at the dermal-epidermal junction. The Journal of Rheumatology. 1986;**13**(2):368-373

[71] Lambova S, Müller-Ladner U. Capillaroscopic findings in primary fibromyalgia. Current Rheumatology Reviews. 2018;**14**(1):36-41

[72] Kurklinsky AK, Miller VM, Rooke TW. Acrocyanosis: The flying Dutchman. Vascular Medicine. 2011;**16**(4):288-301

[73] Baker JS, Miranpuri S. Perniosis a case report with literature review. Journal of the American Podiatric Medical Association. 2016;**106**(2):138-140

[74] Ahrazoglu M, Moinzadeh P, Hunzelmann N. Differential diagnoses of Raynaud's phenomenon. Deutsche Medizinische Wochenschrift. 2014;**139**(20):1064-1069

[75] Rirash F, Tingey PC, Harding SE, Maxwell LJ, Tanjong Ghogomu E, Wells GA, et al. Calcium channel blockers for primary and secondary Raynaud's phenomenon. Cochrane Database of Systematic Reviews. 2017;**12**:CD000467. DOI: 10.1002/14651858.CD000467.pub2

[76] Thompson AE, Pope JE. Calcium channel blockers for primary Raynaud's phenomenon: A meta-analysis. Rheumatology (Oxford, England). 2005;**44**(2):145-150

[77] Thompson AE, Shea B, Welch V, Fenlon D, Pope JE. Calcium-channel blockers for Raynaud's phenomenon in systemic sclerosis. Arthritis and Rheumatism. 2001;**44**(8):1841-1847

[78] Godfraind T. Discovery and development of calcium channel blockers. Frontiers in Pharmacology. 2017;**8**:286. DOI: 10.3389/fphar.2017.00286. eCollection 2017

[79] Maderazo EG, Breaux S, Woronick CL, Krause PJ. Efficacy, toxicity, and pharmacokinetics of pentoxifylline and its analogs in experimental *Staphylococcus aureus* infections. Antimicrobial Agents and Chemotherapy. 1990;**34**(6):1100-1106

[80] Neirotti M, Longo F, Molaschi M, Macchione C, Pernigotti L. Functional vascular disorders: Treatment with pentoxifylline. Angiology. 1987;**38**(8):575-580

[81] Muir AH, Robb R, McLaren M, Daly F, Belch JJ. The use of *Ginkgo biloba* in Raynaud's disease: a double-blind placebo-controlled trial. Vascular Medicine. 2002;**7**(4):265-267

[82] Kowal-Bielecka O, Fransen J, Avouac J, Becker M, Kulak A, Allanore Y, Distler O, et al. Update of EULAR recommendations for the treatment of systemic sclerosis. Annals of the Rheumatic Diseases. 2017;**76**(8):1327-1339

[83] Rademaker M, Cooke ED, Almond NE, et al. Comparison of intravenous infusions of iloprost and oral nifedipine in treatment of Raynaud's phenomenon in patients with systemic sclerosis: A double blind randomised study. BMJ. 1989;**298**:561-564

[84] Kumana CR, Cheung GTY, Lau CS. Severe digital ischaemia treated with phosphodiesterase inhibitors. Annals of the Rheumatic Diseases. 2004;**63**:1522-1524

[85] Roustit M, Blaise S, Allanore Y, et al. Phosphodiesterase-5 inhibitors for the treatment of secondary Raynaud's phenomenon: Systematic review and meta-analysis of randomised trials. Annals of the Rheumatic Diseases. 2013;**72**:1696-1699

[86] Wigley FM, Seibold JR, Wise RA, et al. Intravenous iloprost treatment of Raynaud's phenomenon and ischemic ulcers secondary to systemic sclerosis. The Journal of Rheumatology. 1992;**19**:1407-1414

[87] Wigley FM, Wise RA, Seibold JR, et al. Intravenous iloprost infusion in patients with Raynaud phenomenon secondary to systemic sclerosis. A multicenter, placebo-controlled, double-blind study. Annals of Internal Medicine. 1994;**120**:199-206

[88] Bettoni L, Geri A, Airò P, et al. Clinical systemic sclerosis therapy with iloprost: A prospective observational study of 30 patients treated for a median of 3 years. Clinical Rheumatology. 2002;**21**:244-250

[89] Coleiro B, Marshall SE, Denton CP, et al. Treatment of Raynaud's phenomenon with the selective serotonin reuptake inhibitor fluoxetine. Rheumatology (Oxford). 2001;**40**: 1038-1043

10

Cardiovascular Safety of Anti-TNF and Non-TNF Biological Therapy in Patients with Rheumatoid Arthritis

Codrina Ancuta, Claudia Mihailov and
Eugen Ancuta

Abstract

The association between cumulative inflammatory burden and increased cardiovascular (CV) risk in patients with immune-mediated inflammatory rheumatic disorders, particularly rheumatoid arthritis (RA), is widely recognized. Furthermore, the complex and dynamic interrelation between traditional cardiovascular risk factors, systemic inflammation, early accelerated atherosclerosis, and RA-related factors remains a challenge in routine practice. New European League Against Rheumatism (EULAR) 2016 recommendations have recently highlighted three key trends in cardiovascular risk assessment and management in patients with RA including optimal disease control (early diagnosis, treat-to-target strategy with the dynamic use of antirheumatic synthetic and biologic drugs) and non-pharmacological as well as pharmacological management of risk factors. The present chapter will emphasize excessive cardiovascular morbidity in RA, the optimal strategy to identify and stratify the cardiovascular risk profile, the prime selection of medication from the whole spectrum of non-biologic and biologic (TNF and non-TNF) drugs according to their cardiotoxicity.

Keywords: cardiovascular burden, rheumatoid arthritis, inflammation, TNF inhibitors, tocilizumab

1. Introduction

The association between cumulative inflammatory burden and increased cardiovascular (CV) risk in patients with immune-mediated inflammatory rheumatic disorders, particularly rheumatoid arthritis (RA), is widely recognized [1–5].

Furthermore, the complex and dynamic interrelation between traditional CV risk factors (such as hypertension, diabetes, obesity, abnormal lipid metabolism), chronic systemic inflammation, early accelerated atherosclerosis, and RA-related factors (e.g., C-reactive protein level, CRP, disease activity and severity, medication) taken together in a genetically predisposed background remains a challenge in routine practice [1–5].

European League Against Rheumatism (EULAR) 2015/2016 recommendations for cardiovascular disease management have recently highlighted three key trends in cardiovascular risk assessment and management in patients with RA and spondyloarthropathies (ankylosing spondylitis, psoriatic arthritis) including optimal disease control (early diagnosis, treat-to-target strategy with the dynamic use of antirheumatic synthetic and biologic drugs) and non-pharmacological as well as pharmacological management of risk factors [6, 7].

The present chapter will emphasize excessive cardiovascular morbidity in RA, the optimal strategy to identify and stratify the cardiovascular risk profile in different RA settings, the prime selection of medication from the whole spectrum of non-biologic (methotrexate and non-methotrexate drugs) and biologic (TNF and non-TNF) antirheumatic drugs according to their cardiotoxicity.

2. Cardiovascular risk in patients with RA

2.1. Cardiovascular burden in RA

Patients with systemic autoimmune conditions especially inflammatory joint disorders such as RA are at increased risk to develop cardiovascular comorbidity, in particular subclinical or clinically significant atherosclerotic coronary heart disease [1–5, 8].

Compared to general population, patients with RA experience excessive cardiovascular morbidity and, even, mortality, with an increased risk of about 50% [1, 2, 8, 9]. The rate of global cardiovascular as well as individual events comprising fatal and nonfatal myocardial infarction, congestive heart failure, stroke, and major adverse cardiac events (MACE) is increased in RA, the magnitude of cardiovascular risk in such patient being comparable with that related to diabetes [1, 2, 8].

A comprehensive overview of cardiovascular complications and safety issues indicates that RA develops twice myocardial infarction and features an increased risk (up to 87%) of heart failure as compared to general, non-RA population [1–3, 8–11]. Moreover, congestive heart failure in different RA subtypes has a worsen prognosis compared to non-RA patients; more than half of patients known with RA are prone to undergo diastolic heart failure, while diastolic ventricular failure and pulmonary arterial hypertension are broadly reported in long-standing RA [2, 8–11]. Myocarditis typically associates with active disease subtypes and is rare, clinically non-symptomatic, without influence on cardiac mortality [1, 2]. Conversely, atherothrombosis and clinically significant coronary heart disease are highly expressed (65% increase in cardiovascular risk) and account for premature death [2]. Finally, valvular disease, especially mitral regurgitation, is frequent (80%) but usually asymptomatic, while valve nodules, conduction anomalies, and arrhythmias are uncommon in such patients [2].

Both early RA and established or long-standing RA are characterized by augmented CV risk, with a special emphasis on active status, irrespective of disease duration [1, 2, 4, 11].

Cardiovascular comorbidities of autoimmune disorders are the result of different contributing factors and their synergistic effects [1, 2, 4, 5, 8, 9, 11]. Although the prevalence and influence of traditional risk factors in RA is high, the excess of cardiovascular burden is only partially clarified [1–4, 6, 8, 9, 11]. A wide spectrum of nontraditional meaning RA-associated factors is already considered, including disease activity, severity, as well as antirheumatic drugs [1, 2, 4, 6, 8, 11–13].

2.2. Factors involved in cardiovascular risk in RA

The dynamic link between chronic systemic inflammation and atherosclerosis remains a key point in the pathobiology of cardiovascular involvement in various systemic autoimmune conditions, including inflammatory rheumatic disorders [1, 2, 10–13].

Cardiovascular risk in RA is multifactorial; since traditional risk factors fairly explain, specific issues related to disease activity and medication endorses the cardiovascular disease in RA [1–4, 10–13].

Smoking, diabetes, obesity, hypertension, as well as abnormal lipid pattern (dyslipidemia) are major metabolic risk factors for cardiovascular disease, while seropositivity (rheumatoid factor, RF, and anti-cyclic citrullinated peptide antibodies (ACPA)), systemic extra-articular features, anti-inflammatory (nonsteroidal anti-inflammatory drugs (NSAIDs) and glucocorticoids), and disease-modifying antirheumatic drugs (DMARDs) are specific aspects with precise relevance for cardiovascular outcomes in RA patients (**Figure 1**) [1, 2, 4–6, 10–13].

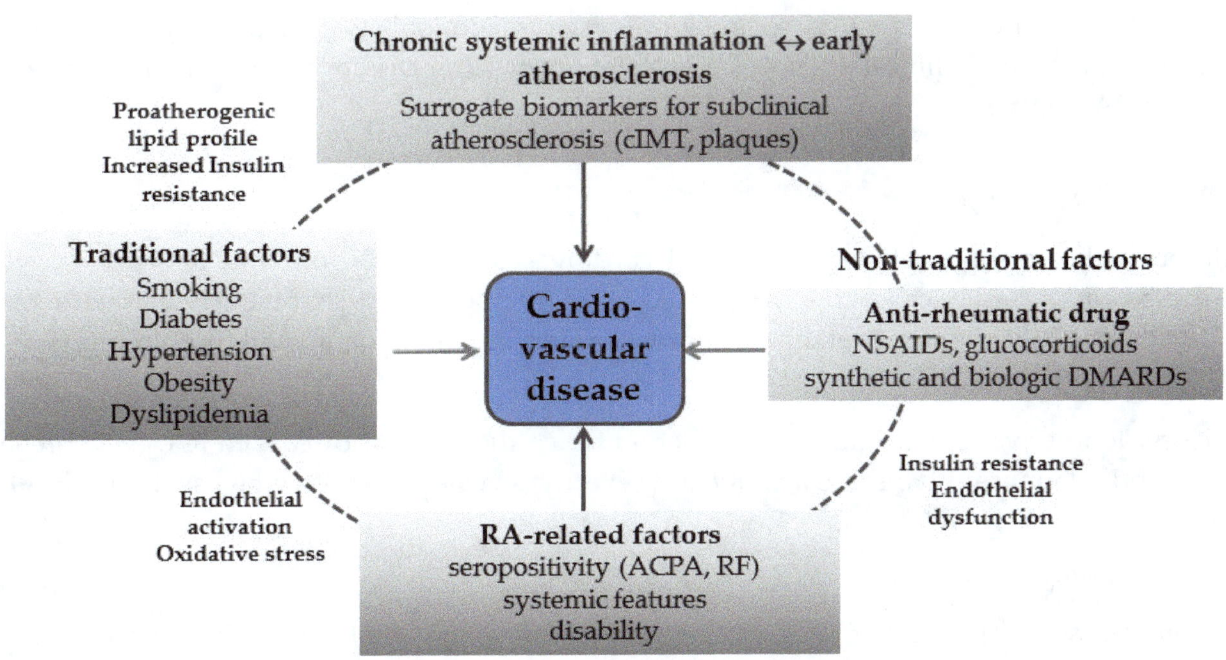

Figure 1. Traditional and non-traditional cardiovascular risk factors in RA (adapted from 8).

Furthermore, it is well established that chronic inflammation represents an independent risk factor for premature atherosclerosis, irrespective of other traditional factors [1, 3, 4], supporting severe, either subclinical or clinical coronary, and carotid disease in patients with RA [10–13].

Inflammation may alter the effect of existing risk or protective factors for cardiovascular disease, leading to an altered cardiovascular profile [1, 2, 6, 10–13].

Potent pro-inflammatory cytokines such as tumor necrosis factor-α (TNF-α) and interleukin (IL)-6 and their signaling pathways play a fundamental role in persistent systemic inflammation and are the main determinants of cardiovascular risk in RA [1–4, 6]; in addition, they may interfere with classic factors resulting in altered endothelial function, insulin resistance, modified lipid spectrum, and the obesity paradox in RA [1, 2, 10–14].

There is a body of evidence showing the proatherogenic role of TNF-α and IL-1 as well as potential dual effect of IL-6 on atherogenesis [2, 3].

Thus, targeting inflammation to reduce the cardiovascular disease risk in inflammatory conditions seems to be a realistic project; additionally, an optimal control of rheumatoid inflammation through specific synthetic and/or biologic antirheumatic drugs always underwrites the decline of cardiovascular comorbidity [1–3, 6, 7].

The exclusive relationship of inflammation, endothelial dysfunction, and surrogate biomarkers of atherosclerosis with risks to cardiovascular disease among RA patients was extensively addressed [1–3, 10–13]. The pathophysiology of endothelial dysfunction is multifactorial, a complex network of interacting factors and mechanisms being emphasized. Not only different metabolic (dyslipidemia, hyperglycemia), non-metabolic (hypertension, smoking, oxidative stress) but also RA-specific factors (systemic inflammation) are associated with vascular dysfunction [1, 2, 9, 15–21].

Early intervention of irreversible vascular damage is strictly related to abnormal vascular tone, upregulation of fibrinolysis, and coagulation systems with subsequent procoagulant imbalance, subclinical and clinical atherosclerosis, and supporting cardiovascular disease development in RA (**Figure 2**) [1, 2, 6, 9–13].

2.2.1. *Traditional risk factors*

Although the relation between traditional cardiovascular risk factors and RA was largely addressed in the last decade, conflicting effects are still open [1–3, 9]. Obviously, classic factors mapping cardiovascular outcomes are more common among patients with autoimmune disorders [1, 2, 9].

A closer look to various traditional risk factors for cardiovascular disease in RA, their prevalence, and relations with disease activity and severity revealed the following aspects (**Table 1**).

2.2.1.1. *Smoking*

Recognized as a risk factor of both autoimmune diseases and accelerated atherosclerosis [1, 2, 15], tobacco smoking is able to modulate the immune system (e.g., induction of the inflammatory

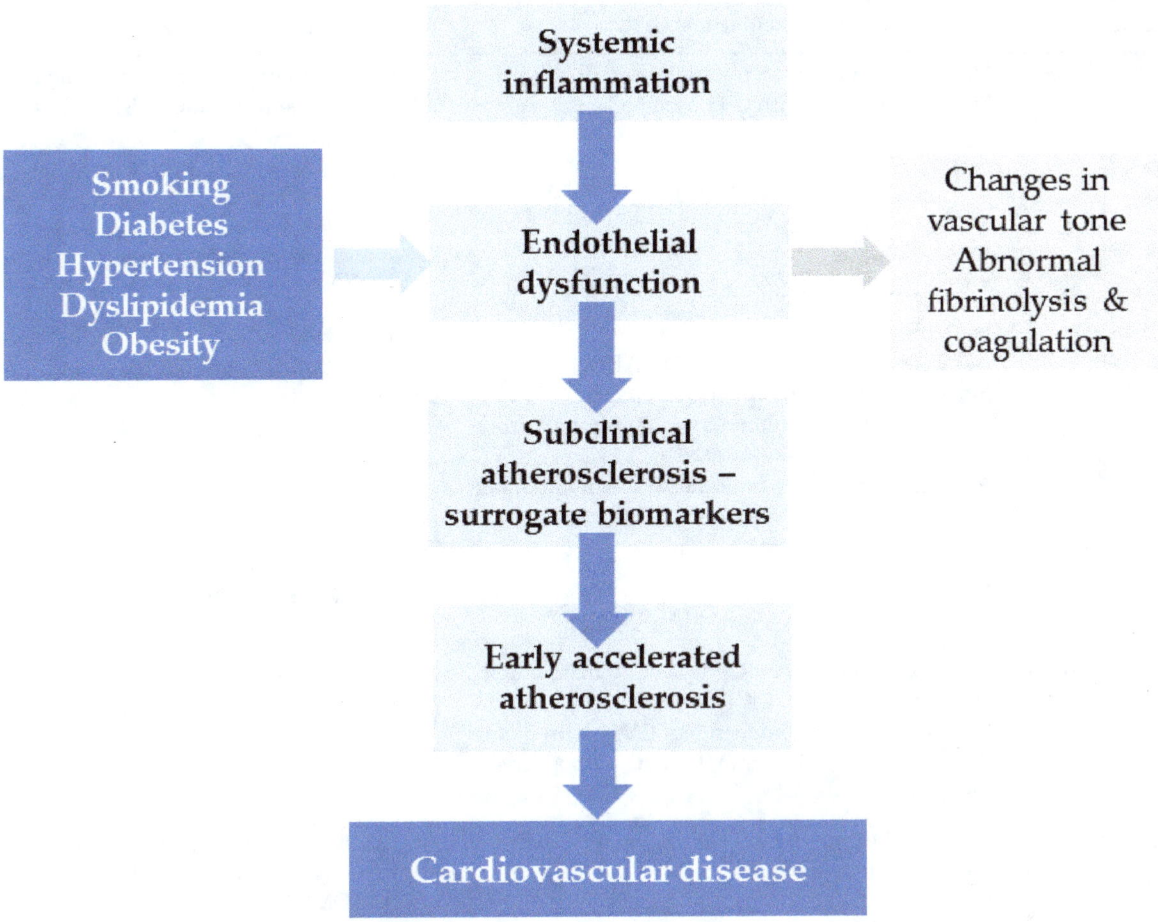

Figure 2. Inflammation, endothelial dysfunction, and atherosclerosis in cardiovascular disease.

responses and apoptosis, cytokine imbalance, DNA damage), to alter endothelial cells (e.g., overexpression of adhesion molecule, endothelial dysfunction), and to promote a procoagulant and inflammatory environment [1, 3, 15].

Smoking has a high prevalence in patients with RA and is classically associated with different predictive factors of the cardiovascular outcomes including seropositivity (for both RF and ACPA), disease severity, disability, and articular damage (erosions) [1, 2, 15]. Various studies have suggested that smoking and second-hand (passive) smoking may limit the therapeutic response in RA, promoting and perpetuating inflammatory aggressive effects on cardiovascular risk [1–3, 6, 15].

2.2.1.2. *Hypertension*

Among classical risk factors, hypertension is an important predictor of cardiovascular events not only in general population but also in patients with systemic autoimmune conditions, with the highest morbidity in RA (up to 40% in CORRONA) [1, 9, 16].

Since the pathobiology of increased blood pressure is multifactorial, blood pressure control in inflammatory autoimmune settings is largely related to chronic inflammation and immune-mediated mechanisms, along with classic mechanical injury of the arterial wall. Strong evidence

CV risk factors	Prevalence and particularities in RA	Relation with RA activity
Tobacco smoking	High prevalence in RA population String association with CV outcome Direct link with • seropositivity (ACPA, RF) • RA severity and activity • disability • articular damage	May impair therapeutic response, modulating inflammation effects on CV risk
Hypertension	High prevalence (COMORA 40%) Associated with NSAIDs and DMARDs increased vascular peripheral resistance interplay between inflammation and hypertension • TNFα results in endothelial vascular damage & oxidative stress • IL-6 alter the arterial tonus	Without evidence Adversely impact with NSAIDs and glucocorticoids
Insulin resistance	High prevalence in RA Promote low-grade chronic inflammation	Irrespective of RA activity
Body mass index & obesity	Paradoxical relation in RA: low body mass index associated with high CA risk Body mass index—independent CV risk predictor Relation obesity—inflammation via adipose tissue metabolism	Irrespective of RA activity
Dyslipidemia	Not only the quantity but also the quality, structure, and function of lipids 55–65% cases—abnormal lipid profile Lipid paradox (low lipids in inflammation associated with high CV risk) LDL-, HDL-, total cholesterol negatively correlates with inflammatory biomarkers Inflammation = consumption + decreased lipoprotein synthesis + defect of lipoprotein synthesis + structural and functional changes (altered HDL)	HDL cholesterol and atherogenic index improvement following non-biologic and biologic DMARDs

Table 1. Traditional cardiovascular risk factors in RA.

indicates the direct association between inflammation and hypertension; TNF-α can exert vascular endothelial damage and oxidative stress, while IL-6 enhances the arterial tonus. Not only blood pressure itself but also arterial inflammation is more prevalent in patients with RA and independently associated with both traditional cardiovascular risk factors and rheumatoid arthritis disease characteristics [1, 16].

There is no clear data suggesting the relation between hypertension and RA activity. However, the deleterious role of NSAIDs and glucocorticoids on hypertension is well established [1, 16].

2.2.1.3. *Insulin resistance*

Although underdiagnosed, especially in RA with longer disease duration, the prevalence of impaired fasting glucose, type 2 diabetes, as well as abnormal insulin resistance is largely increased among patients with autoimmune joint conditions compared to age- and gender-matched controls [1, 13, 18–20]. In addition, the link between diabetes and chronic low-grade inflammation [1–3] is well known, supporting the hypothesis of the interaction between traditional CV risk factors and inflammatory burden in determining diabetes in RA [1, 2, 13, 18–20]. Furthermore, both classic risk factors (e.g., high blood pressure, high body mass index, high total cholesterol, metabolic syndrome) and novel cardiovascular risk factors (RA duration, exposure to glucocorticoids, radiographic damage, CRP levels) significantly correlated with glucose metabolism abnormalities and diabetes [1, 2, 13, 18–20].

2.2.1.4. *Body mass index and obesity*

While in general, non-RA population, body mass index is recognized as an independent predictor for cardiovascular disease, patients with RA are characterized by the paradoxical relation obesity (cardiovascular risk): low body mass index correlates with high cardiovascular events, unrelated to disease activity [1, 2, 6]. Moreover, the relation obesity-inflammation via adipose tissue metabolism is largely applicable in RA patients.

2.2.1.5. *Dyslipidemia and lipid paradox in RA*

Abnormal serum lipid pattern remains one of the main risk factors for cardiovascular morbidity and mortality in general population [1]; overall, modifications in high-density lipoprotein (HDL)-cholesterol as well as total/ HDL-cholesterol and triglyceride/HDL-cholesterol ratios are associated with adverse cardiovascular disease risk [1, 20].

Up to 65% of RA patients display an altered lipid profile [1, 2, 11, 12, 20], comprising modifications in absolute circulating lipid levels that widely reflect the interconnection between inflammatory and metabolic pathways [1, 2, 20].

The well-known lipid paradox, meaning low serum concentration of lipids associated with high cardiovascular burden in autoimmune inflammatory conditions, accounts for a negative correlation between total cholesterol, high-density and low-density lipoprotein (LDL)-cholesterol fractions, and inflammatory biomarkers.

Additionally, chronic inflammation is characterized by excessive consumption and deleterious synthesis of lipoproteins associated with structural (e.g., HDL associated with increased serum amyloid A with a potentially proatherogenic phenotype) as well as functional modifications (e.g., altered HDL phenotype) [1, 20].

Generally, both HDL-cholesterol and LDL-cholesterol are decreased in active RA and may increase with efficient control of inflammation with to non-biologic and biologic drugs [1, 2, 6, 20]. Moreover, small-dense LDL particles, known as more atherogenic than larger particles, are raised not only in metabolic disorders but also in RA [1, 20].

Interestingly, preclinical phase of RA accounts for raised inflammatory biomarkers (CRP) and dyslipidemia, with a negative correlation between the increased inflammation and decreased serum lipids [1, 2, 20]. This paradigm is applicable not only for chronic systemic autoimmune joint pathology but also in cardiovascular disease, postsurgery, or related to antineoplastic therapy [1, 2, 6, 20].

Tight control of inflammation in RA by non-biologic and/or biologic antirheumatic medication usually accounts for the improved lipid level [1, 2, 6, 7].

2.2.2. *RA activity and cardiovascular risk*

Individual inflammatory parameters (erythrocyte sedimentation rate, ESR, and CRP), composite scores reflecting disease activity (such as disease activity score (DAS28) and clinical disease activity index (CDAI)), and disease severity (extra-articular disease) are commonly associated with cardiovascular complications in RA [1, 2, 22–28].

The link between systemic inflammation and cardiovascular outcomes persists even after adjusting according to classical risk factors (obesity, hypertension, hyperlipidemia) [1, 2, 20–22].

Thus, elevated CRP levels at the baseline and the duration of uncontrolled disease correlate with cardiovascular burden in RA [1, 2, 22–28], while very high disease activity over time or high disease activity at RA onset also contributes to the cardiovascular risk [22, 23]. Moreover, it seems that uncontrolled high disease activity promotes the highest risk of developing cardiovascular disease [1, 2, 21–28]. CRP also correlated with acute myocardial infarction, one of the central complications of early accelerated atherosclerosis in RA [1, 22, 23].

Clearly, low disease activity (DAS28 < 3.2) and remission (DAS28 < 2.6) are fundamental in preventing a 10-years risk of cardiovascular events (particularly fatal or nonfatal cases of cardiovascular disease) in RA [1, 22, 23, 29]. In fact, it seems that low stable disease activity is able to reduce the cardiovascular burden and is appropriate to attain a protective effect against cardiovascular disease in RA [1, 22, 23]. Similarly, clinical remission or the absence of inflammation may be associated with a reduced risk of cardiovascular disease in RA [1, 22, 23]; apparently, remission has no additional protective effect against cardiovascular risk profile compared with low disease activity [1, 2, 22, 23].

Thus, it becomes clear that the manipulation of inflammatory response and tight disease control [22, 23, 28] are able to prevent cardiovascular events in RA [3, 26].

2.3. Cardiovascular risk assessment in RA

Different scores designed for the calculation of cardiovascular risk in general population (e.g., Framingham, SCORE, QRISK) underestimate the cardiovascular burden in patients with inflammatory rheumatic conditions, mainly RA [1, 2, 6, 29, 30]; thus, there is no standard or validated model for cardiovascular risk prediction in RA.

In EULAR 2009 has proposed to multiply by 1.5 points the SCORE risk for patients with RA if two out of three RA-related parameters are present: a disease duration more than 10 years, rheumatoid factor or ACPA positivity, and severe extra-articular manifestations [2, 6, 29, 30]. Despite good reliability, this score is not able to reclassify patients with RA in the adequate cardiovascular risk category [2, 6].

QRESEARCH Cardiovascular Risk Algorithm (QRISK) 2 is a prediction model including RA as a specific risk factor, multiplying with 1.4; it overestimates both nonfatal and fatal cardiovascular events [2, 6, 29, 30].

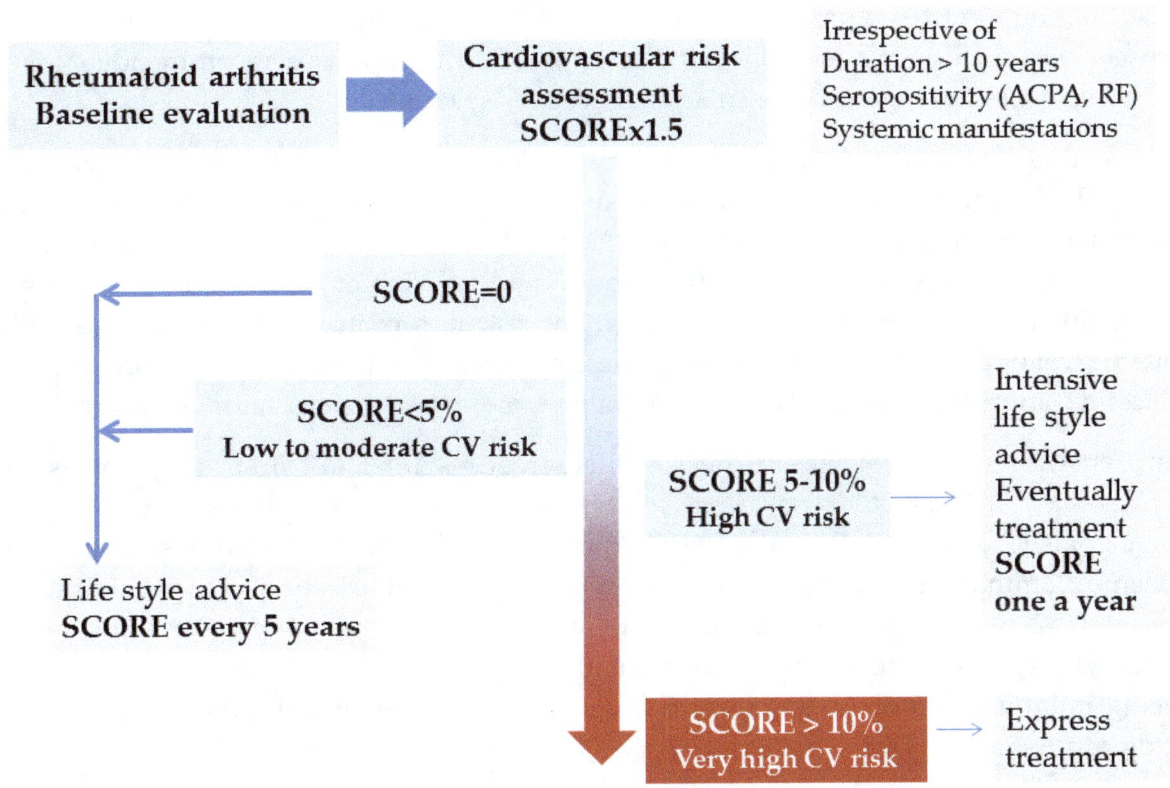

Figure 3. Algorithm for cardiovascular risk assessment in RA (adapted from Gualtierotti [4]).

EULAR 2016 has recommended the use of a modified SCORE adapted for patients with RA, meaning SCORE multiplied by 1.5 irrespective of disease duration, seropositivity, or the presence of systemic features [2, 6, 29, 30].

According to EULAR recommendations [6], the assessment of RA patients should be adapted based on CV risk stratification and several individual factors such as change of specific anti-rheumatic medication [2, 6, 29, 30]. Thus, risk monitoring is warranted once every 5 years if the risk is low to moderate or more often if the patient has an intermediate and high risk or when adapting the therapeutic protocol [2, 6]. An interesting algorithm was recently adapted/ proposed by Gualtierotti et al. (**Figure 3**) [2].

2.4. Recommendations for cardiovascular risk assessment in RA

Cardiovascular risk stratification and further monitoring based on the risk class is essential in RA [1, 2, 6, 29, 30]. EULAR 2009 guidelines have proposed the assessment of the cardiovascular disease on an annual basis, except for patients classified as low risk or low disease activity where the risk is typically monitored as 2–3 years [1–3, 6].

Updated EULAR 2016 guidelines released four new recommendations emphasizing the interval, scores, and protocol for cardiovascular disease screening [6]. Interestingly, cardiovascular risk assessment is no longer recommended annually but every 5 years or following a major change in the DMARD therapy (recommendation 2) [6]. Either local or national guidelines or SCORE are equally accepted for the calculation of CV risk (recommendation 3) [6]. Lipid profile comprising total cholesterol and its HDL fraction should be evaluated during stable disease or remission (recommendation 4) [6]. Finally, surrogate biomarkers for subclinical atherosclerosis such as plaques on Doppler carotid ultrasound are recommended for the extensive screening of the cardiovascular disease in RA patients [6].

Recommendations for the management of CV risk in RA take into account three essential points [1, 2, 6, 14]: (i) control of disease activity meaning early diagnosis and dynamic choice of the antirheumatic drug starting with non-biologic DMARDs followed by biologic DMARDs, with or without glucocorticosteroids until reaching the therapeutic target (remission or low disease activity), (ii) non-pharmacological management of risk factors including smoking cessation, adequate level of physical activity, as well as healthy diet, (iii) pharmacological management of risk factors comprising statins for lipid abnormalities, antihypertensives, antidiabetics, etc.

Optimized disease control within the so-called treat-to-target (T2T) strategy consistently improves the cardiovascular risk in RA, as remission and low disease activity become realistic goals [1, 2, 4, 6, 7]. Recent advances in the pathobiology of the disease and the link between inflammation, RA disease activity, and cardiovascular issues have highlighted the following [1, 2, 6, 7]: (i) disease duration is not an independent cardiovascular risk factor; (ii) disease activity, the number, and duration of flares significantly alter the CV risk; (iii) reducing inflammation obviously improves the CV outcomes; and (iv) long-term DMARD therapy results in lowering the CV risk.

Not only chronic persistent systemic as well as local inflammation and RA disease activity endorse excessive cardiovascular burden in RA but also traditional CV risk factors, e.g., body mass index, lipids, gender, tobacco smoking, and hypertension [1–3, 6].

Aggressive T2T approach in daily clinical practice for patients with RA proved successful in negatively impacted systemic and synovial inflammation, impair cytokine release, and promote quantitative and qualitative lipid changes, significantly decreasing the cardiovascular disease in such patients [1, 2, 6, 7]. Conversely, anti-inflammatory drugs (e.g., not only NSAIDs and COX-2 inhibitors but also steroids) are commonly associated with high cardiovascular safety issues [1, 2, 6].

Regardless of substantial progresses in RA treatment, patients develop and die considerably earlier than the general population mainly related to cardiovascular comorbidities, generally in connection with accelerated atherosclerosis and cardio-metabolic complication [1, 2, 13, 18, 21].

2.5. 2016 EULAR recommendation for CV management

Since broad cardio-metabolic evaluation and optimal strategies for cardiovascular risk reduction are still poorly integrated in routine practice in autoimmune conditions [13, 18, 21], EULAR has recently updated guidelines for cardiovascular disease risk assessment and management in systemic inflammatory conditions including RA, psoriatic arthritis, and ankylosing spondylitis [6]. An extended EULAR task force has reconsidered the old guidelines and released new overarching principles and recommendations in accordance to PRISMA (Preferred Reporting Items for Systematic Reviews and Meta-analysis) statement suggesting an appropriate algorithm for cardiovascular risk management in these patients [6].

Updated EULAR 2015/2016 guidelines for cardiovascular comorbidity in RA are listed below [6]:

1. Lowering the cardiovascular risk in RA largely relies on both early diagnosis and tight control of disease activity as well as the disease flares.

2. The cardiovascular risk reassessment is advised at least every 5 years or when major changes in DMARD therapy are specified.

3. EULAR endorses the application of risk assessment scores according to the general population such as systematic coronary risk evaluation (SCORE) or national guidelines for CVD risk evaluation.

4. A systematic evaluation of lipid profile including non-fasting total cholesterol and low- and high-density lipoprotein fractions is mandatory to further mitigate the cardiovascular risk; however, measurements should be achieved during stable RA or in remission disease.

5. A correct estimate of the increased risk of cardiovascular events in RA encompasses for a modified risk score multiplied by 1.5.

6. Surrogates of subclinical atherosclerosis and cardiovascular disease such as artery plaques identified by carotid ultrasound screening are useful to perceive the increased cardiovascular risk in RA.

7. Several protective measures, e.g., healthy diet, exercise on a daily basis, and smoking cessation, should underline the general approach of RA patients with raised cardiovascular risk.

8. New trends in treating hypertension and dyslipidemia with specific medication including antihypertensives and statins are widely recommended in patients with RA with such comorbidities.

9. Since both traditional nonselective NSAIDs and coxibs have an increased risk of developing cardiovascular toxicity in RA, these drugs are carefully proposed in such patients, especially in those with prior history of or at increased risk to develop further cardiovascular events (congestive heart failure, ischemic heart disease, peripheral arterial or cerebrovascular disease).

10. If mandatory, long-term corticosteroids are managed to minimize the total dosage, with tapering as soon as remission or low disease activity is reached.

3. Cardiovascular safety of non-biologic and biologic anti-rheumatic drugs

Evidence-based medicine provides key insights into the consequences of various classes of antirheumatic drugs on cardiovascular risk in RA, suggesting that TNF inhibitors (TNF-i) and methotrexate decrease the risk of such events, while corticosteroids and IL-6 receptor inhibition via tocilizumab exert a multifaceted intervention on cardiovascular outcomes [1, 2, 26, 31]. Data are summarized in **Table 2**.

Drug	Positive effects	Negative effects	Overall influence on CV safety
Methotrexate	Improved RA activity	High homocysteinemia	Protective
Other csDMARDs Leflunomide Antimalarials	Improved RA activity, improved lipid profile, reduced risk of diabetes	Arterial hypertension May be responsible of cardiomyopathy although rarely	Complex effect Protective
TNF inhibitors	Improved RA activity, reduced insulin resistance	Contraindicated in severe heart failure (class III/IV NYHA)	Protective
Non-TNF inhibitors Tocilizumab Rituximab Abatacept Tofacitinib	Improved RA activity Safe in heart failure Safe in heart failure Safe in heart failure	Abnormal lipids	Complex effect Complex effect Complex effect
Corticosteroids	Reduced inflammation	May increase CV events, BMI, dyslipidemia, insulin resistance, hypertension	Complex effect
NSAIDs		All NSAIDs increase CV risk (prothrombotic effect)	

Table 2. Cardiovascular profile of anti-rheumatic drugs: non-biologic and biologic DMARDs, corticosteroids, NSAIDs.

3.1. Non-biologic DMARDs: methotrexate and non-methotrexate drugs (e.g., sulfasalazine, antimalarials, leflunomide) improve cardiovascular outcomes in RA

Recent meta-analysis as well as real-life data showed that traditional synthetic DMARDs are able to reduce the cardiovascular risk in RA. However, the precise cardioprotective mechanism of classic immunosupressants remains still under debate.

Undoubtedly, methotrexate and non-methotrexate agents efficiently control inflammation and disease activity, alter the lipid spectrum and concentration, and are able to reduce the arterial stiffness, improving cardiovascular risk in different RA scenarios [1–32].

Furthermore, methotrexate, the drug of choice as first-line treatment, is associated with a consistent reduction in mortality (70%), a decline in the rate of total cardiovascular events (around 28%), and up to 18% lower risk of myocardial infarction in patients with RA [31]. Unlike the anti-TNF agents, methotrexate is not related to a significant decrease in strokes and major adverse cardiac events; nevertheless, it seems that the risk of heart failure is also decreased [1, 2, 31, 32].

The interesting hypothesis of inflammatory origin of cardiovascular disease prompted the ongoing randomized Cardiovascular Inflammation Reduction Trial (CIRT) aiming to investigate whether low-dose methotrexate is able to decrease rates of heart attacks, strokes, and cardiovascular death among stable coronary artery disease patients with type 2 diabetes and/or metabolic syndrome, conditions associated with an enhanced pro-inflammatory response [3]. Although the study was designed to perceive a 25% cardiovascular risk decline within the methotrexate group, failure to achieve this magnitude of risk reduction will not degrade the immune inflammatory background of cardiovascular pathology [3].

Data about other synthetic DMARDs are not consistent. Leflunomide has indirect positive effects on cardiovascular outcome through reducing disease activity, while its role in promoting hypertension is a potential limitation, particularly if high blood pressure is documented [1, 2]. Antimalarials, specifically hydroxychloroquine, are able to modulate lipid profile and to reduce the risk of diabetes, although rare cases of cardiomyopathy have been described [1, 2, 31, 33]. Finally, sulfasalazine seems to exert also protective effects, while further studies are required to clearly define its role [2].

3.2. Glucocorticoids enhance the cardiovascular risk in RA

The association between corticosteroids and the rate of total as well as individual cardiovascular events was systematically evaluated in patients with inflammatory rheumatic disorders, principally in RA and systemic lupus. It is widely accepted that corticosteroids are able to shape the cardiovascular risk by two competitive pathways [1, 2, 6, 31, 34]:

- The risk for future cardiovascular disease is increased due to not only metabolic effects, e.g., abnormal lipid metabolism, impaired glucose tolerance, insulin resistance, relative weight gain, or true obesity, but also glucocorticoid-induced hypertension.
- The cardiovascular risk is attenuated through rapid and salutary anti-inflammatory and anti-proliferative effects of corticosteroids.

Their cardiotoxicity as well as cardiovascular mortality is dose-dependent (actual and previous cumulative dose) [1, 2, 6]. Sustained administration of corticosteroids classically accounts not only for an increased risk of myocardial infarction, stroke, and congestive heart failure but also for all major adverse cardiac events in RA patients as suggested by different studies and meta-analyses [1, 2, 6, 31, 34].

The well-known trend in RA is to maintain the lowest dose of corticosteroids for the shortest period of time and tapering as soon as remission or low disease activity (recommendation 10, EULAR 2016) [6]; the benefits of further administration should be deliberated and reconsidered once the disease outcomes have been achieved [6].

Although NSAIDs no longer represent the mainstay of RA therapeutic protocol, both nonselective and COX2-selective medications are still used, even if intermittently, during RA flares and in short-time administration [1, 2, 22, 23, 31, 35]. NSAID safety profile should be emphasized, as their effect on cardiovascular outcomes in RA is challenging. Both nonselective NSAIDs and coxibs increase the cardiovascular risk in general population; however, not all of them exert the same deleterious cardiovascular effect, especially talking about patients with RA [2, 6, 31, 35].

It is widely recognized that long-term NSAIDs increased the risk of all cardiovascular events and stroke in general population, particularly if cardiovascular disease is documented (congestive heart failure, ischemic heart disease, peripheral arterial disease, or cerebrovascular disease) [2, 6, 31]; only few studies have addressed the cardiovascular outcomes of COX2-selective and traditional NSAIDs specifically in RA [1, 2, 6, 31, 35].

3.3. Biologic DMARD: TNF inhibitors decrease the cardiovascular risk in RA

TNF-α, a pivot pro-inflammatory cytokine involved in both systemic and local (synovial microenvironment) persistent inflammations in RA, may also alter lipid metabolism, insulin resistance, and endorse endothelial dysfunction [1, 2, 6, 31, 36, 37]. Moreover, chronic inflammation and atherosclerosis share common pathways, tailoring the basis of amplified cardiovascular risk in inflammatory rheumatic conditions [1, 2].

On the other hand, TNF inhibitors provide multifaceted influences on cardiovascular safety in patients with RA comprising [1, 2, 6, 31, 37]:

- Rapid and effective control of chronic inflammation signaling with significant decrease in inflammatory parameters (serum CRP levels and ESR), RA activity, and delay articular damage articular
- Changes in lipid pattern with increase in HDL-cholesterol fraction, total cholesterol, triglycerides with or without influence on LDL-cholesterol fraction, and with no major impact on the atherogenic index (TC/HDL); in fact, the trend of rising serum lipids under anti-TNF therapy typically reflects the stabilization through the lipid levels before the RA onset
- Improvement of endothelial dysfunction and insulin sensitivity as well as the anti-oxidative response of HDL

Thus, it seems that TNF inhibitors are efficient in reducing cardiovascular comorbidities in RA, comprising not only all cardiovascular events but also some specific stroke, myocardial infarction, and even MACE [1–3, 31, 36, 37].

A meta-analysis of several observational studies and registries in RA patients treated with TNF inhibitors performed by Roubille et al. showed a significant reduction in the risk of all cardiovascular events (up to 30%), myocardial infarctions, strokes, and major adverse cardiac events with biologics vs. non-biologic DMARDs [1–3, 31, 36, 37]. However, no significant effect on heart failure was detected [2, 31]. Interestingly, the risk of future cardiovascular consequences under anti-TNF medication is twice lower that the risk with non-biologic non-methotrexate drugs [1–3, 31, 36, 37].

Besides, Ljung et al. recently published their study investigating the effects of response to anti-TNF agents on short-term (1- and 2-year follow-up) risk of acute coronary syndrome in individuals with active RA and no previous ischemic or congestive heart disease before starting TNF-i as the first biologic agent [37].

RA patients classified as good (but not moderate) EULAR responders (improvement of more than 1.2 points in disease activity score) to anti-TNF therapy showed a 50% risk reduction of acute myocardial infarction or unstable angina pectoris or acute myocardial infarction as the underlying cause of death in short-term follow-up, similarly to the risk of acute coronary events in general population [1, 2, 6, 31, 36, 37].

In fact, the magnitude of coronary event risk reduction was reported irrespective of the baseline risk stratification (by gender, age, cardiovascular risk factors, disease duration), drug exposure, as well as the risk window [2, 31, 36, 37]. Additionally, the ability to achieve optimal control of RA activity instead of simply improved disease control or TNF-i per se theoretically stabilizes the pattern of ischemic heart disease in RA [1–3, 31, 36, 37].

Still considered the "black box" of TNF biologic class, the link between TNF blockade and moderate to severe congestive heart failure (class III/class IV NYHA) remains controversial [1, 2, 31, 36]. Clearly, heart failure in general population is associated with high TNF-α, with consistent correlation between serum levels and clinical significance and severity of cardiac failure [1, 31, 36]. However, TNF inhibitors are able to improve ventricular dysfunction in experimental models of cardiac failure [1, 2, 6, 31, 36, 37].

Overall, TNF inhibitors significantly damper the cardiovascular comorbidity in RA, especially in patients declared responders to such therapies.

3.4. Non-TNF DMARDs: tocilizumab

Data about tocilizumab, a humanized monoclonal antibody acting against the IL-6 receptor (membrane-bound and soluble), and its cardiovascular toxicity are widely accessible from different clinical trials, including ADACTA, TOWARD, MEASURE, and ENTRACTE [38–41].

Although modest increases of LDL- and HDL-cholesterol as well as triglycerides were noticed in RA patients treated with tocilizumab in randomized controlled trials, only ENTRACTE was specifically designed to evaluate the cardiovascular safety and to compare net cardiovascular risk-benefit ratio of anti-IL-6 therapy with biologics with another mechanism of action, such as etanercept, in active seropositive RA [1, 2, 38–41].

As a potent inhibitor of IL-6 signaling, tocilizumab is associated with excellent clinical efficacy essentially related to patent decline in systemic inflammatory biomarkers; in addition, tocilizumab-associated altered lipid profile, mainly increased LDL-cholesterol, is broadly recognized and potentially connected with atherogenesis and atherothrombosis in patients with RA [1, 2, 3, 39–42].

Moderate elevations of LDL-cholesterol, HDL-cholesterol, and triglycerides were faced in RA patients under tocilizumab in phase II and phase III trials, but the atherogenic implications of these changes are still unsettled [1, 2, 38–41].

A summary of trials reflecting the cardiovascular safety profile of tocilizumab in RA comprises the following:

ADACTA, a randomized clinical trial to evaluate tocilizumab monotherapy vs. adalimumab monotherapy for the treatment of RA, suggested that tocilizumab meaningfully decreases systemic inflammation as supported by low ESR and CRP levels and disease activity (DAS28, CDAI). Changes are obviously more evident as compared to adalimumab, a totally humanized monoclonal anti-TNF antibody; however, tocilizumab induces higher LDL-cholesterol levels more than adalimumab do [39].

TOWARD trial, evaluating tocilizumab in combination with traditional DMARD therapy, revealed the role of IL-6 blockade not only in reducing articular and systemic inflammation but also in improving insulin resistance, along with its capacity to promote increased total cholesterol levels in up to one-fourth of cases [38].

Tocilizumab may induce particular changes in lipid pattern, with potential relevance for cardiovascular safety. Persistent increase in mean fasting plasma lipids, within the normal range, is commonly reported with tocilizumab, together with a consistent decrease in serum CRP, suggesting that abnormal lipid levels may, in part, be related to significant decline in inflammation [38].

An increase in total cholesterol was observed in one out of five RA included in the study, while high LDL and altered HDL status from a pro-inflammatory to a significantly low inflammatory status (12 and 15%, respectively) increases of 30% in the total cholesterol:HDL-cholesterol ratio (12% cases) and more frequent in the LDL-cholesterol:HDL-cholesterol ratio (20%) were also reported. Finally, increases in the mean apolipoprotein A-I and apolipoprotein B, within the normal range, without changes in the ApoB:ApoA-I ratio were also commonly described. Only a limited number of patients initiated statin therapy during the study, with positive influence on lipid modifications [38].

MEASURE trial of tocilizumab effects on surrogates of vascular risk in RA was powered to demonstrate the modulation of lipid and lipoprotein particle (LDL, HDL, VLDL) levels and composition (HDL-associated serum amyloid A), alongside other surrogates of vascular risk (markers of coagulation, thrombosis, and vascular function) with IL-6 receptor inhibition vs. placebo in active disease [40, 41].

McInnes et al. [41] not only reported a dramatic decrease in inflammation in such patients but also demonstrated quantitative and qualitative changes in lipid metabolism profile. Overall, tocilizumab prompted the increase in total cholesterol, LDL-cholesterol, and triglycerides by week 12 of administration, while no significant influence on proatherogenic small LDL particle concentration, oxidized (ox)LDL, or HDL-cholesterol levels, in addition to ApoB:ApoA-1 ratio. Furthermore, tocilizumab-based IL-6 signal blockade altered the HDL particle composition toward a less pro-inflammatory phenotype [40, 41].

Besides, HDL-associated serum amyloid A, secretory phospholipase A2-IIA, lipoprotein(a), fibrinogen, and D-dimers presented a sizeable decrease, while the antioxidant enzyme associated with HDL, paraoxonase, and level significantly increased under tocilizumab. Since a prothrombotic status heightened risk for cardiovascular events independently of established risk factors in general population, the reduction of thrombotic potential with tocilizumab in patients with active RA remains of considerable interest [40, 41].

However, the clear benefit of such modifications for cardiovascular risk is still debatable.

ENTRACTE, a randomized clinical trial aiming to evaluate cardiovascular events with either i. v. tocilizumab monthly or etanercept s.c weekly, was designed as a non-inferiority study comparing cardiovascular safety of tocilizumab vs. the TNF receptor, etanercept, in RA. Primary endpoint focused on major cardiovascular adverse events (MACE) (cardiovascular death, nonfatal myocardial infarction, nonfatal stroke), while secondary endpoints were cardiovascular and non-cardiovascular safety of both drugs [1–3].

ENTRACTE has demonstrated a relative increase in the incidence of cardiovascular events among severe active RA patients with a background of cardiovascular risk factors receiving tocilizumab, specifically the hazard of MACE. Additionally, the average level of LDL-cholesterol was consistently higher under tocilizumab as compared with etanercept. Nevertheless, the cardiovascular issues with tocilizumab vs. etanercept should be deliberated/interpreted in the context of its clinical efficacy and general, non-cardiovascular, safety profile.

3.5. Other non-biologic and targeted DMARDs: rituximab, abatacept, and tofacitinib

- **Rituximab**, a B-cell depletory agent, typically indicated as a second-line biologic therapy after failure of at least one anti-TNF agent, showed no significant differences as compared to placebo in terms of cardiovascular events. There is no cardiovascular safety concern related to rituximab; furthermore, it seems that rituximab is able to improve lipid metabolism, alter HDL-cholesterol to a low atherogenic profile, as well decrease prothrombotic biomarkers. Also, rituximab has no influence on arterial stiffness [1–3, 6, 7, 42].
- **Abatacept**, by blocking the T and B costimulation, commonly acts on lipid pattern resulting in high total cholesterol and its fractions (HDL-cholesterol and LDL-cholesterol), without a significant decrease in the atherogenic index; however, abatacept is known to alter the arterial tonus [1–3, 6, 7].
- **Tofacitinib**, a JAK inhibitor already approved for the management of RA, promotes similar changes in lipid profile as tocilizumab do, meaning an increase of both HDL-cholesterol and LDL-cholesterol, with a minimal impact on atherogenic index [1–3, 6, 7, 43].

4. Conclusions

Systemic autoimmune rheumatic conditions, specifically RA, are widely associated with excessive cardiovascular morbidity, with a magnitude similar to that related to traditional cardiovascular risk factors, particularly diabetes.

A multifaceted dynamic interplay between chronic systemic inflammation, RA-specific issues, early accelerated atherosclerosis, and classic cardiovascular risk factors typically highlights the cardiovascular burden in various RA settings.

The optimal strategy to identify patients at increased risk to develop cardiovascular disease as well as the correct assignment of different risk categories is mandatory in routine practice in every RA case. Furthermore, the selection of suitable medication (non-biological, TNF inhibitor, or non-TNF biological antirheumatic drug) according to cardiovascular toxicity is warranted so as to improve cardiovascular outcomes in RA.

Author details

Codrina Ancuta[1]*, Claudia Mihailov[2] and Eugen Ancuta[3]

*Address all correspondence to: codrina_ancuta@yahoo.com

1 2nd Rheumatology Department, Clinical Rehabilitation Hospital, University of Medicine and Pharmacy "Grigore T Popa", Iasi, Romania

2 2nd Medical Department, Clinical CF Hospital of Constanta, Faculty of Medicine, "Ovidius" University of Constanta, Romania

3 "Elena Doamna" Clinical Hospital, Iasi, Romania

References

[1] Nagy G, Németh N, Buzás EI. Mechanisms of vascular comorbidity in autoimmune diseases. Current Opinion in Rheumatology. 2018;**30**(2):197-206. DOI: 10.1097/BOR.0000000000000483

[2] Gualtierotti R, Ughi N, Marfia G, Ingegnoli F. Practical management of cardiovascular comorbidities in rheumatoid arthritis. Rheumatology and Therapy. 2017;**4**:293-308. DOI: 10.1007/s40744-017-0068-0

[3] Welsh P, Grassia G, Botha S, Sattar N, Maffia P. Targeting inflammation to reduce cardiovascular disease risk: A realistic clinical prospect? British Journal of Pharmacology. 2017; **174**:3898-3913. DOI: 10.1111/bph.13818

[4] Gualtierotti R. Understanding cardiovascular risk in rheumatoid arthritis: Still a long way to go. Atherosclerosis. 2017;**256**:123-124

[5] Sen D, Gonzalez-Mayda M, Brasington RD Jr. Cardiovascular disease in rheumatoid arthritis. Rheumatic Disease Clinics of North America. 2014;**40**(1):27-49

[6] Agca R, Heslinga SC, Rollefstad S, et al. EULAR recommendations for cardiovascular disease risk management in patients with rheumatoid arthritis and other forms of inflammatory joint disorders: 2015/2016 update. Annals of the Rheumatic Diseases. 2017;**76**(1):17-28

[7] Burmester GR, Pope JE. Novel treatment strategies in rheumatoid arthritis. Lancet. 2017; **389**:2338-2348

[8] Nurmohamed MT, Heslinga M, Kitas GD. Cardiovascular comorbidity in rheumatic diseases. Nature Reviews Rheumatology. 2015;**11**(12):693-704

[9] Radner H, Lesperance T, Accortt NA, Solomon DH. Incidence and prevalence of cardiovascular risk factors among patients with rheumatoid arthritis, psoriasis, or psoriatic arthritis. Arthritis Care Research (Hoboken). 2017;**69**:1510-1518

[10] Houri Levi E, Watad A, Whitby A, Tiosano S, Comaneshter D, Cohen AD, et al. Coexistence of ischemic heart disease and rheumatoid arthritis patients—A case control study. Autoimmunity Reviews. 2016;**15**(4):393-396

[11] Baghdadi LR, Woodman RJ, Shanahan EM, Mangoni AA. The impact of traditional cardiovascular risk factors on cardiovascular outcomes in patients with rheumatoid arthritis: A systematic review and meta-analysis. PLoS One. 2015;**10**(2):e011e7952

[12] Ambrosino P, Lupoli R, Di Minno A, Tasso M, Peluso R, Di Minno MN. Subclinical atherosclerosis in patients with rheumatoid arthritis. A meta-analysis of literature studies. Thrombosis and Haemostasis. 2015;**113**(5):916-930. DOI: 10.1160/TH14-11-0921

[13] Ruscitti P, Margiotta DPE, Macaluso F, Iacono D, D'Onofrio F, Emmi G, Atzeni F, Prete M, Perosa F, Sarzi-Puttini P, Emmi L, Cantatore FP, Triolo G, Afeltra A, Giacomelli R, Valentini G. Subclinical atherosclerosis and history of cardiovascular events in Italian patients with rheumatoid arthritis: Results from a cross-sectional, multicenter GIRRCS (Gruppo Italiano di Ricerca in Reumatologia Clinica e Sperimentale) study. Medicine (Baltimore). 2017;**96**(42):e8180. DOI: 10.1097/MD.0000000000008180

[14] Turk SA, Heslinga SC, Dekker J, et al. The relationship between cardiac conduction times, cardiovascular risk factors, and inflammation in patients with early arthritis. The Journal of Rheumatology. 2017;**44**:580-586

[15] Hammam N, Gheita TA. Impact of second hand smoking on disease activity in women with rheumatoid arthritis. Clinical Rheumatology. 2017;**36**:2412-2420

[16] Bartoloni E, Alunno A, Gerli R. Hypertension as a cardiovascular risk factor in autoimmune rheumatic diseases. Nature Reviews Cardiology. 2018;**15**:33-44. DOI: 10.1038/nrcardio.2017.118

[17] Geraldino-Pardilla L, Zartoshti A, Bag Ozbek A, et al. Arterial inflammation detected with 18 f-fluoro-deoxyglucose positron emission tomography in rheumatoid arthritis. Arthritis and Rheumatology. 2017;**70**(1). DOI: 10.1002/art.40345

[18] Ruscitti P, Ursini F, Cipriani P, Ciccia F, Liakouli V, Carubbi F, Guggino G, Berardicurti O, Grembiale R, Triolo G, De Sarro G, Giacomelli R. Prevalence of type 2 diabetes and impaired fasting glucose in patients affected by rheumatoid arthritis: Results from a cross-sectional study. Medicine (Baltimore). 2017;**96**:e7896

[19] Ursini F, Russo E, D'Angelo S, Arturi F, Hribal ML, D'Antona L, Bruno C, Tripepi G, Naty S, De Sarro G, Olivieri I, Grembiale RD. Prevalence of undiagnosed diabetes in rheumatoid arthritis: An OGTT study. Medicine (Baltimore). 2016 Feb;**95**(7):e2552. DOI: 10.1097/MD.0000000000002552

[20] Kim JY, Lee EY, Park JK, Song YW, Kim JR, Cho KH. Patients with rheumatoid arthritis show altered lipoprotein profiles with dysfunctional high-density lipoproteins that can exacerbate inflammatory and atherogenic process. PLoS One. 2016;**11**(10):e0164564

[21] Ruscitti P, Ursini F, Cipriani P, et al. Poor clinical response in rheumatoid arthritis is the main risk factor for diabetes development in the short-term: A 1- year, single-Centre, longitudinal study. PLoS One. 2017;**12**:e0181203

[22] Arts EE, Fransen J, Den Broeder AA, van Riel PLCM, Popa CD. Low disease activity (DAS28 < 3.2) reduces the risk of first cardiovascular event in rheumatoid arthritis: A time-dependent cox regression analysis in a large cohort study. Annals of the Rheumatic Diseases. 2017;**76**:1693-1699

[23] Arts EEA, Fransen J, den Broeder AA, et al. The effect of disease duration and disease activity on the risk of cardiovascular disease in rheumatoid arthritis patients. Annals of the Rheumatic Diseases. 2015;**74**:998-1003

[24] Provan SA, Semb AG, Hisdal J, et al. Remission is the goal for cardiovascular risk management in patients with rheumatoid arthritis: A cross-sectional comparative study. Annals of the Rheumatic Diseases. 2011;**70**:812-817

[25] Gonzalez-Gay MA, Gonzalez-Juanatey C, Pineiro A, et al. High-grade C-reactive protein elevation correlates with accelerated atherogenesis in patients with rheumatoid arthritis. Journal of Rheumatology. 2005;**32**:1219-1223

[26] Meissner Y, Zink A, Kekow J, et al. Impact of disease activity and treatment of comorbidities on the risk of myocardial infarction in rheumatoid arthritis. Arthritis Research Therapy. 2016;**18**:183

[27] Myasoedova E, Chandran A, Ilhan B, Major BT, Michet CJ, Matteson EL, et al. The role of rheumatoid arthritis (RA) flare and cumulative burden of RA severity in the risk of cardiovascular disease. Annals of the Rheumatic Diseases. 2016;**75**(3):560-565

[28] Meek IL, Vonkeman HE, van de Laar MAFJ. Cardiovascular case fatality in rheumatoid arthritis is decreasing; first prospective analysis of a current low disease activity rheumatoid arthritis cohort and review of the literature. BMC Musculoskeletal Disorders. 2014;**15**:142

[29] Semb AG, Rollefstad S, van Riel P, et al, Cardiovascular disease assessment in rheumatoid arthritis: A guide to translating knowledge of cardiovascular risk into clinical practice; Annals of the Rheumatic Diseases 2014;**73**:1284-1288. DOI:10.1136/annrheumdis-2013-204792

[30] Crowson CS, Gabriel SE, Semb AG, van Riel PL,Karpouzas G, Dessein PH et al. Rheumatoid arthritis-specific cardiovascular risk scores are not superior to general risk scores: A validation analysis of patients from seven countries. Rheumatology (Oxford). 2017;**56**(7): 1102-1110

[31] Roubille C, Richer V, Starnino T, et al. The effects of tumour necrosis factor inhibitors, methotrexate, nonsteroidal anti-inflammatory drugs and corticosteroids on cardiovascular events in rheumatoid arthritis, psoriasis and psoriatic arthritis: A systematic review and meta-analysis. Annals of the Rheumatic Diseases. 2015;**74**:480-489

[32] Mangoni AA, Baghdadi LR, Shanahan EM, et al. Methotrexate, blood pressure and markers of arterial function in patients with rheumatoid arthritis: A repeated cross-sectional study. Therapeutic Advances in Musculoskeletal Disease. 2017;**9**:213-229

[33] Kerr G, Aujero M, Richards J, Sayles H, Davis L, Cannon G, et al. Associations of hydroxychloroquine use with lipid profiles in rheumatoid arthritis: Pharmacologic implications. Arthritis Care Research (Hoboken). 2014;**66**(11):1619-1626

[34] van Sijl AM, Boers M, Voskuyl AE, Nurmohamed MT. Confounding by indication probably distorts the relationship between steroid use and cardiovascular disease in rheumatoid arthritis: Results from a prospective cohort study. PLoS One. 2014;**9**:e87965. Epub 2014/02/06

[35] Nissen SE, Yeomans ND, Solomon DH, Luscher TF, Libby P, Husni ME, et al. Cardiovascular safety of celecoxib, naproxen, or ibuprofen for arthritis. The New England Journal of Medicine. 2016;**375**(26):2519-2529

[36] Pope JE. TNF inhibitors and cardiovascular risk management in RA. Nature Reviews Rheumatology. 2016;**12**(6):317-318. DOI: 10.1038/nrrheum.2016.67

[37] Ljung L, Rantapää-Dahlqvist S, Jacobsson LTH, Askling J, for the ARTIS Study Group. Response to biological treatment and subsequent risk of coronary events in rheumatoid arthritis. Annals of the Rheumatic Diseases. 2016;**75**:2087-2094

[38] Gabay C, Emery P, van Vollenhoven R, et al, ADACTA Study Investigators. Tocilizumab monotherapy versus adalimumab monotherapy for treatment of rheumatoid arthritis (ADACTA): A randomised, double-blind, controlled phase 4 trial. Lancet. 2013;**381**(9877): 1541-1550. DOI: 10.1016/S0140-6736(13)60250-0

[39] Genovese MC, McKay JD, Nasonov EL, Mysler EF, da Silva NA, Alecock E, Woodworth T, Gomez-Reino JJ. Interleukin-6 receptor inhibition with tocilizumab reduces disease activity in rheumatoid arthritis with inadequate response to disease-modifying antirheumatic drugs: The tocilizumab in combination with traditional disease-modifying antirheumatic drug therapy study. Arthritis and Rheumatology. 2008 Oct;**58**(10):2968-2980. DOI: 10.1002/art.23940

[40] McInnes IB, Thompson L, Giles JT, Bathon JM, Salmon JE, Beaulieu AD, Codding CE, Carlson TH, Delles C, Lee JS, Sattar N. Effect of interleukin-6 receptor blockade on surrogates of vascular risk in rheumatoid arthritis: Measure, a randomised, placebo-controlled study. Annals of the Rheumatic Diseases. 2015;**74**(4):694-702. DOI: 10.1136/annrheumdis-2013-204345

[41] Gualtierotti R, Ingegnoli F, Griffini S, Grovetti E, Meroni PL, Cugno M. Prothrombotic biomarkers in patients with rheumatoid arthritis: The beneficial effect of IL-6 receptor blockade. Clinical and Experimental Rheumatology. 2016;**34**(3):451-458

[42] Benucci M, Saviola G, Manfredi M, Sarzi-Puttini P, Atzeni F. Factors correlated with improvement of endothelial dysfunction during rituximab therapy in patients with rheumatoid arthritis. Biologics. 2013;**7**:69-75

[43] Souto A, Salgado E, Maneiro JR, Mera A, Carmona L, Gomez-Reino JJ. Lipid profile changes in patients with chronic inflammatory arthritis treated with biologic agents and tofacitinib in randomized clinical trials: A systematic review and meta-analysis. Arthritis Rheumatology. 2015;**67**(1):117-127

11

Cytokines in Rheumatoid Arthritis (RA)

Selim Nalbant and Ahmet Merih Birlik

Abstract

Cytokines are cell molecules that are secreted by immune cells and aid cell to cell communication in immune responses and stimulate the movement of cells towards sites of inflammation, infection and trauma. So, the cytokines are the main part of the immune network to provide the communication in rheumatoid arthritis (RA) too. In RA, cytokines may be classified into four groups: pro-inflammatory cytokines, inflammatory cytokines in joints, anti-inflammatory cytokines and natural cytokine antagonists. After the initial stimuli have occurred, cytokines play a role in communication between the parts of immune system in every step of the pathophysiology process of RA. The differentiation of narve T cells into Th17 cells results in inflammation (synovitis) in joints. B cells further the pathogenic process through antigen presentation and autoantibody and cytokine production. The release of cytokines, especially tumor necrosis factor (TNF)-α, interleukin (IL)-6 and IL-1, causes synovial inflammation. In addition to their articular effects, pro-inflammatory cytokines promote the development of systemic effects (anemia, cardiovascular disease, fatigue and depression). So, cytokines are the main molecules contributing to all facets of the disease.

Keywords: cytokines, effector cells, rheumatoid arthritis, anti-cytokine treatment

1. Cytokine and rheumatoid arthritis

Rheumatoid arthritis (RA) is a progressive inflammatory disease, which is characterized by symmetrical polyarthritis. As an inflammatory disease, RA is characterized by increased levels in pro-inflammatory cytokines. In this complex cytokine environment, apart from arthritis, systemic manifestations also occur. Genetic and environmental factors are contributory to this complex nature of RA process. T cells, B cells and their cytokines play key roles in the pathophysiology of RA. Today's modern RA treatment basically targets these cytokines. While we do this, we are generally treat the *"normal and abnormal cytokine response"* at the same time, because we do not know the main etiology of this abnormal cytokine response. To better manage RA, we should understand the role of cytokines and the relation between the effector cells [1–6].

The term "**cytokine**" is derived from a combination of two Greek words–"cyto" **meaning** cell and "kine" **meaning** move. **Cytokines** are cell molecules that are secreted by immune cells and aid cell to cell communication in cases of inflammation, infection and injury. So, the cytokines are vital part of the immune network to provide communication [7].

2. What is the origin of this complex cytokine response?

RA is an autoimmune disease. The term autoimmunity usually means a lot information that defines ***the way*** but not ***the origin of the process***, and this stands for RA too. On the other hand, autoimmunity also means autoantibody production. In RA, there are two autoantibodies, rheumatoid factor and anti-cyclic citrullinated peptide antibodies, which contribute to inflammation. In the end, chronic inflammatory arthritis and the organ damage occur [8, 9].

The very early events of RA pathogenesis get into motion by breaking T-cell and/or B-cell tolerance and/or ignorance. However, this mechanism was poorly defined. After, shaping of this autoimmune background, some subsequent events intervene to perpetuate the process of synovial inflammation. What directs this process to the joints is unknown and it probably includes biomechanical factors, neuro-immuno-endocrinological interactions and altered articular microvascular microenvironment. Several factors have been proposed to have an association with the susceptibility and severity of rheumatoid arthritis [1–10].

These factors are as follows:

(1) Genetic loci:

- HLA-DR4 alleles
- *PTPN22* (protein tyrosine phosphatase, nonreceptor type 22)
- *PADI4* (peptidyl arginine deiminase, type IV)
- *CTLA4* (cytotoxic T-lymphocyte antigen 4)
- FcγRs (Fc receptors for IgG)
- Various cytokine and cytokine-receptor loci.

(2) Environmental factors (smoking, stress, hormonal factors, etc.)

(3) Infectious organisms

The earliest event in RA pathogenesis perhaps is activation of the innate immune response. In this first step, cytokines play a role in communication between the parts of immune system. In second step, antigen-presenting cells present arthritis-associated antigens to T cells. This step is the starting point of the cytokine effect, which augments the inflammation and stimulate the other systems (such as lipid mediators, nitric oxide, RANKL-RANK signaling, etc.) that cause joint destruction and the organ damage [11–13].

3. How can we classify this cytokine network in RA

Actually to make classification of cytokines for rheumatoid arthritis is not feasible. Because many of them have some pleotropic effect at the same time. However, we may basically, classify cytokines four groups in the pathogenesis of rheumatoid arthritis. Actually, this classification is not a real one, it is just for the establishment of understanding the whole mechanism [10] (**Table 1**).

1. Pro-inflammatory cytokines: IL-1 and TNF-alpha cytokine role in

IL-1

- Increased synovial fibroblast cytokine, chemokine, MMP and PG release
- Increased monocyte cytokine, reactive oxygen intermediate and PG release
- Osteoclast activation
- Endothelial cell adhesion molecule expression
- Acute-phase protein production
- Cardiovascular disease promotion
- HPA axis dysregulation (fatigue and depression) [2, 14, 15]

TNF-alpha

- Increased monocyte activation, cytokine release, prostaglandin release
- T-cell clonal regulation
- Increased endothelial cell adhesion molecule expression, cytokine release
- Acute-phase protein production and fatigue-depression [2, 16]

2. Inflammatory cytokines in joints: IL-1 and TNF-alpha, IL-6, IL-15, IL-16, IL-17, IL-18, IFN-gamma, granulocyte macrophage-colony stimulating factor

IL-6

- Osteoclast and B-cell activation
- T-cell proliferation and differentiation
- Acute-phase protein and hepcidin (anemia) production [17, 18]

IL-15

- Structural similarities to IL-2,4 produced primarily by macrophages
- Regulation of synovial inflammation [19–21]

IL-16

- Suppression of IFN-γ, TNF-α and IL-1β expression
- Anti-inflammatory effect by regulation of Tregs [22]

IL-17

- Increase local chemokine production
- Augmentation of immune response (increase IL-6 production)
- Cartilage damage
- Promotes the effect of IL-1b, TNF-a and IFN-g [20, 23, 24]

IL-18

- Increase the production of pro-inflammatory cytokines, chemokines, adhesion molecules and RANKL which are the main molecules of joint destruction
- Increase the production of fibroblast-like synoviocytes and chondrocytes [25, 26]

IL-21

- Activate TH17 cells
- Induces osteoclastogenesis
- Plasma levels shows correlation with DAS28 [2]

IFN-gamma

- Immune modulation (both protection and activation) [27, 28]

Granulocyte macrophage-colony stimulating factor (GM-CSF)

- Promotes existing RA [29]

3. Anti-inflammatory cytokines

IL-10

- Inhibit Th1 cell activity by suppressing IFN-γ expression
- Direct inhibitory effect on the macrophage activity in the synovium
- Elevated levels in the synovial fluid
- Dominant suppressive cytokine effect
- Protection against cartilage destruction combination with IL-4 [2, 7]

IL-4

- Increased level in synovial fluid during only synovial inflammation
- Preventing collagen type I breakdown in RA [30–33]

IL-13

- Synergistic or inhibitory roles during the arthritis with IL-10, IL-21R, galectin-3 and TGFβ [34]

IL-20

- Regulates osteoclast differentiation [35]

4-Natural cytokine antagonists

IL-1 receptor antagonist (IL-1ra)

- Low levels of IL-1 receptor antagonist (IL-1ra) causes erosive disease in patients and [36]

Soluble type 2 IL-1 receptor

- Cause competitive inhibition by binding interleukin-1α (IL1A), interleukin-1β (IL1B) and interleukin 1 receptor antagonist (IL1Ra), and acts as a pseudo receptor activity that inhibits the activity of its ligands [37, 38]

Soluble TNF receptor (sTNF-RI)

- It is not well-known; possible effect is to cause cleavage of TNF alpha [39]

IL-18 binding protein

- Protect against the joint destructive effect by binding IL-18 in RA [40]

Table 1. Actions of cytokines that play major roles in RA pathobiology.

3.1. Pro-inflammatory cytokines

Interleukin (IL)-1 and tumor necrosis factor (TNF)-alpha are the main pro-inflammatory cytokines involved in RA. The influx and/or local activation of mononuclear cells and the formation of new blood vessels are main findings in synovial membrane. Differentiation of naive T cells into Th17 cells contributes to synovitis. B cells further the pathogenic process through antigen presentation and autoantibody and cytokine production. Enzymes secreted by synoviocytes and chondrocytes degrade cartilage. The release of cytokines, especially TNF-alpha and IL-1, have multiple detrimental effects on cartilage and bone. Pro-inflammatory cytokines act locally but also have systemic effects, such as production of acute-phase proteins, anemia of chronic disease, cardiovascular disease, osteoporosis, etc. [1–7, 11, 12].

3.2. Inflammatory cytokines in joints

These cytokines are basically cytokine found in higher levels in the joints of patients with RA than in the serum. Most are pro-inflammatory cytokines. They cause mostly local joint destruction and also systemic effects of the disease and include IL-1, TNF-alpha, IL-6, IL-15, IL-16, IL-17, IL-18, interferon (IFN)-γ, granulocyte macrophage-colony stimulating factor) [10–12].

3.3. Anti-inflammatory cytokines: (IL-4, IL-10, IL-11, IL-13 and IL-20)

In case of an inflammatory state, such as RA, the immune system utilizes anti-inflammatory cytokines to restrict the inflammatory reaction. In RA synovitis, there is an imbalance between pro-inflammatory and anti-inflammatory cytokines due to insufficient local concentrations of anti-inflammatory cytokines, IL-10, IL-11 and IL-13 to mediate counter-regulatory activity against the dominant pro-inflammatory cytokines. This is almost valid for the T-cell-derived cytokines, which are IL-2 and IL-4. They are also absent, which may impair Treg-cell generation and favor TH1-cell or TH17-cell immune responses [1, 2, 10].

3.4. Natural cytokine antagonists

Immune system is the most complex system, which has a self-limiting or self-controlling mechanism. The known molecules for this purpose are IL-1 receptor antagonist (IL-1ra), soluble type 2 IL-1 receptor, soluble TNF receptor (sTNF-RI) and IL-18 binding protein. However, current information about them is not entirely known. It is suggested that TNFR1 and the type II IL-1R have a regulatory role in sequestering soluble TNF and IL-1 away from their cell-bound receptors. Their detected levels in synovial tissues and fluid are insufficient to counteract the inflammatory cytokines and bring cytokine homeostasis. We currently use these natural anti-inflammatory molecules for therapeutic reasons [1–6].

4. Conclusion

As a result, cytokine effects do not occur with a single cytokine signalling cascade. There are many factors effecting the cytokine response. These are not only to control the equilibrium between inflammatory and anti-inflammatory cytokines but also the pleotropic and individual effects of cytokines. Here, we describe the topics of cytokine network only. It will be crucial to select cytokine targets based not on one single inflammatory pathway but rather on a biosystematic approach to pathogenesis. Implicit in this will be the recognition of pivotal checkpoints that facilitate the progression from autoimmunity to chronic inflammation [1, 11–13].

As it was seen, cytokines are the main molecules at all these stages. However, they are not only the origin of the all cascade but also the last point which is occurring the damage. So, this fact makes the cytokine as a target molecule to treat.

Author details

Selim Nalbant[1,*] and Ahmet Merih Birlik[2]

*Address all correspondence to: nalbantselim@hotmail.com

1 Department of Internal Medicine, Medical Faculty of Maltepe University, Istanbul, Turkey

2 Department of Immunology and Rheumatology of Medical School of Dokuz Eylul Universty, Izmir, Turkey

References

[1] Feldmann, M., Brennan, F. M. & Maini, R. N. Rheumatoid arthritis. Cell 1996; **85**: 307–310.

[2] Feldmann, M., Brennan, F. M. & Maini, R. N. Role of cytokines in rheumatoid arthritis. Annu. Rev. Immunol. 1996; **14**: 397–440.

[3] Firestein, G. S. Evolving concepts of rheumatoid arthritis. Nature 2003; **423**: 356–361.

[4] McInnes, I. B. & Liew, F. Y. Cytokine networks—towards new therapies for rheumatoid arthritis. Nat. Clin. Pract. Rheumatol 2005; **1**: 31–39.

[5] Venkatesha, S. H., Dudics, S., Acharya, B. & Kamal D. Moudgil. Cytokine-modulating strategies and newer cytokine targets for arthritis therapy. Int. J. Mol. Sci. 2015; **16**: 887–906.

[6] Ponchel, F., Goéb, V., Parmar, R., El-Sherbiny, Y., Boissinot, M., El Jawhari, J., Burska, A., Vital, E. M., Harrison, S., Conaghan, P. G., Hensor, E & Emery, P. An immunological biomarker to predict MTX response in early RA. Ann. Rheum. Dis. 2014; **73**(11): 2047–2053.

[7] Kasama, T., Isozaki, T., Takahashi, R. & Miwa, Y. Clinical effects of tocilizumab on cytokines and immunological factors in patients with rheumatoid arthritis. Int. Immunopharmacol. 2016; **35**: 301–306.

[8] Burmester, G. R. et al. Emerging cell and cytokine targets in rheumatoid arthritis. Nat. Rev. Rheumatol. 2014; **10**: 77–88.

[9] van der Helm-van Mil, A. H., Wesoly, J. Z. & Huizinga, T. W. Understanding the genetic contribution to rheumatoid arthritis. Curr. Opin. Rheumatol. 2005; **17**: 299–304.

[10] Choy, E. Understanding the dynamics: pathways involved in the pathogenesis of rheumatoid arthritis. Rheumatology 2012; **51**: 3–11.

[11] Jimenez-Boj, E. et al. Interaction between synovial inflammatory tissue and bone marrow in rheumatoid arthritis. J. Immunol. 2005; **175**: 2579–2588.

[12] Chabaud, M. et al. Human interleukin-17: a T cell-derived proinflammatory cytokine produced by the rheumatoid synovium. Arthritis Rheum. 1999; **42**: 963–970.

[13] Joosten, L. A. et al. IL-32, a proinflammatory cytokine in rheumatoid arthritis. Proc. Natl. Acad. Sci. 2006; **103**: 3298–3303.

[14] Dayer, J. M. & Bresnihan, B. Targeting interleukin-1 in the treatment of rheumatoid arthritis. Arthritis Rheum. 2002; **46**: 574–578.

[15] Horai, R. et al. Development of chronic inflammatory arthropathy resembling rheumatoid arthritis in interleukin 1 receptor antagonist-deficient mice. J. Exp. Med. 2000; **191**: 313–320.

[16] Redlich, K. et al. Osteoclasts are essential for TNF-α-mediated joint destruction. J. Clin. Invest. 2002; **110**: 1419–1427.

[17] Nishimoto, N. & Kishimoto, T. Interleukin 6: from bench to bedside. Nat. Clin. Pract. Rheumatol. 2006; **2**: 619–626.

[18] Alonzi, T. et al. Interleukin 6 is required for the development of collagen-induced arthritis. J. Exp. Med. 1998; **187**: 461–468.

[19] McInnes, I. B., Leung, B. P., Sturrock, R. D., Field, M. & Liew, F. Y. Interleukin-15 mediates T celldependent regulation of tumor necrosis factor-α production in rheumatoid arthritis. Nat. Med. 1997;**3**: 189–195.

[20] Ferrari-Lacraz, S. et al. Targeting IL-15 receptor bearing cells with an antagonist mutant IL-15/Fc protein prevents disease development and progression in murine collagen-induced arthritis. J. Immunol. 2004; **173**: 5818–5826.

[21] Baslund, B. et al. Targeting interleukin-15 in patients with rheumatoid arthritis: a proof-of-concept study. Arthritis Rheum. 2005; **52**: 2686–2692.

[22] Suzuki, M., Konya, C., Goronzy, J. J. & Weyand, C. M. Inhibitory CD8+ T cells in autoimmune disease. Hum. Immunol. 2008; **69**(11): 781–789.

[23] Lubberts, E., Koenders, M. I. & van den Berg, W. B. The role of T-cell interleukin-17 in conducting destructive arthritis: lessons from animal models. Arthritis Res. Ther. 2005; **7**: 29–37.

[24] Weaver, C. T., Hatton, R. D., Mangan, P. R. & Harrington, L. E. IL-17 family cytokines and the expanding diversity of effector T cell lineages. Annu. Rev. Immunol. 2007; **25**: 821–852.

[25] Gracie, J. A. et al. A proinflammatory role for IL-18 in rheumatoid arthritis. J. Clin. Invest. 1999; **104**: 1393–1401.

[26] McInnes, I. B., Liew, F. Y. & Gracie, J. A. Interleukin-18: a therapeutic target in rheumatoid arthritis? Arthritis Res. Ther. 2004; **7**: 38–41.

[27] Manoury-Schwartz, B. et al. High susceptibility to collagen-induced arthritis in mice lacking IFN-γ receptors. J. Immunol. 1997; **158**: 5501–5506.

[28] Vermeire, K. et al. Accelerated collagen-induced arthritis in IFN-γ receptor-deficient mice. J. Immunol. 1997; **158**: 5507–5513.

[29] Di Franco, M., Gerardi, M. C., Lucchino, B. & Conti, F. Mavrilimumab: an evidence based review of its potential in the treatment of rheumatoid arthritis. Core Evid. 2014; 9: 41–48.

[30] Krabben A, Wilson AG, de Rooy DP, Zhernakova A, Brouwer E, Lindqvist E, Saxne T, Stoeken G, van Nies JA, Knevel R, Huizinga TW, Toes R, Gregersen PK, van der Helm-van Mil AH. Association of genetic variants in the IL4 and IL4R genes with the severity of joint damage in rheumatoid arthritis: a study in seven cohorts. Arthritis Rheum. 2013; **65**: 3051–7.

[31] Schulze-Koops, H. & Kalden, J. R. The balance of Th1/Th2 cytokines in rheumatoid arthritis. Best Pract. Res. Clin. Rheumatol. 2001; **15**: 677–691.

[32] Raza, K. et al. Early rheumatoid arthritis is characterized by a distinct and transientsy-novial fluid cytokine profile of T cell and stromal cell origin. Arthritis Res. Ther. 2005; **7**: R784–R795.

[33] Nalbant, S., Koc, B., Top, C., Kucukardali, Y., Baykal, Y., Danaci, M. & Kocer, I. Hypersensitivity vasculitis and cytokines. Rheumatol. Int. 2002; **22**(6): 244–248.

[34] Steven J. Van Dyken & Richard M. Locksley. Interleukin-4-and interleukin-13-mediated alternatively activated macrophages: roles in homeostasis and disease. Annu. Rev. Immunol. 2013; **31**: 317–343.

[35] Hsu, Y. H. & Chang, M. S. IL-20 in rheumatoid arthritis. Drug Discov Today. 2015; **19**. pii:S1359-6446(15)00312-8. doi:10.1016/j.drudis.2015.08.002 [Epub ahead of print]

[36] Cantagrel, A., Navaux, F., Loubet-Lescoulié, P., Nourhashemi, F., Enault, G., Abbal, M., Constantin, A., Laroche, M. & Maziéres, B. Interleukin-1β, interleukin-1 receptor antagonist, interleukin-4, and interleukin-10 gene polymorphisms: relationship to occurrence and severity of rheumatoid arthritis. Arthritis Rheum. 1999; **42**(6): 1093–1100.

[37] McMahan, C. J., Slack, J. L., Mosley, B., Cosman, D., Lupton, S. D., Brunton, L.L., Grubin, C. E., Wignall, J. M., Jenkins, N. A. & Brannan, C. I. A novel IL-1 receptor, cloned from B cells by mammalian expression, is expressed in many cell types. EMBO J. 1991; **10**(10): 2821–2832.

[38] Dripps, D. J., Verderber, E., Ng, R. K., Thompson, R. C. & Eisenberg, S. P. Interleukin-1 receptor antagonist binds to the type II interleukin-1 receptor on B cells and neutrophils. J. Biol. Chem. 1991; **266**(30): 20311–20315.

[39] Galvani, V. Soluble tumor necrosis factor receptor I (sTNFRI) as a prognostic factor in melanoma patients in Slovene population Article Pflügers Archiv. Eur. J. Physiol. 2000; **440**(5 Suppl): R61–R63.

[40] Bresnihan, B., Roux-Lombard, P., Murphy, E., Kane, D., FitzGerald, O., Dayer, J. M. Serum interleukin 18 and interleukin 18 binding protein in rheumatoid arthritis. Ann. Rheum. Dis. 2002; **61**: 726–729.

12

Rheumatoid Arthritis and Periodontal Disease: A Complex Interplay

Codrina Ancuta, Cristina Iordache,
Eugen Ancuta and Claudia Mihailov

Abstract

Recent advances in understanding the dynamic pathways involved in the pathogenesis of rheumatoid arthritis have emphasized the pivotal role of pro-inflammatory cytokines, inflammatory cells, endothelial cell activation and matrix degradation, acting in a genetically predisposed environment. On the other hand, there are significant amounts of data highlighting the potential role of bacteria (leading periodonthopatic pathogen *Porfiromonas gingivalis*) in promoting different types of arthritis, as well as the influence of periodontis (an infectious-inflammatory condition) as etiological or modulating factor in different pathologies, including cardio-vascular disorders, diabetes, respiratory disease and inflammatory rheumatic disorders (such as rheumatoid arthritis, ankylosing spondylitis and lupus). The present chapter deals with the possible association between rheumatoid arthritis and periodontitis as entities with common pathological events.

Keywords: rheumatoid arthritis, periodontitis, *Porfiromonas gingivalis*, citrullination, anti-citrullinated antibodies

1. Introduction

Rheumatoid arthritis (RA) and periodontitis are chronic inflammatory disorders that share a complex, multifaceted host-mediated pathobiology promoted by significant levels of inflammatory mediators that are able to induce synovium and periodontal tissues inflammation, joint damage and alveolar bone loss, respectively [1–7].

RA, a chronic inflammatory autoimmune disease with articular as well as systemic consequences, is outlined by a dynamic pathobiology with chronic synovitis as the epicenter of immunologic responses, inflammation and tissue destruction, occurring as a response to an initiating event (microbial exposure) or a putative antigen in genetically predisposed host [1–11].

On the other hand, known as a destructive, dysbiotic inflammatory condition that concerns gums, periodontal disease or periodontitis is typically characterized by rapid tooth loss directed by local anaerobic bacterial colonization (the "red complex" microorganisms with leading *Porphiromonas gingivalis*), biofilm-related periodontal inflammation, subsequent neutrophilic and immune activation, soft tissue destruction and alveolar bone loss [1–12].

The bidirectional relationship between periodontitis and RA is governed by common genetic (HLA-DR) and environmental influences (smoking), chronic inflammatory events with immunoregulatory imbalance (excessive TNF-α, IL-1β, IL-6, IL-11, IL-17 activation, prostaglandin E2, nitric oxide, matrix metalloproteinases), osteoclast activation (RANKL overregulation) promoting active bone destruction and periodontal lesions, bacterial factors, persistence of antigens, citrullination of endogenous proteins by the means of peptidyl arginine deiminase as second inflammatory event [1–13].

Furthermore, the association among periodontal disease and RA has been extensively addressed in recent years, emphasizing the role of gingival microorganisms, particularly *Porphyromonas gingivalis* (*P. gingivalis*), as the underlying link between dental and rheumatic pathology via citrullination [1–10].

We systematically reviewed data from literature focusing on inflammation and tissue-damaging aspects, oral microbiota, antibodies against bacteria and autoantibodies and treatment for both RA and periodontitis, aiming to explore the relationship between both diseases.

2. A closer look to periodontitis

2.1. Pathobiology of periodontitis

As a chronic immuno-inflammatory disease and a consequence of an infectious trigger that originally involves gingival soft tissue, periodontitis is classically characterized by the destruction of periodontium and surrounding connective tissue matrix [1–11]. It is a complex, dynamic and progressive condition, resulting from a continuing cross-talk between microbial challenge and host inflammatory and immune response [1–7].

The extent and severity of periodontitis, as well as disease staging covers a sequence of pathobiologic steps comprising gingivitis, plaque accumulation and chronic inflammation, colonization by periodontopathogenic anaerobes, loss of connective tissue attachments to teeth, bone resorption and, ultimately, tooth loss [1–10].

The oral cavity behaves as a perpetual source of infectious, generally nonpathogenic agents; however, subgingival microbiota may accumulate to shape this biofilm through particular settings, and favor networking between pathogens and host tissues, with or without direct dissemination [1–11].

The pathways underlying chronic periodontitis encompass for an intricate array of events, starting with gingival colonization by *P. gingivalis*, chronic inflammation, immune-mediated periodontal damage and alveolar bone loss, local citrullination, host immune response [1–11].

A schematic overview of the microbial and host-associated pathology in periodontal disease is represented in **Figure 1**.

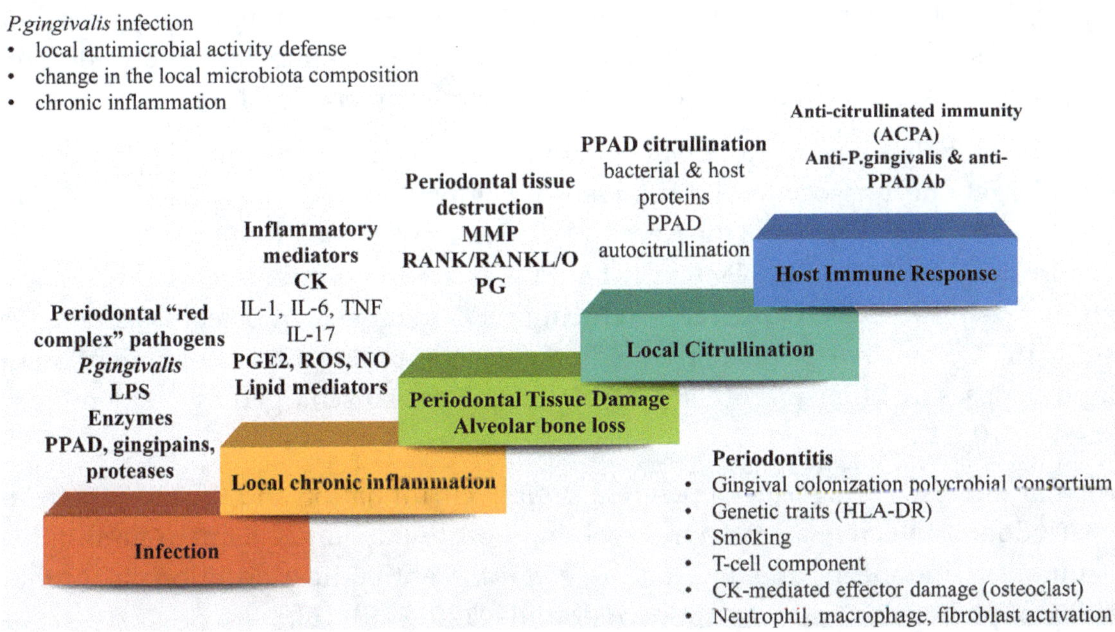

Figure 1. Sequence of events in chronic periodontitis.

It is widely recognized that the oral microbiota arising in a tolerant genetic background is involved in the initiation and extension of periodontal disease [1–12]. Several bacterial species, e.g., *P. gingivalis, Treponema denticola (T. denticola), Tannerella forsythia (T. forsythia)* and *Aggregatibacter actinomycetemcimtans*, the so-called red complex [1–12], remain of particular relevance as they are true pathogens and late colonizers of the oral biofilm, act synergistically and by co-aggregation with the support of attaching bacteria through specific adhesion molecules [1–10].

Further, *P. gingivalis* is able to release pathogen-associated molecular patterns, specifically lipopolissacharides (LPS), peptidoglycans, proteases and lytic enzymes, engaging local immune cell trafficking and activation—neutrophils (acting to protect the host from periodontal pathogens as the first-line defenders), macrophages (as potent antigen-presenting cells), T-cells and B-cells (perpetuating and amplifying inflammatory response and antibody synthesis) [1–11].

However, *P. gingivalis* escapes the local antimicrobial defense as a result of delayed neutrophil apoptosis and complement system manipulation with subsequent change in the gingival bacterial composition [11].

To better understand, *P. gingivalis* encourages the immune subversion by several strategies including: IL-8 inhibition, complement manipulation and toll-like receptor 4 (TLR4) antagonism, leading to impaired host defense. Symbiotic gingival microbiota with tissue homeostasis swaps to dysbiotic environment, with inflammation and bone loss as main attributes of periodontal disease [1, 8, 11, 12].

Locally recruited cells release a wide range of factors, such as pro-inflammatory cytokines (TNF-α, IL-1β, IL-6, IL-8, IL-12, IL-11, IL-17), reactive oxygen species, prostaglandin E2, nitric oxide, and other inflammatory mediators in the gingival tissue and gingival crevicular fluid as well [1–5, 11–14]. Otherwise, anti–inflammatory cytokines including IL-10 and TGF-β1 are down regulated in active periodontal lesions, demonstrating an imbalance between pro- and anti-inflammatory systems in the periodontal microenvironment [1, 11].

Although the initial trigger of gingival inflammation is microbial, the cytokine-mediated damage is largely host-associated [1–10]. Hence, augmented TNF-α, IL-1β, IL-6, IL-11, and, particularly, IL-17 directly control the Receptor Activator of NF-κB/Receptor Activator of NF-κB Ligand/osteoprotegerin (RANK/RANKL/OPG) system and stimulate osteoclastogenesis through increasing RANKL expression reducing OPG synthesis in osteoblasts and stromal cells [1–11, 15]. Connective tissue matrix degradation is supplementary dependent on matrix metalloproteinases (MMPs) and other proteolytic enzymes discharged by resident activated fibroblasts [1, 10, 11].

Of particular interest, *P. gingivalis*-dependent protein citrullination and the immune response to the periodontal infective aggression involving both innate and adaptive immunity (e.g., anti-citrullinated immunity and IgG anti-*P. gingivalis* antibodies) additionally outline the complexity of pathogenic pathways in periodontitis [1–5, 7–10, 15].

Periodontis is a multifactorial condition, where environmental factors (including oral hygiene, gingival bacterial plaque, smoking, stress), and genetic polymorphism (HLA-DR alleles, IL-1 gene promoter, IL-6 and IL-10 genes) perform critical role in the expression of the disease [1, 4, 10, 11, 15, 16].

Recent data agreed that chronic periodontitis is a risk factor for many multisystem diseases including rheumatoid arthritis and other auto-inflammatory rheumatic conditions, cardio and cerebrovascular disease (atherosclerosis, myocardial infarction, stroke), diabetes, osteoporosis, respiratory and neurodegenerative disorders, adverse pregnancy outcomes [1, 17, 18]. In fact, locally exacerbated and ongoing systemic inflammation, specific tissue damage, mutual triggers (smoking, iatrogenic factors) acting in a genetic vulnerable individuals (HLA-DRβ1) uphold a modulating bidirectional relationship between periodontitis and the above mentioned entities [1–18].

It is obvious that chronic periodontitis remains an authentic infection of the oral cavity; biofilm-associated specific microorganisms are essential but not sufficient, as the bacterial eradication does not spontaneously manage to resolution of periodontitis [1–18].

2.2. *Porphyromonas gingivalis* as a key player in periodontitis

Chronic periodontitis is, therefore, typically initiated by the colonization of dental plaque by a core set of periodontal pathogens, specifically *P. gingivalis, T. forsythia* and *T. denticola*, documented as the "red complex", prototype of polybacterial pathogenic consortium in periodontitis [1–5, 7–11, 19].

P. gingivalis, a leading microorganism in this dysbiotic setting, is a gram-negative anaerobic bacteria, involved in the onset of inflammation and tissue destruction during periodontal disease [1–11]. It is ordinarily found in small number in a healthy oral cavity [11], but the pathology occurs when *P. gingivalis* binds to and accumulates on the tooth surface, leading to the development of a mixed biofilm, the expansion of the bacteria into the gingival sulcus and the formation of a periodontal pocket [11, 19].

P. gingivalis is an outstanding example of a bacteria able to shape the periodontal microenvironment and to destabilize the homeostatic immune system endorsing chronic inflammation and tissue damage as well [11].

At least four mechanisms currently advocate for its essential role in the pathobiology of periodontal disease: (i) the release of specific virulence factors such as specific lipopolysaccharide (LPS), fimbrae, hemagglutins and several enzymes, mainly cysteine proteases (gingipains), but also collagenase, gelatinase, hyaluronidase promoting a chronic inflammatory setting and local invasion [2, 3, 11, 20]; (ii) the expression of peptidyl arginine deiminase (PAD) involved in tissue citrullination, loss of tolerance against neo-epitopes and subsequent activation of adaptive immune response [1, 2, 3, 20]; (iii) auto-citrullination of its own PAD [1, 2, 3, 11, 20]; and (iv) enable other co-aggregating pathogenic bacteria to remain in the periodontal tissue [2].

P. gingivalis expresses atypical LPS, proceeding either as a weak TLR4 agonist or even a TLR4 antagonist, enabling the colonization and invasion of periodontal pockets as it becomes immunologically silent [1, 2, 8, 11, 21]. Furthermore, *P.gingivalis* invades gingival epithelial cells via binding through its fimbriae to β1 integrin on the host epithelial cell surface [4, 5, 11] and blocks apoptosis through the PI3K/Akt and JAK/Stat pathways, allowing intracellular bacterial proliferation [11].

The true virulence of *P. gingivalis* is, however, associated with its proteolytic enzymes, particularly extracellular arginine and lysine-specific cysteine endopeptidases (gingipain R and gingipain K, respectively) [1–5, 11]. Gingipains are skilled to facilitate the evasion of host defense and cause tissue injury by activation of MMPs (1, 3, 9) and further degradation of host proteins (laminin, fibronectin and collagen) [1, 2, 8 11, 22–24]. Moreover, these enzymes are responsible for the resistance of *P. gingivalis* killing by complement [1, 2, 8, 11]. Remarkably, the degradation of microbial peptides by gingipains allows other pathogenic bacteria co-aggregating with *P. gingivalis* to persist in the gingiva [2, 8, 11, 15, 20, 25]. Finally, gingipains affect proinflammatory signaling pathways by cleavage and activation of the proteinase-activated receptor-2 on human neutrophils [2, 11, 15, 20]. Futile attempts by the host immune response to eliminate infection subsequently lead to connective tissue damage, including alveolar bone resorption [22].

P. gingivalis is a particular periodontal pathogen that expresses endogenous peptidyl-arginine deiminase (PPAD), a citrullinating enzyme bearing potential to generate antigens driving autoimmunity in susceptible individuals [1, 2, 8, 10, 11].

It is worth mentioning that the switching of a charged arginine residue to an uncharged citrulline results in evident, irreversible posttranslational protein modifications, meaning changes in the three-dimensional conformation and abnormal function [8, 10, 17]. Citrullinated antigens as neo-epitopes in the periodontal tissues may selectively activate adaptive immune response and break the self-tolerance leading to severe aggressive periodontitis, anti-cyclic citrullinated peptides, anti-*P. gingivalis* antibodies as well, and, potentially, to the development of RA in genetically predisposed hosts [1–3, 20, 25].

PAD-mediated citrullination is also responsible for evading host defense against *P. gingivalis* by two additional mechanisms: generation of ammonia that result in a favorable microenvironment for anaerobic bacteria and inactivation of certain chemokines contributing to neutrophil recruitment into the gingiva [8, 10, 11, 17].

Besides, *P. gingivalis* stimulates a true "local chemokine paralysis" by inhibiting the expression of IL-18 on epithelial cells [8, 11], delaying the traffic of neutrophils and, therefore, permitting its persistence and/or proliferation in the periodontal tissue with subsequent modification of the subgingival microbiota [11, 25].

2.3. *P. gingivalis* peptidyl-arginine deiminase (PPAD) *versus* peptidyl-arginine deiminase (PAD) biology

There is accumulating evidence to outline the citrullination status and biology of PPAD *versus* human PAD, supporting the hypothesis that PPAD is a reliable challenger for inducing autoimmunity, with particular relevance to the pathogenesis of RA [1, 2, 10, 11, 17, 20, 22, 26, 27].

This apparently distinctive bacterial enzyme is effective in generating citrullinated proteins (bacterial and human) and, furthermore, has the ability to autocitrullinate, eliciting the loss of immune tolerance and synthesis of autoantibodies in susceptible individuals [1–5, 7–11, 22].

To date, five isoforms of human PADs (PAD1, 2, 3, 4/5, and 6) are described, with specificities for different tissues and different physiological functions [2, 3, 10]; however, none of them present strict homology with bacterial PAD [1, 2, 10, 11, 17, 27], and only PAD2 and PAD4 are expressed at the synovial level and involved in RA [1, 3, 10, 26].

The main differences between human and bacterial PAD focus on the mechanism of activation and substrates undergoing citrullination [1, 10, 11]. Thus, PPAD is a calcium-independent enzyme that becomes active at higher pH that PAD; its action is facilitated by the co-localization with arginine-specific gingipains in the outer membrane of *P. gingivalis* [1, 2, 10, 11, 20, 25]. PPAD act specifically on C-terminal arginine residues and free arginine [1, 2], events enabled by the proteolytic activity of gingipains. In fact, we talk about a two-step process in the inflamed-infected periodontal sites, initiated by cysteine protease gingipains that cleave protein chains and expose the C-terminal arginine, facilitating the secondary intervention of PPAD [1, 2, 10, 11, 25].

Other substrates citrullinated by PPAD include peptides resulted from fibrinogen and α-enolase degradation by gingipains [2, 10], fibrin and vimentin, bradykinin with the potential impairment of kinin proinflammatory activity [2, 10, 20, 25], and the C-terminal arginine residue of the epidermal growth factor influencing its biologic activity [2, 10, 25, 27, 28].

Finally, PPAD allows, either directly or indirectly (via enhancement of inflammatory reactions and release of host PADs), the abnormal citrullination of bacterial and human proteins with the assembly of the so-called cryptic-epitopes and subsequent antibody production [1, 2, 10, 11, 20, 25].

2.4. PPAD and PAD autocitrullination

Although PPAD preferentially citrullinates different bacterial and/or host peptides bearing C-terminal arginine, it becomes clear that this enzyme may undergo autocitrullination and, hence, stimulate a specific pattern of autoimmunity and request for autoantibody response in permissive genetic background (carriers of HLA-DRB1 shared epitope) [2, 10, 20]. There is a heightened immune response to *P. gingivalis* and IgG specifically targeting autocitrullinated PPAD in chronic periodontal disease and rheumatoid arthritis which could perpetuate the immune response through epitope spreading and cross-reactivity with citrullinated human proteins suggesting a potential mechanistic linkage between the two disorders [10, 11, 25, 29, 30]. Of interest, PAD4 also experiences autocitrullination, and antibodies recognizing this isoform of human PAD embrace predictive value in RA [10, 11, 26, 27, 31].

To summarize, the infection with *P. gingivalis* triggers a broad spectrum of local and systemic inflammatory, destructive and immune events in susceptible individuals. Strategic steps in the complex pathobiology of periodontitis comprise early release of a true arsenal of specialized virulence factors and bacteria-danger signals (LPS, fimbriae, peptidoglycan, various proteolytic enzymes) exerting both direct and indirect effects (via stimulation of inflammatory and immune pathways, release of host PAD), followed by aberrant PPAD-dependent citrullination of different substrates such as host-derived and bacterial proteins, as well as PPAD-autocitrullination, with subsequent generation of criptic epitopes and autoantibody synthesis. Finally, the immune subversion endorses loss of tolerance to structurally similar host proteins and outcomes the induction of anti-cyclic citrullinated antibodies suggesting the relationship between chronic periodontitis and rheumatoid arthritis [1, 2, 10, 13, 17, 19, 20, 25].

3. Role of citrullination in rheumatoid arthritis development

Citrullination is a posttranslational modification of proteins at arginine residues reported in a wide range of tissues and settings, holding relevant physiologic as well as pathologic implications [10, 17, 27, 32]. Although considered a critical event in different inflammatory conditions, currently available data emphasize the link between citrullination and autoimmune diseases, suggesting that immunity towards citrullinated self-proteins rather than citrullination itself is a specific event in RA [10, 17, 27].

3.1. Citrullination and inflammation

Abnormal citrullination of endogenous proteins is typically acknowledged as an initial, tactical process in the complex pathobiology of RA, driving the induction of altered self-epitopes and extensive autoimmune response [10, 17, 27].

Moreover, immunogenicity of these new antigens explains the presence of antibodies against citrullinated peptides (ACPA) considered not only diagnostic biomarkers for RA and prognostic factors for severe aggressive disease, but also consuming a pathogenic role [10, 17, 27]. Nevertheless, only individuals with definite HLA polymorphisms, such as the conserved region of HLA-DRB1 alleles are at risk to recognize as "nonself" such citrullinated proteins and to develop RA [1, 2, 10, 17, 27].

Along with glycosylation and carbamylation, citrullination is basically involved in many physiological processes in a variety of tissues, biochemical enzymatic reactions leading to structural and functional protein/peptide modification [2, 10, 17, 27]. Conversely, dysfunctional posttranslational protein modifications are often reported during autoinflammatory pathology, particularly RA, evading the immunological tolerance and stimulating a specific profile of humoral response [2, 10, 17, 26, 27].

As mentioned before, citrullination or deamination strictly encompass for a change of arginine with citrulline, meaning that an imine nitrogen of arginine-residues is replaced by an atom of oxygen; accordingly, histone modification, genomic regulation and neutrophils extracellular trap (NET) formation are described and engaged in development of newly citrullinated antigens [10, 17, 27].

It is well-known that citrullination constantly requires the activation and intervention of PAD-family enzymes at intra and/or extracellular levels in a Ca^{2+}-dependent manner, and only two out of the five human PAD subtypes (PAD 2 and PAD4) are relevant for RA based on their expression in joints, immune cells, neutrophils and mast cells [1, 10, 11, 12, 17, 26, 27]. Thus, PAD-mediated citrullination could be easily classified as a basic cellular damage but also an inflammatory process occurring in a range of inflammatory backgrounds such as synovial tissue, gingival and periodontal sites and lungs, challenging local immunity [10, 17, 27].

On the other hand, recent advances in understanding the pathophysiology of chronic periodontal infection with *P. gingivalis*, and the potential connection between periodontitis and systemic disorders including RA, have reemphasized the role of this periodonthopathic microbe as one of the risk factors for RA in a permissive genetic context [1–11, 17, 27].

P. gingivalis is the only known periodontal bacteria in the gingival microbiota that expresses a PPAD able to initiate and perpetuate a gradual autoimmune process through epitope-spreading by peptide citrullination (bacterial, PPAD itself as a citrulllinated bacterial protein), cross-reactivity with citrullinated human proteins and ACPA synthesis [1, 2, 10, 11, 25].

The break of tolerance to one citrullinated epitope predisposes to break of tolerance to additional citrullinated epitopes; the initial mechanism might be more related to recognition of citrullinated antigen per se than to a particular citrullinated autoantigen [10, 11, 26, 32, 33].

3.2. Smoking, citrullination and rheumatoid arthritis

Environment-triggered citrullination (smoking, bacterial infections) in articular and extra-articular locations essentially progress to specific immunity and disease in genetic predisposed individuals [1, 2, 10, 12, 16, 32, 34, 35]. Smoking is a well-known risk factor for RA, particularly, in ACPA-positive subsets. Cigarette smoking leads to a sequence of events responsible for local increase in PAD enzyme expression and consequent generation of protein citrullination in the lung [10, 12, 17, 27]. Chronic exposure to self-citrullinated epitopes could further contribute to the loss of immune tolerance and gradual occurrence of humoral immune response towards some of the citrullinated autoantigens (ACPA) [10, 17, 27]. However, smoking and other risk factors might lead to breaking of immune tolerance only in the presence of genetic risk factors for ACPA positive RA [10, 12, 17, 26, 27, 36].

3.3. Anti-citrullinated proteins/peptide antibodies (ACPA) pathobiology

ACPAs, the autoimmune signature of RA, are sensitive and specific diagnostic, prognostic and therapeutic biomarkers in RA; they are detected from very early phases of the disease, up to a decade prior to the RA clinical onset, and feature a dynamic correlation with RA severity, clinical outcomes and efficacy of synthetic and biologic therapies [10, 37, 38]. In fact, ACPAs are a family of partly cross-reactive antibodies which target citrullinated self-proteins and peptides abundant in inflamed joints, such as fibrinogen, fibronectin, vimentin and vinculin, β-enolase, histone, biglycan, clusterin, collagen type II, keratin. So far, 53 such citrullinated members are identified, an assembly called "citrullinome" [10, 12, 17, 27].

According to the ACPA status, RA could be classified in two distinct clinical phenotypes with particular genetics, risk factors, immunopathology, clinical and treatment outcomes; thus, ACPA-positive RA is defined by a specific genetic (HLA-DRB1*0401 and *0404)- environmental interface (e.g., smoking and *P. gingivalis* infection), higher disease severity (erosive RA, extra-articular involvement, comorbidities) and poor remission rates. Besides, high ACPA titers could predict clinical response with B-cell depletive agents (rituximab) or selective co-stimulation modulators (abatacept), independently of disease activity and, therefore, might help to define therapeutic RA profiles [10, 11, 16, 17, 27, 28, 36].

Interestingly, ACPA specificities may also account for distinctive clinical RA subtypes: anti-citrullinated vimentin antibodies may be better prognostic factors for radiographic progression, while anti-citrullinated enolase antibodies predict clinical outcomes [10, 17, 27].

ACPAs are detected as antibodies against cyclic citrullinated proteins (anti-CCP antibodies) which are detectable by specific assays in RA patients, and their screening performance largely varies with different tests: sensitivity and specificity significantly improved with third-generation assays, as well as the ability to identify those subjects with undifferentiated arthritis who are likely to develop RA [10, 17]. Conversely, second-generation tests are classically more specific for longstanding, established disease [10, 17, 39].

The exact molecular pathways of anti-citrullinated immunity in RA are still obscure, but it is clear that ACPAs encourage the perpetuation of synovial inflammation via binding to citrullinated proteins positioned in the cellular membrane, attached to a variety of cellular receptors (such as TLR4 or FcγR) or incorporated in NETs [1–4, 10, 11, 17]. Furthermore, complement binding and activation may enhance local inflammation [7, 12, 17, 27].

ACPAs are constantly produced in the inflamed synovial microenvironment by locally activated B cells [17, 27] and stimulate TNFα production, as well as direct bone injury by osteoclast activation [6, 10, 17, 27, 39, 40].

Overall, the effector functions of different well-defined ACPA may adjust according to antibody specificities. Thus, reactivity towards citrullinated vimentin as well as anti-cartilage-specific protein collagen II antibodies directly bind to osteoclast surface and modulate their activation, determining subchondral bone erosive lesions and osteoporosis [10, 12, 40]. On the other hand, antibodies to autoantigenic enolase and histones focus on local inflammation [10, 12, 17, 27], as ACPAs are able to induce NETs.

3.4. The paradigm of citrullination and ACPA in the development of ACPA positive rheumatoid arthritis

The environmental exposure (such as smoking, silica and other nanomaterials of air pollution, bacterial infection, e.g., *P. gingivalis*) and the genetic determinants (MHC class II alleles) enable abnormal citrullination and support immunity against citrullinated proteins in certain extra-articular sites (lung, periodontal tissue). The relationship between the emergence of local ACPAs as the first sign of autoimmunity and RA is further supported by the documentation of shared citrullinated peptides in the lungs, periodontal sites and joints as potential ACPA epitope bearing proteins [10, 17, 27].

A second event might promote aberrant synovial citrullination, local impaired immunity, generation of ACPA for several immune-dominant citrullinated peptide, chronic inflammation and tissue-specific damage [10, 17, 27].

4. The biological link between periodontitis and rheumatoid arthritis

Continuing periodontal disease as a trigger for chronic arthritis in susceptible individuals via dysregulation in oral microbiota and host immune barriers is a reliable, but still debatable concept [1, 2, 8, 10–12]. The old paradigm indicates that RA could be a consistent risk factor for chronic periodontitis: impaired periodontal health labels the multifactorial and synergistic result of compromised joint functionality (hand as well as temporomandibular joint), oral dryness (secondary Sjogren's) and specific RA medications [8].

In contrast, newer theories emphasize that periodontal disease is a risk factor for RA: both are multifaceted disorders with shared pathogenic mechanisms such as local and systemic excess of inflammation, irreversible bone injury, aberrant activation of the immune system with an extra dose of autoimmunity and a common genetic background [1–5, 8, 41–45].

4.1. Evidences relating periodontitis and rheumatoid arthritis

Substantial amount of research trying to clarify the potential relationship between RA and periodontitis was published during the last decade [1–13]. Nevertheless, the true prevalence, causality, significance, related factors (e.g., smoking habits, oral hygiene, ACPA positivity), together with therapeutic intervention (periodontal host modulation therapy, synthetic remissive drugs, biologics) to mitigate both RA and periodontal disease are still controversial [1–13, 17, 27].

Overwhelming evidence coming from cross-sectional studies [1–13, 10, 40, 46–48] showed a statistically significant correlation between RA and periodontitis (prevalence and/or severity); nevertheless, other cohort-based or case-control studies noticed no association between oral health and rheumatic inflammatory pathology [1, 2, 10, 12]. The conflicting reports may be explained by differences between study populations, sample size, adjustments for confounders (age, gender, race/ethnicity, smoking status, RA activity and medication) and lack of uniformity in disease classification criteria for periodontal disease [49].

The probability of periodontitis among RA is higher compared to healthy individuals [1–4, 8, 47], while the severity greater [1–4, 8, 15, 47], meaning that subjects diagnosed with RA experience more periodontal disease and more periodontal destruction [1, 8, 15]. Furthermore, moderate to severe periodontitis is characteristically described in different settings of RA [1, 8], and vice-versa, higher RA prevalence among patients with advanced periodontitis [1, 8, 15, 47, 49]. Both early and established RA are characterized by substantial periodontal disease compared with presumably healthy non-RA controls [1–4, 6, 8, 44, 45]: higher prevalence of self-reported periodontal symptoms [8], significant more gingival bleeding on probing [1–4, 6, 8], a greater number of missing teeth [1–4, 6, 8], deeper periodontal pockets [1–4, 6, 8], more clinical attachment loss [1–4, 6, 8] and increased alveolar bone injury [1–4, 6, 8] versus healthy controls with comparable oral hygiene [1–4, 6, 8, 44, 45].

More specifically, a meaningful positive correlation between measures of RA activity and extent and severity of periodontitis was reported: high disease activity (DAS28 scores) is generally demonstrated in RA with aggressive periodontitis as compared to RA without or with moderate periodontitis, even after adjusting for multiple confounders [4, 8, 47].

A systematic review of cross-sectional trials further strengthens the evidence addressing periodontitis in relation to autoimmunity damage in RA. Overall, significantly higher ACPA, rheumatoid factor and antibodies to *P. gingivalis* were described among RA with periodontitis than those without periodontal disease [4, 8, 11, 47], whereas increased alveolar bone loss was significantly associated with ACPA positivity in the same patient population [4]. Similarly, detailed analysis of ACPA specificities (citrullinated vimentin and histone) showed increased levels in RA associated with both moderate and high alveolar loss, without differences based on smoking status [4, 15, 16, 26, 48–50]. It seems that periodontitis is a strong predictor of ACPA positivity in RA [8], whereas IgG and IgM ACPA subtypes are highly associated with antibodies against *P. gingivalis* [2, 3, 8, 29]. Additionally, in refractory RA with periodontitis the most powerful anaerobes identified in synovial fluid are *P. intermedia, P. gingivalis* and *T. denticola* [1, 40, 41]. However, no difference in ACPA or rheumatoid factor levels for RA participants with mild periodontal lesions as compared to moderate or severe periodontitis were found among other studies, suggesting that ACPA status might not influence the prevalence and severity of periodontal disease [1, 8, 11, 49].

Regarding smoking as a risk factor for both conditions, subgroup analysis showed an association between RA and periodontitis irrespective to smoking behavior [4, 6, 8, 15, 16, 48, 49]; increased risk of periodontitis was demonstrated in nonsmoking RA [1, 6, 8, 11].

In particular, only a small number of studies focused on periodontitis as a primary event, occurring before clinical onset of RA *versus* periodontitis as comorbidity, described after the diagnosis of rheumatic condition [1, 8, 11].

Finally, effective treatment strategies for periodontal disease (e.g., nonsurgical treatment) on RA activity and systemic inflammation are commonly reported [1, 3, 4, 50, 51].

4.2. A parallel between chronic periodontal disease and rheumatoid arthritis

Exploring the association between chronic periodontal disease and RA has demonstrated striking similar immunological, biological and genetic underlying processes [1, 2, 4, 12, 22], although apparently totally different etiologies (autoimmune RA, infective periodontitis respectively) [10]. **Figure 2** offers a detailed synopsis of similarities between RA and periodontitis.

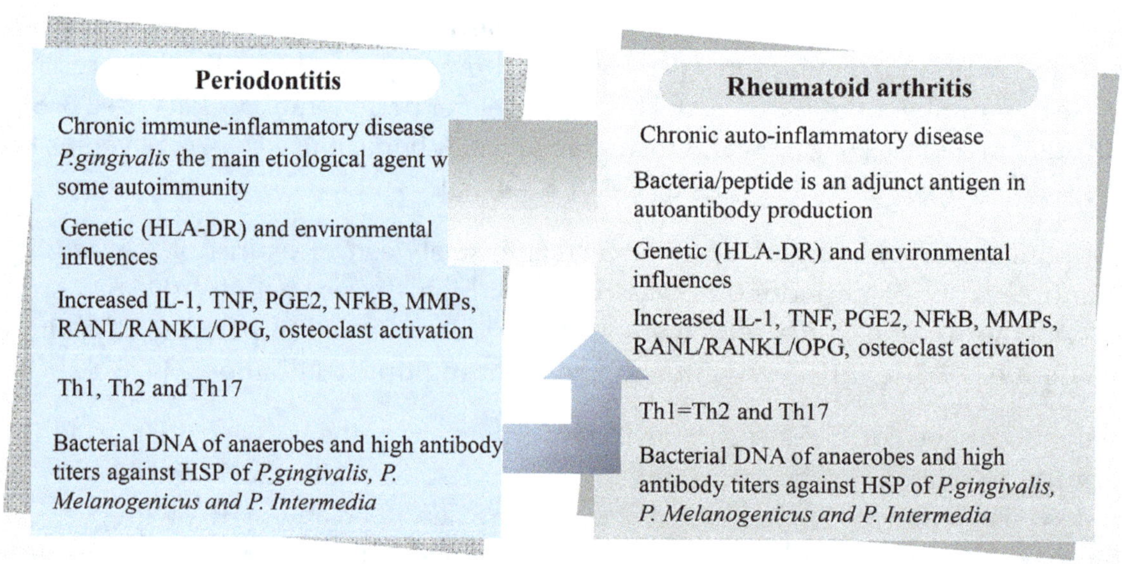

Figure 2. Similarities between PD and RA pathobiology.

Both are complex multifactorial disorders, characterized not only by a dysfunction of basic inflammatory and tissue destructive mechanisms, but also by an altered adaptive and innate immune response in individuals at risk (genetic traits) [1, 2, 8, 10, 12, 22].

The excess of local (periodontal tissue and gingival crevicular fluid in periodontitis, synovial microenvironment in RA) along with systemic chronic inflammation is driven by an imbalance between pro-inflammatory and anti-inflammatory cytokines, with persistent up-regulated pro-inflammatory signaling pathways (mainly IL-1, IL-6, TNFα, NF-kB) and higher amounts of inflammatory mediators including reactive oxygen species, nitric oxide and lipid mediators [1–3, 8, 10–12, 22]. In addition, altered connective tissue and bone homeostasis with irreversible damage of collagen-rich structures (gingiva, periodontal ligament and alveolar bone in periodontitis, subchondral bone and cartilage in RA) is essentially related to augmented activity of collagenolytic matrix metalloproteinases and other enzymes (elastase, bacterial cysteine proteases, neutrophil associated enzymes), but also to overexpression of the RANK/RANKL/OPG system [1–3, 8, 10, 12, 13, 45].

The validity of the relationship between periodontitis and RA is, furthermore, supported by a particular genetic predisposition and related environmental risk factors (e.g., smoking) [1, 8, 10, 12]; both entities share a common genetic profile (shared epitope HLA-DRB1 alleles) [1, 10, 12], while polymorphism of genes encoding inflammatory cytokines as well as IL-1 combined risk alleles which may cause a synergistic effect on bone destruction in joints and the periodontium might also confer susceptibility for RA and periodontitis [1, 8, 10, 12, 15, 16].

Finally, abnormal PAD and PPAD-mediated citrullination of the synovial and host periodontium peptides/proteins (vimentin, keratin, α-enolase), respectively, with sequential loss of tolerance against neo-epitopes account for altered local and systemic immune reactions in susceptible patients with either periodontitis or RA; the generation of citrullinated new autoantigens and patterns of antibody response by ACPA, anti-autocitrullinated PPAD, anti-autocitrullinated PAD4 and anti-heat shock proteins of *P. gingivalis* (anti-hsp70) antibodies are frequently encountered in both RA and periodontitis [1, 10, 12, 15, 25, 30, 45].

Overall, gingival citrullination and local induction of ACPA, as well as cross-reactivity between antibodies to *P. gingivalis* and ACPA may explain the link periodontitis—RA [1, 10, 12, 27].

4.3. Hypothetical model of biological link Between rheumatoid arthritis and periodontitis

A potential scenario exploring the relation between periodontitis and RA could be depicted as follows:

- oral infection with *P. gingivalis* may induce a Th17 polarization with subsequent activation of Th17 signaling pathway, synthesis of pro-inflammatory cytokines (preferentially IL-1β, IL-6, IL-22, TNF-α, TGFβ and IL-23), expression of PPAD with atypical PPAD- and PAD-dependent citrullination of gingival proteins, bacterial peptides and PPAD as well, synthesis of specific antibodies such as ACPA, anti-citrullinated PPAD and anti-*P. gingivalis* antibodies [1, 4, 8, 10–13, 19, 52];
- periodontopathic microbial biofilm and its metabolic products (lipopolysaccharides, matrix degrading enzymes and endotoxins) originally stimulate a localized inflammatory-destructive response branded by augmented levels of tissue destructive proteinases (MMP 8, 9, 13 and neutrophil elastase) and RANK/RANKL/OPG system, as well as resident cells activation (osteoclasts, fibroblasts) [1, 4, 8, 12];

- systemic inflammation and immune dysregulation particularly autoimmunity targeting self-citrullinated synovial peptides delineate one of the first events in RA [1, 4, 8, 10, 12].

Figure 3 presents the paradigm of RA—periodontitis pathogenic link.

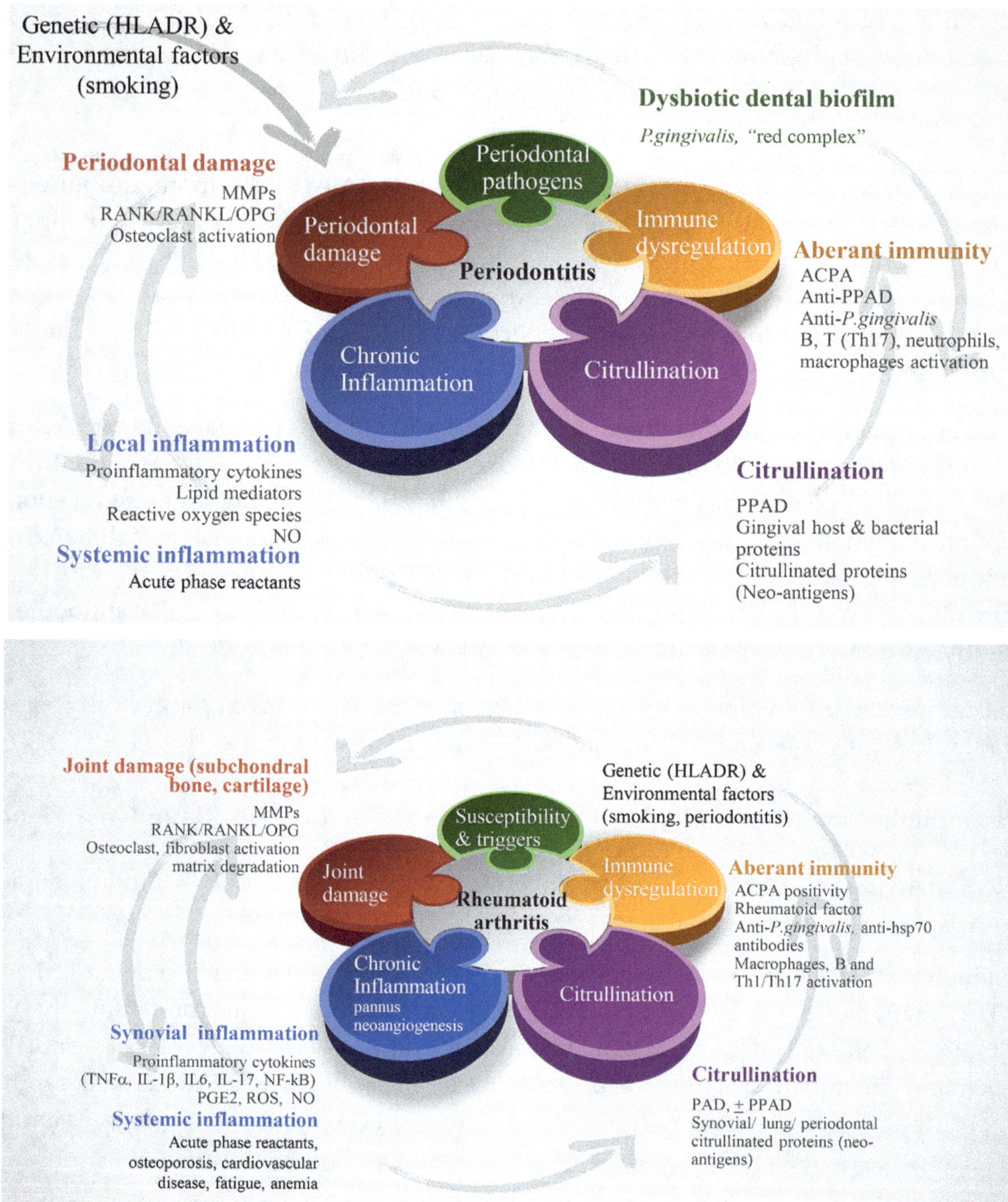

Figure 3. The paradigm of RA—periodontitis pathogenic link.

A 'two-hit' model for the link between periodontitis and systemic diseases including RA have already been proposed by Gloub et al. [4] and recently modified, evoking a sharp cascade of events: induction of severe chronic periodontitis by local and systemic factors in relation to RA ('first hit'), and their mitigation by periodontal host modulating therapy ('second hit') [4].

4.4. Therapeutic interferences in rheumatoid arthritis and chronic periodontitis

Current evidences suggests that periodontal treatment may influence clinical outcomes of RA and vice-versa, stipulating the potential advantage of host-modulating therapy to concomitantly control both disorders [1, 4, 8, 48, 50, 53–57].

4.4.1. Effects of therapy for periodontitis on rheumatoid arthritis disease activity and systemic inflammation

It was advocated that specific therapies for periodontitis not only improve disease activity and severity in RA by removing periodontal infection and gingival inflammation, but also improve patient response to therapeutic drugs [1, 8, 50, 53, 54].

Thus, nonsurgical periodontal therapy was directed to improve both signs and symptoms of active RA as well as periodontal status [1, 8, 12]. Similarly, advanced periodontal treatment with scaling and root planning significantly ameliorated gingival infection and severity of periodontitis, while promoting consistent reduction in acute phase reactants, mainly erythrocyte sedimentation rate, in the RA population [1, 8, 12, 53, 54]. The impact of periodontal treatment on RA seems to be greater in patients with substantial amount of systemic inflammation, particularly if periodontitis intervention therapy combined with adjunctive periodontal host-modulating therapy [4, 12, 53, 54].

Furthermore, a positive influence on RA activity scores, rheumatoid factor and ACPA levels, but also on anti-*P. gingivalis* antibodies was reported following supportive periodontal therapy in patients having concomitant RA and chronic periodontitis [1, 12, 52, 54–56].

The consequences of therapy for periodontal disease on RA status actually reflect on the decrease in systemic inflammation, removal of joint exposure to the infectious trigger and the decline in microbial immune subversion [1, 8, 12].

4.4.2. Effects of conventional therapy for rheumatoid arthritis on periodontal status

On the other hand, different authors concluded that early aggressive RA management with synthetic disease modifying anti-rheumatic drugs (DMARDs) and/or biologic agents aiming to achieve and maintain disease remission according to treat-to-target strategies might also restrict periodontal damage in active periodontitis [1, 8, 12, 54].

It is widely accepted that systematic DMARDs ameliorate periodontal disease burden in RA patients with periodontitis, i.e., they decrease gingival inflammation and periodontal destruction [1, 8, 12, 54]. Moreover, glucocorticoids and TNF antagonists are able to clinically improve periodontal disease in RA patients [1, 8, 12, 54]. Anti-cytokine therapy, specifically anti-TNF agents, may play dual role on synovitis as well as periodontal disease [1, 8, 12, 54, 55], reducing inflammation and mitigating both conditions [1, 4, 8, 12]. However, the role of TNF inhibition on periodontitis outcomes in the absence of periodontal treatment is still controversial [1, 8, 12].

5. Conclusions

There is a significant interplay between periodontitis and rheumatoid arthritis as supported by emerging evidences. Despite common T cell activation, the imbalance between pro-inflammatory and anti-inflammatory cytokine profile, citrullination of endogenous proteins and the resultant bone destruction in specific environments (synovium and gingival tissue), further research is required to assess the exact mechanisms and causative link, as well as to define top therapy.

Author details

Codrina Ancuta[1*], Cristina Iordache[2], Eugen Ancuta[3] and Claudia Mihailov[4]

*Address all correspondence to: codrina_ancuta@yahoo.com

1 2nd Rheumatology Department, Clinical Rehabilitation Hospital, "Grigore T. Popa" University of Medicine and Pharmacy, Iasi, Romania

2 Ergonomics Department, School of Dentistry, "Grigore T. Popa" University of Medicine and Pharmacy, Iasi, Romania

3 Research Department, "Elena Doamna" Clinical Hospital, Iasi, Romania

4 2nd Medical Department, Clinical Port Hospital of Constanta, Faculty of Medicine, 'Ovidius' University of Constanta, Romania

References

[1] Joseph R, Jose Raj MG, Sundareswaran S, et al. Does a biological link exist between periodontitis and rheumatoid arthritis? World J Rheumatology. 2014;4(3):80–87.

[2] Koziel J, Mydel P, Potempa J. The link between periodontal disease and rheumatoid arthritis: an updated review. Curr Rheumatol Rep. 2014;16:408.

[3] Batool H, Afzal N, Shahzad F, Kashif M. Relationship between rheumatoid arthritis and chronic periodontitis. J Med Radiol Pathol Surg. 2016;2:11–14.

[4] Payne JB, Gloub LM, Thiele GM, et al. The link between periodontitis and rheumatoid arthritis: a periodontist's perspective. Curr Oral Health Rep. 2015;2:20–29.

[5] Araujo VM, Melo IM, Lima V. Relationship between periodontitis and rheumatoid arthritis: review of the literature. Mediat Inflam. 2015;259074:1–15.

[6] Fuggle NR, Smith TO, Kaul A, Sofat N. Hand to mouth: a systematic review and metaanalysis of the association between rheumatoid arthritis and periodontitis. Front Immunol. 2016;7(80):1–10.

[7] Saini R. Periodontitis and rheumatoid arthritis: inflammatory relationship. J Pharm Bioallied Sci. 2011;3(3):464–465.

[8] Bingham CO. Round 34: periodontal disease and rheumatoid arthritis [Internet]. 2010 [Updated: 2011]. Available from: http://www.hopkinsarthritis.org/physician-corner/rheumatology-rounds/r. [Accessed: 01-aug-2016]

[9] Detert J, Pischon N, Burmester GR, et al. The association between rheumatoid arthritis and periodontal disease. Arthritis Res Ther. 2010;12:218 (1–7).

[10] Valesini G, Gerardi MC, Iannuccelli C, et al. Citrullination and autoimmunity. Autoimmun Rev. 2015;14(6):490–497.

[11] Hussain M, Stover CM, Dupont A. P. gingivalis in periodontal disease and atherosclerosis—scenes of action for antimicrobial peptides and complement. Front Immunol. 2015;6(45):1–6.

[12] Hein C. A closer look at the association between periodontal disease and rheumatoid arthritis. Dimens Dent Hyg. 2008;6(3):30–33.

[13] van Dyke TE. Commentary: periodontitis is characterized by an immuno-inflamatory host-mediated destruction of bone and connective tissues that support the teeth. J Periodontol. 2014;85:509–511.

[14] Gümüş P, Buduneli E, Başak B, et al. Gingival crevicular fluid, serum levels of receptor PArheumatoid arthritis and osteoporosis and with periodontal disease. J Periodontol. 2013;84(11):1627–1637.

[15] Kobayashi T, Yoshie H. Host responses in the link between periodontitis and rheumatoid arthritis. Curr Oral Health Rep. 2015;2:1–8.

[16] Klareskog L, Malmström V, Lundberg K, et al. Smoking, citrullination and genetic variability in the immunopathogenesis of rheumatoid arthritis. Semin Immunol. 2011;23:92–98.

[17] Catrina AI, Ytterberg AJ, Reynisdottir G, et al. Lungs, joints and immunity against citrullinated proteins in rheumatoid arthritis. Nat Rev Rheumatol. 2014;10:645–653.

[18] Badran Z, Strillou X, Verner C, et al. Periodontitis as a risk factor for systemic disease: are microparticles the missing link? Med Hypotheses. 2015;84(6):555–556.

[19] Mysak J, Podzimek S, Sommerova P, et al. Porphyromonas gingivalis: Major periodontopathic pathogen overview. J Immunol Res.2014;2014:476068.

[20] Maresz KJ, Helvard A, Sroka A, et al. Porphyromonas gingivalis facilitates the development and progression of destructive arthritis through its unique bacterial peptidylarginine deiminase (PAD). PLoS Pathog. 2013;9:81003627.

[21] Hajishengallis G, Liang S, Payne MA, et al. Low-abundance biofilm species orchestrates inflammatory periodontal disease through the commensal microbiota and complement. Cell Host Microbe. 2011;10:497–506.

[22] Leech MT, Bartold PM. The association between rheumatoid arthritis and periodontitis. Best Pract Res Clin Rheumatol. 2015;29:189–201.

[23] Scher JU, Abramson SB. Periodontal disease, Porphyromonas gingivalis, and rheumatoid arthritis: what triggers autoimmunity and clinical disease? Arthritis Res Ther. 2013;15:122(1–3).

[24] Scher JU, Bretz WA, Abramson SB. Periodontal disease and subgingival microbiota as contributors for rheumatoid arthritis pathogenesis: modifiable risck factors? Curr Opin Rheumatol. 2014;26:424–429.

[25] Konig MF, Paracha AS, Moni M, et al. Defining the role of Porphyromonas gingivalis peptidylarginine deiminase (PPAD) in rheumatoid arthritis through the study of PPAD biology. Ann Rheum Dis. 2015;74(11):2054–2061.

[26] Harvey GP, Fitzsmmons TR, Dhamarpatni AA, et al. Expression of peptidylarginine deiminase-2 and-4, citrullinated proteins anti citrullinated protein antibodies in human gingiva. J Periodontal Res. 2013;48:252–261.

[27] Hensvold A-H, Reznisdottir G, Catrina A. From citrullination to specific immunity and disease in rheumatoid arthritis. Protein Deimin Human Health Dis. 2014;2:25–42.

[28] Abdukkah SN, Farmer EA, Spargo L, et al. Porphromonas gingivalis peptidylarginine deiminase substrate specificity. Anaerobe. 2013;23:102–108.

[29] Amara K, Steen J, Murray F, et al. Monoclonal IgG antibodies generated from joint derived B cells of RA patients have a strong bias towards citurllianted autantingen recognition. J Exp Med. 2013;3:445–455.

[30] Quirke AM, Lugli EB, Wegner N, et al. Heightened immune response to autocitrullinated Porphyromonas gingivalis peptidylarginine deiminase: a potential mechanism for breaching immunologic tolerance in rheumatoid arthritis. Ann Rheum Dis. 2014;73(1):263–269.

[31] Andrade F, Darrah E, Gucek M, et al. Autocitrullination of human peptidylarginine deiminase type 4 regulates protein citrullination during cell activation. Arthritis Rheum. 2010;62(6):1630–1640.

[32] Baka Z, György B, Géher P, et al. Citrullination under physiological and pathological conditions. Joint Bone Spine. 2012;79:431–436.

[33] Mikuls TR, Payne JB, Yu F, et al. Periodontitis and porphromonas gingivalis in patients with rheumatoid arthritis. Arthr Rheumatol. 2014;66(5):1090–1100.

[34] Wegner N, Lundberg K, Kinloch A, et al. Autoimmunity to specific citrullinated proteins gives the first clues to the etiology of rheumatoid arthritis. Immunol Rev. 2010;233:34–54.

[35] Arnson Y, Shoenfeld Y, Amita H. Effects of tabacco smoke on immunity, inflammation and autoimmunity. J Autoimmun. 2010;34:258–265.

[36] Lappin DF, Apatzidou D, Quirke AM, et al. Influence of periodontal disease, Porphyromonas gingivalis and cigarette smoking on systemic antic-citrullinated peptide antibody titres. J Clin Periodontol. 2013;40:907–915.

[37] Manivelavan D, Vijayasamundeeswari CK. Anti-cyclic citrullinated peptide antibody: an early diagnostic and prognostic biomarker of rheumatoid arthritis. J Clin Diagn Res. 2012;6(8):1393–1396.

[38] Gottenberg JE, Ravaud P, Cantagrel A, et al. Positivity for anti-cyclic citrullinated peptide is associated with a better response to abatacept: data from the "Orencia and Rheumatoid Arthritis" registry. Ann Rheum Dis. 2012;7(11):1815–1819.

[39] Demoruelle MK, Parish MC, Derber LA, et al. Performance of anti-cyclic citrullinated peptide assazs differs in subjects at increased risk of rheumatoid arthritis and subjects with established disease. Arthritis Rheum. 2013;65:2243–2263.

[40] Gonzales SM, Payne JB, Yu E, et al. Alveolar bone loss is associated with circulating anti-citrullinated proteins antibody (ACPA) in patients with rheumatoid arthritis. J Periodontol. 2015;86(2):221–231.

[41] Ishi PE, Barros Bertolo M, Rossa Jr C, et al. Periodontal condition in patients with rheumatoid arthritis. Braz Oral Res. 2008;22(1):72–77.

[42] Pischon N, Pischon T, Kroger J, et al. Association among rheumatoid arthritis, oral hygiene, and periodontitis. J Periodontol. 2008;79:979–986.

[43] Dissick A, Redman RS, Jones M, et al. Association of periodontitis with rheumatoid arthritis: a pilot study. J Periodontol. 2010;81:223–230.

[44] Joseph R, Rajappan S, Nath SG, et al. Association between chronic periodontitis and rheumatoid arthritis: a hospital-based case-control study. Rheumatol Int. 2013;33(1): 103–109.

[45] Hendler A, Mulli TK, Hughes FJ, et al. Involvement of autoimmunity in the pathogenesis of aggressive periodontitis. J Dent Res. 2010;89:1389–1394.

[46] Seror R, David-Gall S, Bonnaure-Mallet M, et al. Association of anti-Porphromonas gingivalis antibody titers with nonsmoking status in early rheumatoid arthritis: results from the prospective French cohort of patients with early rheumatoid arthritis. Arthr Rheumatol. 2015;67(7):1729–1737.

[47] Kaur S, Bright R, Proudman SM, et al. Does periodontal treatment influence clinical and biochemical measures for rheumatoid arthritis? A systemic review and meta-analysis. Semin Arthr Rheum 2014;44:113–22.

[48] Potikuri D, Dannana KC, Kanchinadam S, et al. Periodontal disease is significantly higher in nonsmoking treatment-naïve rheumatoid arthritis patients: results from a case-control study. Ann Rheum Dis. 2012;71:1541–1544.

[49] Eriksson K, Nise L, Kats A, et al. Prevalence of periodontitis in patients with established rheumatoid arthritis: a Swedish population based case-control study. PLoS One. 2016;11(7):e0155956.

[50] Pinho Mde N, Oliveira RD, Novaes Jr AB, et al. Relationship between periodontitis and rheumatoid arthritis and the effect of non-surgical periodontal treatment. Braz Dent J. 2009;20:355–364.

[51] Bryrkoglu B, Buduneli N, Aksu K, et al. Periodontal therapy in chronic periodontitis lowers gingival crevicular fluid interleukin-1beta and DAS 28 in rheumatoid arthritis patients. Rheumatol Int. 2013;33:2607–2616.

[52] Moutsopoulos NM, Kling HM, Angelov N, et al. Porphromonas gingivalis promotes Th 17 inducing pathways in chronic periodontitis. J Autoimmun. 2012;39:294–303.

[53] Monsarrat P, Vergnes JN, Cantagrel A, et al. Effect of periodontal treatment on the clinical parameters of patients with rheumatoid arthritis: study protocol of the randomized, controlled ESPERA trial. Trials. 2013;14:253(1–9).

[54] Ortis P, Bissada NF, Paloma L, et al. Periodontal therapy reduces the severity of active rheumatoid arthritis in patients treated with or without tumor necrosis factor inhibitors. J Periodontal. 2009;80:535–540.

[55] Okada M, Kobayashi T, Ito S, et al. Periodontal treatment decreases levels of antibodies to porphryromonas gingivalis and citrulline in patients with rheumatoid arthritis and periodontics. J Periodontol. 2013;84(12):e74–e84.

[56] Erciyas K, Sezer U, Ustün K, et al. Effects of periodontal therapy on disease activity and systemic inflammation in rheumatoid arthritis patients. Oral Dis. 2013;19:394–400.

[57] Fisher BA, Cartwright AJ, Quirke AM, et al. Smoking, Porphyromonas gingivalis and the immune response to citrullinated autoantigens before the clinical onset of rheumatoid arthritis in a Southern European nested case-control study. BMC Musculoskelet Disord. 2015;16:331(1–11).

13

Role of MicroRNAs in Rheumatoid Arthritis

Merih Birlik, Ayşe Koçak and Duygu Harmancı

Abstract

Rheumatoid arthritis (RA) is a common autoimmune disease. The hallmarks of RA are synovial inflammation and hyperplasia, autoantibody production, systemic features, and deformity. A lot of researchers have paid attention to the possibility that microRNAs (miRNAs) play a role in the pathogenesis of RA. miRNAs are a class of small noncoding RNAs, which have 18–25 nucleotides. These small RNAs modify gene expression by binding to target messenger RNA (mRNA), and they block the translation or induce the degradation of target mRNA. Biological relevance of miRNAs has been investigated in physiological and pathological conditions. A growing body of evidence suggests that miRNAs participate in the inflammatory disorders including RA. In this chapter, an overview of biogenesis and function of miRNAs has been presented to introduce researchers to the changes and functional regulation of the key miRNAs in RA and to provide current knowledge in miRNA and RA. It is important to understand the relationship between the key miRNAs and RA pathology as modulation of specific miRNA alterations could be of great pharmaceutical interest in the future.

Keywords: microRNA, miRNA, small noncoding RNA, rheumatoid arthritis, pathogenesis

1. Introduction

Rheumatoid arthritis (RA) is an autoimmune disease characterized by chronic synovial inflammation exemplified by cell hyperplasia, autoantibody production, systemic features, and deformity [1–3]. It affects approximately 0.36–2.0% of the human population worldwide and roughly three to four times more females than males [2, 4]. RA progression is a complex process and consists of many genes and environmental factors [3]. Accumulating clinical and experimental evidence points out that the immune system plays a key role in disease pathogenesis. However, pathogenesis of RA is not entirely clear [1–3]. Generally, RA progression leads to joint destruction, functional disability, and cardiovascular comorbidities [5]. The immune system and different cell types such as macrophages, T and B cells, and synovial fibroblasts participate in the pathogenesis of RA. RA synovial fibroblasts and "fibroblast-like synoviocytes" (FLS) play an important role in RA [6, 7].

Genetic and environmental factors are associated with RA. These factors include infectious agents, exposure to cigarette smoke, air pollution, insecticides, and occupational exposures to mineral oil and silica. But so far, smoking is the only environmental risk factor that has been extensively studied and widely accepted [3]. When environmental factors are considered some of them can be controlled, but the control of genetic and epigenetic regulation is highly complex and difficult to predict. The contribution of epigenetic gene regulation is considerably less well established. Epigenetics is a mechanism that regulates gene expression independently of the underlying DNA sequence. In early 2000s, with the discovery of micro RNAs (miRNAs), researchers have started to discuss their roles in physiological and pathologic processes [8]. miRNAs are small noncoding RNAs 18–25 nucleotides in length that block the translation or induce the degradation of target mRNA [9]. The clinical application of epigenomic information has improved in recent years. A growing body of evidence suggests that miRNAs participate in the inflammatory disorders including RA [10–12].

In this chapter, we summarize the biogenesis and function of miRNA, with an emphasis of its role in the pathogenesis and the importance of miRNA in RA as a potential biomarker.

2. What are microRNAs?

The small RNAs are crucial for the cellular gene regulatory systems. Over the last decade, these small RNAs have become important regulators in eukaryotic genomes. These noncoding RNAs regulate genes and genomes. This regulation includes chromatin structure, transcription, RNA processing, RNA stability, and translation. Generally, the small RNAs show inhibitory activity on gene expression. One type of these small RNAs is microRNAs [13].

MicroRNAs (miRNAs) are small endogenous noncoding RNAs [13]. In 1993, Ambros and his collaborators discovered the first miRNA, lin-4 from *Caenorhabditis elegans*. Researchers studied the postembryonic development of *C.elegans* and found two noncoding RNAs which were produced by lin-4 with complementary sequences to the 3′UTR (un-translated region) of lin-14 mRNA [14]. These small transcripts could bind the 3′UTR of lin-14 mRNA and decrease protein levels without affecting mRNA stability. In early 2000s, Reinhart (and) et al discovered the second miRNA, let-7, and following this discovery, more than a dozen miRNAs were found in plant and animal species in 2000s [15–18]. The name "microRNA" was first used in 2001, and papers published in science reported that there were up to 50 miRNAs [19–22]. The brief history of miRNAs is reviewed in **Figure 1**.

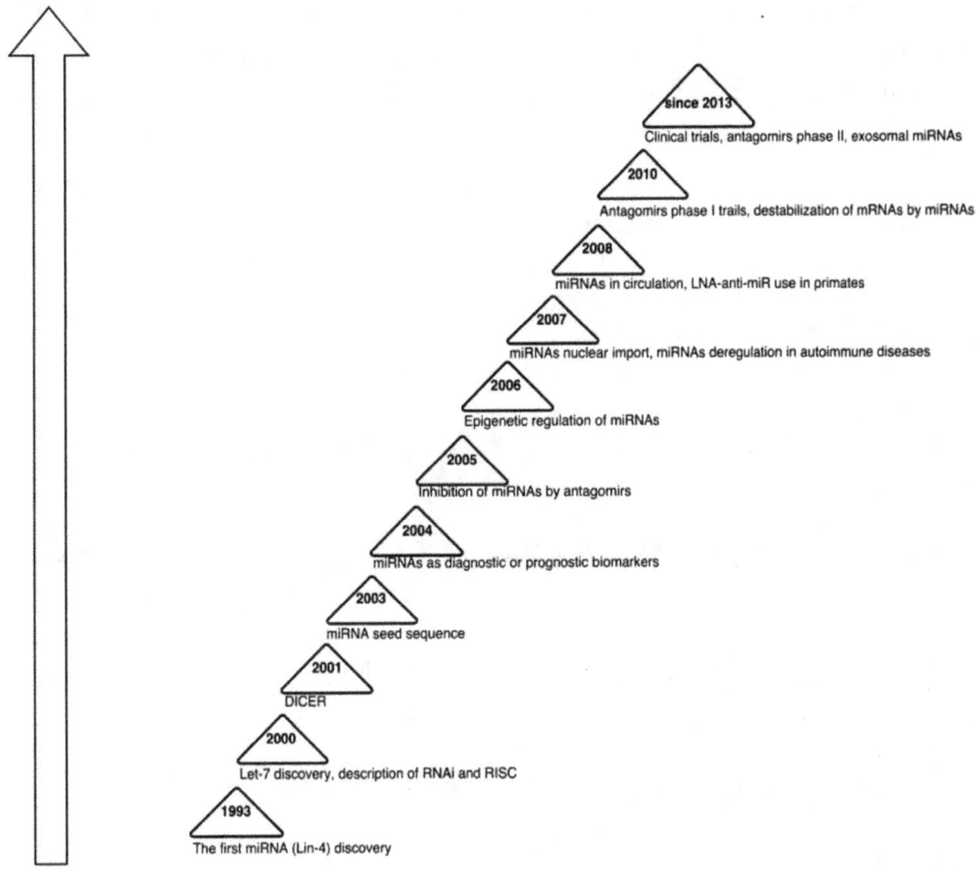

Figure 1. The brief history of miRNAs.

miRNAs are short (about 18–25 nucleotides long) noncoding RNAs that can affect messenger RNA (mRNA) processing at the post-transcriptional level [15]. They are endogenous and goal-oriented expressed products of an organism's own genome [13]. Chromosomal locations of miRNAs affect the expression and function themselves [23]. According to their genomic localizations, miRNAs can be classified into five groups [24]:

1. Intergenic miRNAs (miRNA genes are located between two consecutive protein-coding genes).
2. Intronic miRNAs in noncoding transcripts (miRNA genes are located in any intron of a noncoding RNA gene).
3. Intronic miRNAs in protein-coding transcripts (miRNA genes are located in any intron of a protein-coding RNA gene).
4. Exonic miRNAs in noncoding transcripts (miRNA genes are located in any exon of a noncoding RNA gene).
5. Exonic miRNAs in protein-coding transcripts (miRNA genes are located in any exon of a protein-coding RNA gene).

Some miRNAs are located in every second group because of alternative splicing [9]. Intergenic miRNAs are transcribed from their own promoters but intragenic miRNAs generally located in the same orientation as the host genes [24] (**Figure 2**).

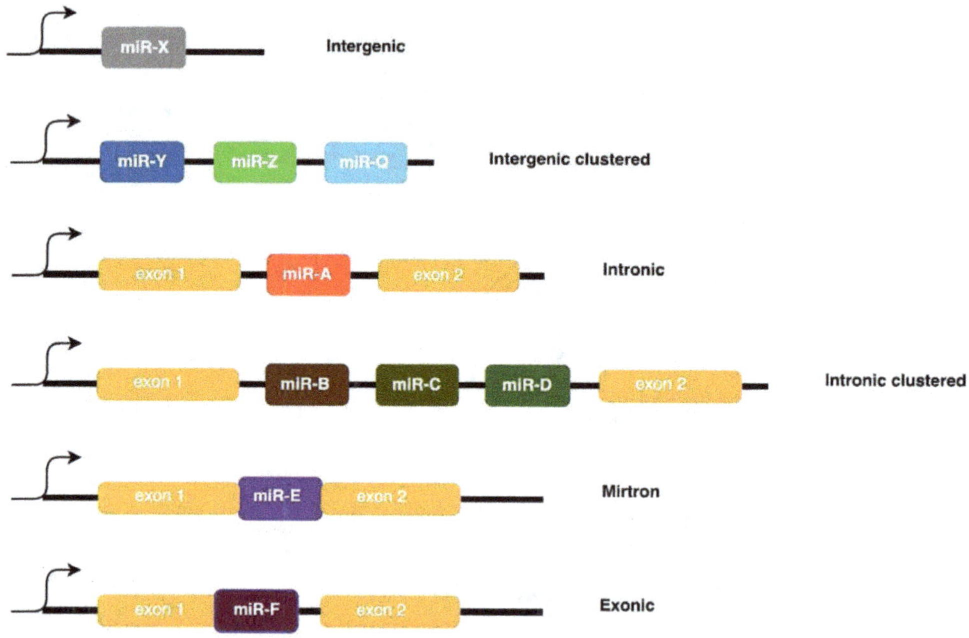

Figure 2. The genomic organization of miRNAs.

The scientific denomination rule is simple for the miRNAs. The mature miRNA is abbreviated with a capitalized "miR-" while the uncapitalized "mir-" indicates both the gene locus and precursor miRNA (pre-miRNA and pri-miRNA). Every miRNA is named according to discovery order, and "MIR" refers to the gene that encodes them. The numbering of miRNA genes is simply sequential. For example, miR-21 was discovered before the miR-155 [10]. In addition, three letters specific for each species precede each name. Thus "hsa-miR155" means that this miR origins from *Homo sapiens* while ggo-mir-155 is an example of gorilla's miRNA name. A letter after the number in the suffix is used to differentiate among multiple members of the same family (e.g., hsa-mir-155a and hsa-mir-155b). Today, miRNAs is still a popular subject for the researchers and have been studied in many organisms. Some miRNA databases (http://www.mirbase.org/, http://mirdb.org/miRDB/, http://www.microrna.org/microrna/home.do and so forth) are available and every moment the miRNA list is updated [25, 26].

3. miRNA biogenesis

In the early 2000s, the scientific world discovered small RNAs. They work as gene regulators, but their biogenesis is still unclear. Most mammalian miRNA genes are located in the intron region; some are located in the exon region and also approximately 30% are located in the intergenic regions. Since 2000, the miRNA biogenesis pathway has been studied and in 2001, Mello and his colleagues obtained the first data [17].

Generally, mammalian miRNA biogenesis pathway can be divided into two main parts with regard to processing pri-miRNAs: canonical and noncanonical [27]. In the canonical miRNA biogenesis pathway, the pri-miRNA is processed to pre-miRNA in the nucleus. In the noncanonical miRNA biogenesis pathway, mirtrons participate in microprocessor processing as alternative miRNA precursors. There are some differences between pri-miRNAs and mirtrons. Mirtrons arise from the spliced-out introns and lack lower stem loop structure and the flanking single-stranded segments thus the mirtrons bypass Drosha processing [28, 29].

The canonical miRNA biogenesis pathway is Drosha and Dicer dependent. Drosha is a member of ribonuclease III enzyme family, and the core nuclease that initiates miRNA processing in the nucleus [16]. Dicer is also a member of RNAse III family. It cleaves double-stranded RNA (ds-RNA) and precursor miRNA (pre-miRNA) into short dsRNA fragments. Dicer forms the mature miRNA in the cytoplasm [16, 18]. The noncanonical miRNA biogenesis pathway is Drosha independent/Dicer dependent. Here, microprocessor is not required. Mirtrons are a type of miRNA that are direct Dicer substrates. A number of noncanonical pathways have been described, but most pathways remain unclear. Besides, mirtrons comprise small part of the miRNAs, so generally miRNAs are processed via canonical pathway [16, 18, 27].

Microprocessor components, Drosha, DiGeorge critical region 8 (DGCR8, also known as Pasha), and Dicer, are essential for the canonical miRNA biogenesis, and the biogenesis pathway is compartmentalized and stepwise [27]. The canonical mRNA biogenesis pathway starts with RNA Pol II-mediated transcription of genomic region containing miRNA genes. Transcripts (pri-miRNAs) are capped (at the 5′ end) and polyadenylated (at the 3′ end). The pri-miRNAs are cleaved to pre-miRNA hairpins by RNAse III enzyme Drosha in the nucleus. DGCR8 (Pasha) proteins accompany this processing. Then, pre-miRNAs are exported from the nucleus to cytoplasm by exportin-5 (XPO-5) via Ran-GTP–dependent mechanism. In the cytoplasm, pre-miRNA is processed into a mature miRNA. RNAse III Dicer cleaves the pre-miRNA together with trans-activation response RNA binding protein (TRBP)/protein activator of PKR (PACT) proteins to produce unstable, 18–22 nt asymmetric miRNA:miRNA* duplex.

miRNA represents guide RNA strand, and the other miRNA* means passenger RNA strand. The guide RNA strand incorporates into RNA-induced silencing complex (RISC), and passenger RNA strand is discarded. Argonaute (AGO) is one of the key components of RISC for this process [18, 27]. The canonical miRNA biogenesis pathway is summarized in **Figure 3**.

The alternative miRNA biogenesis pathways are named noncanonical pathways. These pathways do not require all enzymes and protein factors of the canonical pathway. Some miRNAs differ from the others in terms of structure and function and these miRNAs bypass one or more steps of miRNA canonical biogenesis [27, 29]. Dicer is required for both pathways—canonical and noncanonical, but Drosha and DGCR8 are only needed for the canonical pathway. If there is a mutation or deficiency of these enzymes, miRNA biogenesis goes on via the noncanonical pathway. The noncanonical miRNA biogenesis pathway can be divided mainly into two classes [27, 30].

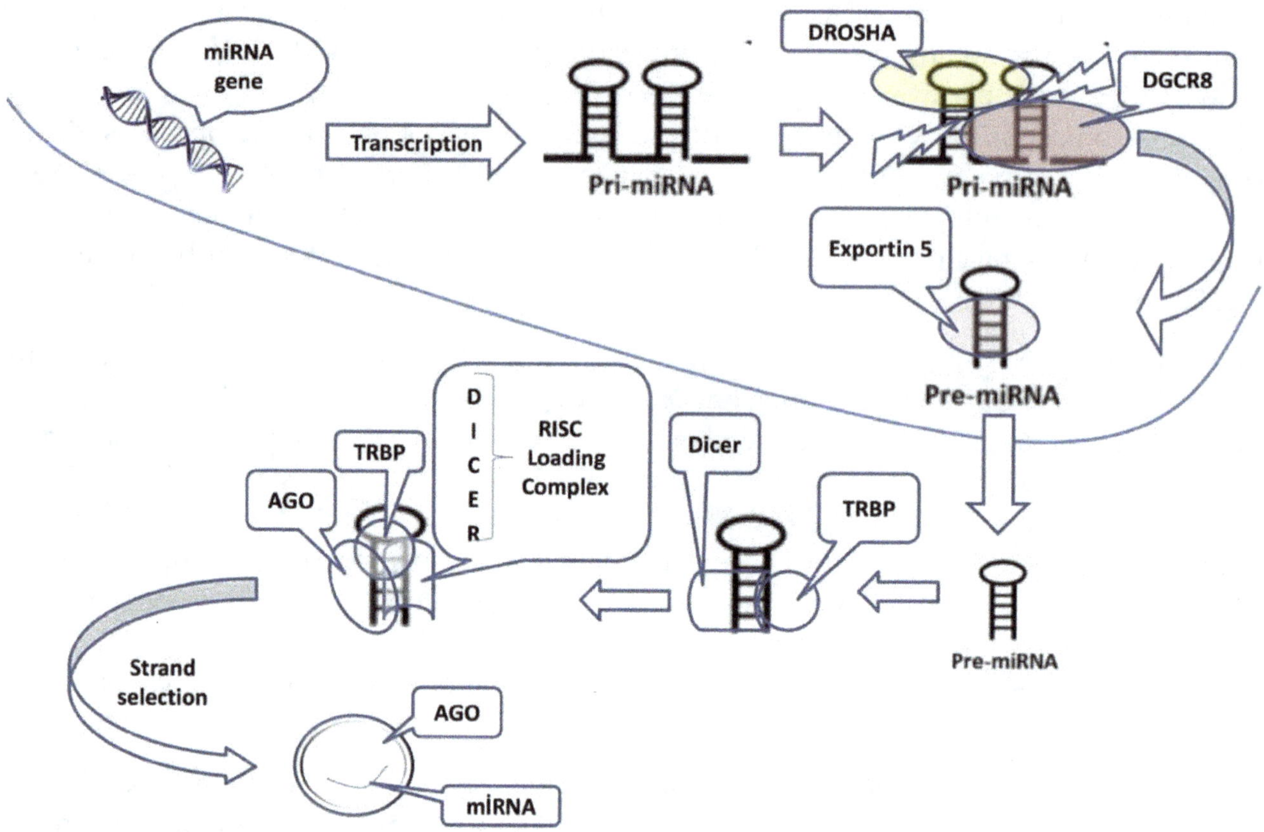

Figure 3. The canonical miRNA biogenesis pathway.

3.1. Drosha/DGCR8-independent/Dicer-dependent pathways

3.1.1. Mirtron pathway

Some introns form short RNA hairpins, and they are termed "mirtrons" that can be spliced resulting in a nonlinear intermediate. Investigations of the data of small RNAs from Drosophila melanogaster and Caenohabditis elegans led to the discovery of mirtrons [28]. They can be debranched into pre-miRNA hairpins and form the duplex. After this step, this product can join he (the) canonical pathway and is ready to be transported to the cytoplasm by exportin-5 (EXP-5) [29].

Depending on the splice donor and acceptor site, mirtrons can be categorized into three groups: 5′-tailed mirtron, regular mirtron, and 3′-tailed mirtron. Generally, 3′-tailed mirtrons have been found in Drosophila, and 5′-tailed mirtrons have only been described in vertebrates [28, 29]. Mirtrons being a new research area, there are many unanswered questions.

3.1.2. snoRNA-derived RNAs (sdRNAs)

Small-nucleolar RNAs are a class of noncoding RNAs. Generally, they show similar properties and structures to miRNAs. They are dependent on Dicer and can be bound with AGO acting as a miRNA [29, 31].

3.1.3. miRNAs from tdRNAs

The first (tdRNA) tRNA-derived RNA species to be discovered were isoleucine tRNA-derived miRNA [27]. Normally, they differ from regular miRNAs but they have RNA silencing function. tRNA-derived (tdRNA) precursors can be a potential substrate of Dicer because of their different folding form [29, 31]. In the light of this information, they have different properties from typical mammalian miRNAs, and their pattern of behavior remains a puzzle.

3.1.4. miRNAs from endogenous short hairpin RNAs (shRNAs)

Several studies have shown that some shRNAs could join the noncanonical miRNA-processing pathway. Normally, in the canonical miRNA pathway, pre-miRNAs hairpins are conserved and thus can be recognized by microprocessor complex. However, shRNA-derived miRNAs do not have the microprocessor sequence. For this reason, they are DiGeorge critical region-8 (DGCR-8) independent [27, 29]

3.2. Drosha/DGCR8-dependent/Dicer-independent pathways

Some miRNAs mature in a different way. One of them is miR-451. MiR-451 maturation occurs without Dicer. Initially, pri-miR-451 is cleaved by Drosha/DGCR8 to form pre-miRNA duplex. But it is too short to present to Dicer as a substrate, so directly it interacts with AGO proteins [29, 31]. The miRNA biogenesis pathways and their regulation have been studied extensively in last 10 years, but further information is required for miRNA processing.

4. miRNA function

The functions of miRNAs are post-transcriptional repression and degradation of mRNAs [13]. They have different expression patterns and regulate several biological and pathological processes [16, 32, 33]. The major function of miRNAs is protein synthesis inhibition. They can maintain this function either by inhibition of translation or by mRNA degradation [34, 35]. The miRNA-mRNA interaction is important for miRNA function, and each mature miRNA interacts with specific miRNA/miRNAs. Generally, the interaction takes place between the miRNA seed region and 3′ UTR of mRNA for the inhibition of target mRNA. There are a few exceptions about miRNA binding sites. In some cases, the miRNA-mRNA interaction occurs at the 5′-UTR. The second issue is miRNA's tissue specificity. MiRNAs are expressed in a tissue-specific fashion, and also, the action of miRNA is tissue specific [36–39].

Identification of miRNA target genes is crucial for the functional characterization of miRNAs. Recently, we can predict the target gene with the help of some bioinformatics algorithms and software. The most popular software is TargetScan [5, 10]. If *in silico* analysis is insufficient, further analysis can be needed. Some genetic or biochemical methods are preferable. The success of the prediction is important to understand miRNA function.

The miRNAs have a part as an adaptor for miRISC to recognize and regulate target mRNAs. MiRISC regulates the translation of AGO proteins by introducing silencing through mRNA deadenylation, degradation, or translation [13]. miRNAs which are integrated into the RISC complex control the gene expression the level of post-transcription by reducing miRNA stability or inhibiting translation of mRNA [9, 32, 40]. Besides, miRNAs can affect several epigenetic regulators (DNA methyltransferases and histone deacetylases) [16].

In addition to mRNAs repression, some miRNAs have positive effects on gene expression [9]. This can occur directly or indirectly. For instance, miR-373 binds to the promoter of E-cadherin directly and increases the function of RNA polymerase. If its target mRNA does not consist of poly (A)-tail, AGO2 activates the gene expression [8, 9].

The selectivity in gene regulation mechanism depends on the degree of the match occurred between target mRNA and miRNA. Exact match is usually found in plants. miRISC complex which make partial matches is required to make an exact match with the seed region in the related to miRNA to inhibit the translation [41, 42]. Although many miRNAs cause of gene silencing by reducing the target mRNA stability, some miRNAs lead to gene silencing by inhibiting target mRNA translation, but there is not enough evidence about what stage they repress. In general, studies suggest that miRNAs repress the translation with four different mechanisms: (1) suppression of protein synthesis, (2) a drop of premature mRNAs in ribosomes, (3) slowing down during the alongation step of protein synthesis, (4) in parallel with protein synthesis the fragmentation of protein [40, 43, 44].

The function of miRNAs has been studied since the first two microRNAs discovered. miRNAs are considered key regulators to physiological processes, such as cellular and tissue differentiation, apoptosis, innate, and adaptive immune responses and development [13, 17, 35, 45, 46]. Thus, miRNAs are crucial for the regulation of biological processes [17]. Deregulation of this regulatory network can lead to the initiation of undesired pathological processes, such as cancer, fibrotic diseases, and autoimmune diseases [17, 35, 45, 46].

miRNAs have essential roles in immune system as they arrange innate and adaptive immune systems and have pivotal roles in the regulation of inflammation, by controlling the differentiation of B cells, conventional T cells, and regulatory T cells [11, 39].

4.1. Innate immunity and miRNAs

The innate immune system fights microorganisms. It has many cell types, which are physical epithelial barriers, phagocytic leukocytes, dendritic cells, natural killer (NK) cells, and circulating plasma proteins. Pattern recognition receptors (PRRs) recognize microorganisms and include toll-like receptors (TLRs), C-type lectin-like receptors (CLRs), retinoic acid-inducible gene (RIG)-I-like-receptors (RLRs) and nucleotide-binding oligomerization domain (NOD)-like receptors (NLRs). This process starts to intracellular signaling pathways. TLR has 10 subtypes such as TLR1, TLR2, TRL3, TLR4, TLR5, TLR6, TRL7, TRL8, TRL9, and TLR10 [47–50]. TLR4 identify lipopolysaccharides (LPSs). miR-146a/b, miR-132, and miR-155 are overexpressed for the LPS-mediated inflammatory responses. miR-146 upregulation causes interleukin-1 receptor-associated kinase (IRAK) 1 and genes expression and tumor necrosis factors receptor–associated factor (TRAF) 6 [51]. miR-146 was investigated in *in vitro* model of mouse macrophages, and it is a negative regulator of IRAK1, IRAK2 and TRAF6 [52]. On the other hand, miR-155 and miR-125b levels are related to TNF-α secretion in mouse macrophages. Regulation of miR-155 and miR-125b is LPS/TNF-α dependent; therefore, it is suggested that they are new targets of drug design. miR-155 increases TNF-α translation, Fas-associated death domain protein (FADD), IkappaB kinase epsilon (IKKepsilon), and TNFR superfamily-interacting serine–threonine kinase 1 (Ripk1) [53]. One study showed that miR-147 increased in murine macrophages after stimulation with TLR2, TLR3, and TLR4 ligands and in the lungs of mice after LPS exposure [54]. Also, NF-κB is regulated by miR-1303. Mir-1303 regulates the process of autophagy related to mycobacteria by targeting Atg2B [55]. Besides, miR-146a and miR-155 affect IFN-type I synthesis by TLR-7 and TLR-9, some miRNAs such as miR-126, miR-21, miR-146a, miR-155, and miR-1246 can mediate regulation with epigenetic modification [56].

4.2. Adaptive immunity and miRNAs

T and B-lymphocytes are major cellular components of the adaptive immunity. As previously described, Dicer enzymes are important in the biogenesis of miRNA. In B cells, miR-181b and miR-148a play role as miR-148a inhibits the expression of the autoimmune suppressor Gadd45α [57, 58]. In T cell early development, decrease of Dicer leads to reduction of T cell numbers both in the thymus and peripheral lymphoid organs [59]. In early B cell development, miR-17 deficiency induced by ablation of Dicer in pro-B cells affected B cell antibody diversity and B cell survival [60]. miR-326 and miR-155 are related to IL-17 [61]. Moreover, miR-155 expression related to Th17 cell production and miR-155 downregulated the LPS-induced inflammatory process [62, 63]. miR-146 has an essential role in the adaptive immune system. In the Treg cells miR-146 is an activator of STAT1 transcription that is associated with Th1-mediated autoimmunity [64].

Many studies in animal (many researches on animal olabilir) models and clinical studies showed that miRNAs participate in the inflammation and autoimmune diseases mechanisms. In humans, loss of miRNA expression related of the many autoimmune conditions. Especially, multiple sclerosis (MS), osteoarthritis, and rheumatoid arthritis (RA) are most studied (are the most).

5. Expression profiles of miRNAs in rheumatoid arthritis patients

RA, characterized by chronic joint inflammation, is an autoimmune disease. Small joints of the hands and feet are affected most (more or the most) often; however, the disease is known to vary among individuals. In the general population, RA affects roughly three times more women (females) than men (males) and is more common between 35 and 50 years and in older individuals [65–68]. Persistent inflammation over time leads to joint damage and disability [69]. This disease is characterized by autoimmunity with multiple joint lesions and systemic inflammation. Also, patients can develop complications, which result in lifelong disability and increased mortality. Accordingly, RA is a growing public health concern as it is associated with significant social and economic burden [70].

In genetically susceptible people, various environmental factors can act as a trigger for inducing autoimmunity [71]. Recent experimental data showed that the pathogenesis of RA is associated with epigenetic regulation. Over the past few years, it has become clear that different microRNAs (miRNAs) expression levels, particularly in RA, contribute to the development of autoimmunity. miRNAs plays (play) multiple roles in regulation of pro-inflammatory cytokine secretion and development of immune cells, and they work in the induction or suppression of autoimmunity and ECM remodeling. Thus, dysregulated miRNA expression seems to promote the molecular mechanisms of the RA process [72–77]. Stanczyk et al. described for the first time the dysregulation of miRNAs in RA in 2008 [78]. They reported increased miR-155 and miR-146a expression in RA synovial fibroblasts compared to those in osteoarthritis (OA) patients. miRNAs expression is detected in several cell types in RA, and miRNAs expression profiles can regulate many physiological actions in RA (**Table 1**) [79, 80].

Cell type	**miRNA**		**Refs.**
	Downregulated	**Upregulated**	
Synovial tissue	miR-22	miR-146a	[80–86]
	miR-23b	miR-146b	
	miR-30a	miR-150	
		miR-155	
		miR-223	
Synovial fibroblasts	miR-124a	miR-133a	[85–91]
	miR-34a	miR-142-3p	
	miR-22	miR-142-5p	
	miR-152	miR-146a	
	miR-375	miR-155	
		miR-203	
		miR-221	
		miR-222	
		miR-323-3p	
Synovial fluid	miR-152	miR-16	[86, 92, 93]
	miR-375	miR-146a	
		miR-155	
		miR-223	
Synovium macrophages		miR-146a miR-155	[81, 94]
Whole blood		miR-99	[95, 96]
		miR-100	
		miR-125b	
		miR-146a	

Cell type	miRNA		Refs.
	Downregulated	Upregulated	
		miR-155	
Peripheral blood mononuclear cells (PBMCs)	miR-21	miR-26a	[82, 96–98]
		miR-132	
		miR-146a	
		miR-146b	
		miR-150	
		miR-155	
		miR-16	
Plasma and serum	miR-16	miR-16	[91, 95, 98–100]
	miR-125a-3p	miR-21	
	miR-126-3p	miR-24	
	miR-132	miR-26a	
	miR-146a	miR-125a-5p	
	miR-155	miR-125b	
		miR-126-3p	
		miR-223	
		miR-451	

Table 1. Expression of miRNAs in RA.

6. The roles of miRNAs in RA

Several miRNAs are found to be upregulated or downregulated in synovial tissue and cells of joint or blood compartment of patients with RA. The bone and joint destruction occurring in RA is accompanied by specific changes in cellular miRNAs that can affect epigenetic regulation. The current literature demonstrates that a variety of miRNAs is frequently dysregulated in RA patients.

miR-15/miR-16: miR-15a/16-1 and miR-15b/16-2 are highly protected in mammalian species. miR-15a is downregulated in arthritic synovial tissue, which has a potential role in apoptosis [95]. Nagata et al showed that in synovium miR15a, expression levels are lower in diseased mice than in healthy controls [101]. miR-15 plays a role in apoptosis; it has a negative regulatory effect on Bcl-2. Sera of patients with early RA show differential levels of miR-16-1 and miR-16-2, which are increased in peripheral blood mononuclear cells (PBMC) of RA patients [86, 95, 98]. Besides, miR-16 is a good candidate as a marker of disease activity. It is one of the key pro-inflammatory (proinflammatory) mediators in RA: mir-16 being able to target "tumor necrosis factor-α" (TNF-α) may be the biomarker of the RA.

miR-17-92 cluster: It is a controller of apoptosis, lots of research groups found de-regulated expression of miRNAs within this cluster in the context of RA [102].

miR-18: miR18a is upregulated in fibroblast-like synoviocytes (FLS) of RA patients. It is important in inflammation, because miR-18 contributes to NFκBmediated cartilage destruction and chronic inflammation in the joint through a positive feedback loop involving silencing of the "nuclear factor kappa-light-chain-enhancer of activated B cells" (NFκB) inhibitor TNFinduced protein-3 [103].

miR-21: In RA patients, levels of miR-21 are raised in plasma [99]; on the other hand, one study showed that miR-21 level is decreased in peripheral blood mononuclear cells (PBMCs). Downregulation of miR-21 is related to upregulation of "signal transducer and activator of transcription 3" (STAT-3) expression and decreased "forkhead box P3" (FOXP 3) mRNA levels in RA patients [104].

miR-22: Lin and his colleagues showed that expression of miR-22 is down regulated and negatively correlated with Cyr61 expression in synovial tissue of RA patients [85]. CYR61 expression is high in RA FLS and stimulates RA synovial fibroblast proliferation and interleukin (IL)-6 secretion in an autocrine-paracrine manner [85]. CYR61 may encourage synovial tissue hyperplasia alongside IL-6-dependent Th17 differentiation, which is critical for joint lesions in RA.

miR-23b: miR-23b is reported to be decreased in RA. miR-23b expression level is reduced and correlated with the high concentration of IL-17 in tissue samples from RA patients [83]. IL-17 suppresses the expression of miR-23b in human primary FLS. miR-23b regulates IL-1β, TNF-α, and IL-17 signaling and decreased levels of miR-23b in RA may be responsible for the induction of autoimmune inflammation.

miR-24: In RA, increased levels of plasma miR-24 have been reported, also its level significantly increased compared to OA [100]. Furin enzyme is important for the processing of latent TGF-β1, which may increase the inflammation by miR-24. Furin is a protein that is encoded by the FUR gene in humans. It was named FUR because it is in the upstream region of FES oncogene. Furin is also known as paired basic amino acid cleaving enzyme (PACE).

miR-26a: Murata and Nimoto worked with this molecule, and they showed that miR-26a is overexpressed in PBMCs and plasma of RA patients. Thus, it may be biomarker for the diagnosis of RA [82, 100]. miR-26a is upregulated during differentiation of IL-17 and generation of CD4+ cells. CD4+ cells are very important in the pathology of RA [82].

miR27a and miR27b: These miRNAs' expression is decreased in OA chondrocytes and coincides with increased expression of "Insulin Like Growth Factor Binding Protein 5" (IGFBP5) and Matrix Metallopeptidase-13 (MMP13) [105, 106].

miR-30a: miR-30a has been shown to be downregulated in RA synovial tissue and miR-30a-3p has a critical role in the regulation of "B lymphocyte activating factor of the tumor necrosis factor family" (BAFF) expression, which has a major impact in the regulation of the autoimmune responses occurring in RA [107].

miR-34a/miR-34b: miR-34a and miR-34b family are investigated in RA. miR34a is downregulated in RA synovial fibroblasts. The "X-linked inhibitor of apoptosis protein" (XIAP) is identified as a direct target of miR-34a [89]. So, miR-24 may contribute to the impaired apoptosis of activated RA synovial fibroblasts. On the other hand, miR-34b is overexpressed in RA T cells.

miR-124a: In 2009, Nakamachi et al. identified decreased expression levels of miR-124 in RA FLS. They showed that miR-24a targets the "monocyte chemoattractant protein-1" (MCP-1) mRNA expression and "cyclin-dependent kinase-2" (CDK-2) and decreases their protein levels [88]. miR-124 controls inflammatory process in RA, indirectly. The curtailed expression of miR-124a can contribute to RA pathogenesis via increased RA synovial fibroblast proliferation, angiogenesis, and leukocyte chemotaxis [89].

miR-125a-3p/miR-125a-5p/miR-125b: The family of miR-125 is dysregulated in the peripheral blood of RA patients. Kim et al. found that miR-125a-5p and miR-125b activate the proinflammatory NF-κB signaling pathway [108]. Thus, they may have roles in the induction of excessive inflammation in RA. Because of that, miRNA levels are monitored in serum from RA patients [95]. MiR-125b has a specific role in the regulation of normal and abnormal immune functions. Hruskova et al. suggested that the expression of miR-125b in those patients may present a novel biomarker for monitoring the treatment outcome during the early phase of RA [109].

miR-126-3p: miR-126-3p is significantly irregular in the plasma of RA patients. There is conflicting evidence regarding miR-126-3p. Wang et al. showed that miR-126-3p is lower in the plasma of RA patients [99], while another research group showed that the expression level of circulated miR-126-3p is markedly elevated in RA [100]. miR-126 can inhibit PI3K/AKT signaling pathway. It may clinically be helpful for RA patients [110].

miR-132: The expression of miR-132 of PBMCs from RA patients was twice higher as compared to controls [45]. However, miR-132 concentrations were found to be lower in RA plasma than in the plasma of healthy individuals [86]. Plasma concentrations of miR-132 differentiated patients with RA or OA from healthy controls, though plasma and synovial fluid miR-132 failed to differentiate RA from OA. Besides, plasma miR-132 or its SF/PB ratio (ratio of concentration of synovial fluid miRNA to plasma miRNA) correlated with tender joint count. These results indicate that miR-132 may have a role in systemic conditions with joint inflammation, such as RA [86]. miR-132 studies have mainly focused on central nervous system and neurotransmission; however, further analyses are required to determine the importance of miR-132 in inflammatory diseases [111].

miR-133a: MiR-133a is upregulated in RA synovial fibroblasts. Also, miR-133a is known as a negative regulator of the "Runt-related transcription factor 2" (Runx2), which is essential for the osteoblast differentiation [112].

miR146a/miR-146b: Studies showed that miR-146 is upregulated in all RA samples. One study found an increased basal expression of miR-146a in RA synovial fibroblasts compared with OA synovial fibroblasts [81, 87, 113]. In addition, increased expression levels of miR-146a have been observed in synovial fluid [85, 86, 97], synovial tissue [82, 83, 99], PBMCs [96, 97, 99, 114, 115], and whole blood [96] of RA patients. Expression of miR-146a is detected in many cell types, T cells, B cells, monocytes, macrophages, and IL-17 producing CD4+ cells [81, 82, 97, 114, 115]. However, plasma or serum miR-146a levels in patients with RA are comparable to that seen in healthy controls [86, 98], and two studies demonstrated that miR-146a was markedly decreased in plasma from patients with established RA [99]. miR-146a can inhibit T-helper 1-mediated responses and is required for the suppressive activity of Treg cells, which are both important in RA pathogenesis [64, 115]. Nevertheless, the increasing expression of miR-146a is not specific to RA, as it is also reported in OA cartilage after stimulation by IL-1b [116].

Pauley and Abou-Zeid found that peripheral blood mononuclear cell expression of miR-146a was positively correlated with CRP, ESR, DAS28 index, and TNF-α concentration [97, 115]. There are two known gene targets of miR-146a, that is, TNF-α/TNF receptor-associated factor 6 (TRAF6) and IL-1 receptor-associated kinase 1 (IRAK1). Also, miRNA-146a can regulate genes such as FAF1, IRAK2, FADD, IRF-5, STAT-1, and PTC-1. However, miR-146a has also been reported to correlate inversely with the tender joint count [97, 115]. In addition, miRNA-146a expression levels in the peripheral blood of RA patients were comparable to the levels seen in synovial tissue and fibroblastic cells of those patients [97]. miR-146a/b is induced in response to a variety of microbial components and pro-inflammatory cytokines, such as LPS, CpG, IFN-β, and TNF-α [51]. miR-146a in PBMCs enhances the function of Th1 cells and induces the expression of TNF-α, MCP-1, and NFκB p65 [117]. miR-146b was reported to increase in RA synovial tissue and in PBMCs of RA patients [82]. Upregulated miR-146b is related with infiltration of IL-17-producing T cells in RA synovium and higher expression of IL-17 within T cells expanded from RA PBMCs. So, it suggested that miR-146a and miR-146b are strongly implicated in RA development.

miR-152: Decreased expression of miR152 is reported in FLS of arthritic rats. It leads to activation of the Wnt-signaling pathway through direct targeting of "DNA (cytosine-5)-methyltransferase-1" DNMT1 and "encoding Frizzled8" (FZD8) by turn [92, 93].

miR-155: This is the most widely studied miRNA in RA. miR-155 expression profiles in RA synovial fibroblasts can also be induced by TNF-α [118]. The first miRNAs found to be abnormally expressed in FLS with RA were miR146a and miR155, both previously known as important regulators of inflammation. Also, miR146a and miR155 are two miRNAs, which are negative and positive regulators of inflammatory responses, respectively. miR-155 has been shown to express strongly in RA synovial tissue, synovial fluid and synovial fluid CD14+ cells [118]. Nonetheless, miR-155 concentrations are significantly lower as compared to controls in RA serum [98, 99]. The increased level of miR-155 in synovial fluid CD14+ cells and in synovial tissue macrophages is associated with decreased expression of the miR-155 target, a potent inhibitor of inflammation, called Src homology 2-containing inositol phosphatase-1 (SHIP-1), in patients with RA [94]. In addition, targets of miR-155 are the genes ZNF652, matrix metalloproteinase (MMP)-1 MMP-3, SHIP-1, c-Maf, PU.1, CEBP, ZIC3, HIVEP2, ARID2, SMAD5, and Bach-1. These pathways are all play a role in RA.

miR-203: One study showed that miR-203 is higher in RA synovial fluid in comparison with OA synovial fluid. Expression of miR-203 in the RA and OA synovium may be explained by differences in cellular composition of synovial tissue among RA patients [67, 78, 91]. Overexpression of miR-203 in RA synovial fluid resulted in higher release of MMP-1 and secretion of IL-6 via the NF-κB pathway and NF-κB-dependent production of IL-6, thus contributing to the RA synovial fluid activated phenotype and joint inflammatory state. Also, miR-203 plays a role in oncogenic transformation, proliferation, migration, and invasiveness of tumor cells. This mechanism is unknown in RA.

miR-221/miR-222: miR-221 and miR-222 are expressed together. miR-221/miR-222 are overexpressed in synovial fluids, blood serum, and synovial tissues of RA patients. MiR-221 plays a role in increasing production of pro-inflammatory cytokines, RA synovial fibroblast activation and migration. It also has a role in increasing resistance to apoptosis [119].

miR-223: miR223 is increased in T cells from patients with RA compared to levels in T cells from healthy donors [120]. miR-223 overexpressed in peripheral blood CD3+ and CD4+ naive T-lymphocytes of RA patients contributes to pathogenesis of the disease. CD14+ monocytes from RA synovia also overexpress miR223 and modulate differentiation of myeloid precursors into osteoclasts [121].

miR-323-3p: miR-323-3p expression is higher in RA synovial fibroblasts than OA synovial fibroblasts [90]. This miRNA may increase the Wnt-cadherin pathway and decrease the levels of target protein "β-transducin repeat containing E3 ubiquitin protein ligase" (BTRC) that contains an inhibitor of β-catenin [90]. It has been shown that miR-323-3p may have pro-inflammatory role in RA.

miR-375: miR-375 regulates the pathogenesis of adjuvant-induced arthritis rat model through the canonical Wnt signaling pathway [93].

miR-451: miR451, most preserved in vertebrates, regulates cell proliferation, invasion, and apoptosis. Neutrophils are important players in RA pathogenesis. miR451, significantly overexpressed in RA serum, peripheral blood T cells from patients with active RA and downregulated in neutrophils from patients with RA. Besides, it negatively regulates the migration of neutrophils by silencing CPNE3 (encoding copine3) and RAB5A (encoding Rasrelated protein Rab5A) [122]. In RA, miR-451 may reduce neutrophil chemotaxis through p38 MAPK (p38 mitogen-activated protein kinases) [122].

miR-455-3p: miR-455-3p can drive cartilage degradation by suppressing the expression of key molecules involved in cartilage formation. Increased expression of miR4553p in OA cartilage contributes to its destruction by targeting ACVR2B (encoding activin receptor type2B), SMAD2 (encoding MAD homology 2), CHRDL1 (encoding chordinlike protein 1), and by suppressing TGF-β signaling [118].

miR-498: miR-498 is associated with neurotransmission and inflammation. miR-498 is downregulated in CD4+ T cells from synovial fluid and peripheral blood [85].

miR-886-3p: A recent study reported that the combination of low expression of miR-22 and high expression of miR-886-3p were predictive of a good clinical response to adalimumab treatment in patients with early RA [123].

7. The importance of miRNAs in RA

MicroRNAs (miRNAs) are involved in the pathophysiological mechanisms underlying human diseases states. During the last decade, researchers have obtained a growing body of evidence regarding miRNAs in many human autoimmune diseases, such as RA, multiple sclerosis, psoriasis and systemic lupus erythematosus. miRNAs-mediated regulation is very clear from all of the present data and can play an important role in the development of various inflammatory conditions. So, dysregulation of miRNA expression (loss or downregulation of miRNA because of mutation, miRNA promoter region mutation, or overexpression of miRNA, epigenetic activation etc.) can lead to a variety of diseases.

For example, upregulation of miR-146 and miR-203 were observed in psoriasis [11]. Also, serum miR-1266 levels were highly significant in patients with psoriasis [124, 125]. Aberrations of miR-223, miR-143, miR-142, miR-378, miR-100, miR-21, and miR-31 levels were also found in these patients [126–128]. In systemic lupus erythematosus, some miRNAs, miR-146, miR-17-5p, miR-112, miR-141, miR-184, miR-196a, miR-383, and miR-409-3p, are downregulated, but miR-21, miR-61, miR-78, miR-142-3, miR-189, miR-198, miR-298, miR-299-3p, and miR-342 are upregulated in PBMCS from patients as compared to healthy controls [11, 127–131]. In multiple sclerosis, miR-18b, miR-599, and miR-96 are dysregulated in PBMCs in those patients [11, 132].

RA is a polygenic disease with multiple effects and miRNAs are post-transcriptional regulators of gene expression. In RA, high miRNA expressions (high mirna expressions mı olacak?) have been identified in different sites and cells, such as synovial tissue, synovial fibroblasts, PBMCs, plasma, synovial fluid, and activated immune cells within injured joints. The identified miRNA candidates for RA play a substantial role for key molecular mechanisms. These mechanisms are especially cytokine signaling pathways and inflammation. So, miRNAs are upregulated or downregulated in RA patients, relative to other diseases and healthy controls.

miRNAs, as diagnostic tools for RA, have many advantages. As such, miRNAs are stable and can be isolated from different parts of bodies (synovial fibroblasts, blood, plasma). miRNAs can be detected in circulating blood without the need for biopsies. Finally, miRNAs expression levels can be estimated by PCR.

8. Conclusion and perspectives

Since the discovery that microRNAs (miRNAs) take part in biological and pathological processes, it has become important to determine the roles.

In this chapter, we have summarized the role of miRNAs in RA. RA is a systemic autoimmune disorder characterized by chronic inflammation of the synovial tissue, and many studies suggest that miRNAs play role on autoimmunity in RA, as miR-16, miR-146b, miR-132, and miR-155 are upregulated in RA circulation. This suggests that miRNAs contribute to

RA pathogenesis. miR-124a is downregulated in RA synovium tissue [88] while miR-146a, miR-155 and miR-203 are upregulated in RA synovium tissue [51, 91, 133]. As we mentioned above, miR-146 and miR-203 are also upregulated in psoriasis; for this reason, they are questionable as possible biomarkers. miR-16, miR-132, miR-146, and miR-155 are upregulated in RA PBMCs, and miR-223 is upregulated in CD4+ naïve T-lymphocytes of RA patients [121].

Recently, the understanding of the molecular mechanism, prediction, or identification of miRNA targets is the main subjects of research in this area. This contribution may be lead to consider miRNAs as therapeutic targets. However, some miRNAs mentioned above are not specific for RA, as they are also dysregulated in the other immune disorders or cancers.

In the past few years, some experimental models have been used to study the therapeutic potential of miRNAs in RA, but still they are insufficient. Further studies are necessary.

In summary, each miRNA that is identified for RA opens the door slightly in terms of diagnostic and/or prognostic marker. Today, the available evidence shows that miRNAs are not diagnostic markers yet, but they can be used for therapy in the future.

Author details

Merih Birlik[1*], Ayşe Koçak[2] and Duygu Harmancı[2]

*Address all correspondence to: birlikm@gmail.com

1 Department of Internal Medicine, Division of Rheumatology, Faculty of Medicine, Dokuz Eylül University, Izmir, Turkey

2 Department of Molecular Medicine, Graduate School of Health Sciences, Dokuz Eylül University, Izmir, Turkey

References

[1] Klareskog, L., A.I. Catrina, and S. Paget, *Rheumatoid arthritis.* Lancet, 2009. **373**(9664): p. 659–72.

[2] Scott, D.L., F. Wolfe, and T.W. Huizinga, *Rheumatoid arthritis.* Lancet, 2010. **376**(9746): p. 1094–108.

[3] Chung, I.M., et al., *Rheumatoid arthritis: The stride from research to clinical practice.* Int J Mol Sci, 2016. **17**(6).

[4] Akar, S., et al., *The prevalence of rheumatoid arthritis in an urban population of Izmir-Turkey.* Clin Exp Rheumatol, 2004. **22**(4): p. 416–20.

[5] McInnes, I.B. and G. Schett, *The pathogenesis of rheumatoid arthritis.* N Engl J Med, 2011. **365**(23): p. 2205–19.

[6] Vicente, R., et al., *Deregulation and therapeutic potential of microRNAs in arthritic diseases.* Nat Rev Rheumatol, 2016. **12**(4): p. 211–20.

[7] Turner, J.D. and A. Filer, *The role of the synovial fibroblast in rheumatoid arthritis pathogenesis.* Curr Opin Rheumatol, 2015. **27**(2): p. 175–82.

[8] Lai, E.C., *microRNAs: runts of the genome assert themselves.* Curr Biol, 2003. **13**(23): p. R925–36.

[9] Carthew, R.W. and E.J. Sontheimer, *Origins and mechanisms of miRNAs and siRNAs.* Cell, 2009. **136**(4): p. 642–55.

[10] Ceribelli, A., et al., *MicroRNAs in rheumatoid arthritis.* FEBS Lett, 2011. **585**(23): p. 3667–74.

[11] Furer, V., et al., *The role of microRNA in rheumatoid arthritis and other autoimmune diseases.* Clin Immunol, 2010. **136**(1): p. 1–15.

[12] Duroux-Richard, I., et al., *MicroRNAs as new player in rheumatoid arthritis.* Joint Bone Spine, 2011. **78**(1): p. 17–22.

[13] He, L. and G.J. Hannon, *MicroRNAs: Small RNAs with a big role in gene regulation.* Nat Rev Genet, 2004. **5**(7): p. 522–31.

[14] Lee, R.C., R.L. Feinbaum, and V. Ambros, *The C. elegans heterochronic gene lin-4 encodes small RNAs with antisense complementarity to lin-14.* Cell, 1993. **75**(5): p. 843–54.

[15] Almeida, M.I., R.M. Reis, and G.A. Calin, *MicroRNA history: discovery, recent applications, and next frontiers.* Mutat Res, 2011. **717**(1–2): p. 1–8.

[16] Bhaskaran, M. and M. Mohan, *MicroRNAs: history, biogenesis, and their evolving role in animal development and disease.* Vet Pathol, 2014. **51**(4): p. 759–74.

[17] Orellana, E.A. and A.L. Kasinski, *MicroRNAs in cancer: a historical perspective on the path from discovery to therapy.* Cancers (Basel), 2015. **7**(3): p. 1388–405.

[18] Riaz, A., R. Dalziel, V.M. Venturina, M.A. Shah, *MicroRNAs: History, biogenesis and modes of action to regulate gene expression.* Veterinaria, 2015. **2**: p. 14–20.

[19] Ruvkun, G., *Molecular biology. Glimpses of a tiny RNA world.* Science, 2001. **294**(5543): p. 797–9.

[20] Lagos-Quintana, M., et al., *Identification of novel genes coding for small expressed RNAs.* Science, 2001. **294**(5543): p. 853–8.

[21] Lau, N.C., et al., *An abundant class of tiny RNAs with probable regulatory roles in Caenorhabditis elegans.* Science, 2001. **294**(5543): p. 858–62.

[22] Lee, R.C. and V. Ambros, *An extensive class of small RNAs in Caenorhabditis elegans.* Science, 2001. **294**(5543): p. 862–4.

[23] Bushati, N.and S.M. Cohen, *microRNA functions.* Annu Rev Cell Dev Biol, 2007. **23**: p. 175–205.

[24] Jiu, S., X. Zhu, J. Wang, C. Zhang, Q. Mu, C. Wang, J. Fang, *Genome-wide mapping and analysis of grapevine microRNAs and their potential target genes.* The Plant Genome, 2015. **8**: p. 1–16.

[25] Lewis, B.P., et al., *Prediction of mammalian microRNA targets.* Cell, 2003. **115**(7): p. 787–98.

[26] Liu, B., J. Li, and M.J. Cairns, *Identifying miRNAs, targets and functions.* Brief Bioinform, 2014. **15**(1): p. 1–19.

[27] Ha, M. and V.N. Kim, *Regulation of microRNA biogenesis.* Nat Rev Mol Cell Biol, 2014. **15**(8): p. 509–24.

[28] Westholm, J.O. and E.C. Lai, *Mirtrons: microRNA biogenesis via splicing.* Biochimie, 2011. **93**(11): p. 1897–904.

[29] Abdelfattah, A.M., C. Park, and M.Y. Choi, *Update on non-canonical microRNAs.* Biomol Concepts, 2014. **5**(4): p. 275–87.

[30] Krol, J., I. Loedige, and W. Filipowicz, *The widespread regulation of microRNA biogenesis, function and decay.* Nat Rev Genet, 2010. **11**(9): p. 597–610.

[31] Havens, M.A., et al., *Biogenesis of mammalian microRNAs by a non-canonical processing pathway.* Nucleic Acids Res, 2012. **40**(10): p. 4626–40.

[32] Ameres, S.L. and P.D. Zamore, *Diversifying microRNA sequence and function.* Nat Rev Mol Cell Biol, 2013. **14**(8): p. 475–88.

[33] Stenvang, J., et al., *Inhibition of microRNA function by antimiR oligonucleotides.* Silence, 2012. **3**(1): p. 1.

[34] Miao, C.G., et al., *Critical roles of microRNAs in the pathogenesis of systemic sclerosis: New advances, challenges and potential directions.* Int Immunopharmacol, 2015. **28**(1): p. 626–33.

[35] Lai, E.C., *miRNAs: whys and wherefores of miRNA-mediated regulation.* Curr Biol, 2005. **15**(12): p. R458–60.

[36] Chen, X.M., et al., *Role of Micro RNAs in the Pathogenesis of Rheumatoid Arthritis: Novel Perspectives Based on Review of the Literature.* Medicine (Baltimore), 2015. **94**(31): p. e1326.

[37] Sharma, A.R., et al., *miRNA-regulated key components of cytokine signaling pathways and inflammation in rheumatoid arthritis.* Med Res Rev, 2016. **36**(3): p. 425–39.

[38] Luo, X., et al., *Evidence for microRNA-mediated regulation in rheumatic diseases.* Ann Rheum Dis, 2010. **69 Suppl 1**: p. i30–36.

[39] Dai, R. and S.A. Ahmed, *MicroRNA, a new paradigm for understanding immunoregulation, inflammation, and autoimmune diseases.* Transl Res, 2011. **157**(4): p. 163–79.

[40] Filipowicz, W., S.N. Bhattacharyya, and N. Sonenberg, *Mechanisms of post-transcriptional regulation by microRNAs: Are the answers in sight?* Nat Rev Genet, 2008. **9**(2): p. 102–14.

[41] Doench, J.G. and P.A. Sharp, *Specificity of microRNA target selection in translational repression.* Genes Dev, 2004. **18**(5): p. 504–11.

[42] Alipoor, S.D., et al., *The roles of miRNAs as potential biomarkers in lung diseases.* Eur J Pharmacol, 2016. **791**: p. 395–404.

[43] Nilsen, T.W., *Mechanisms of microRNA-mediated gene regulation in animal cells.* Trends Genet, 2007. **23**(5): p. 243–9.

[44] Vidigal, J.A. and A. Ventura, *The biological functions of miRNAs: lessons from in vivo studies.* Trends Cell Biol, 2015. **25**(3): p. 137–47.

[45] Pauley, K.M., S. Cha, and E.K. Chan, *MicroRNA in autoimmunity and autoimmune diseases.* J Autoimmun, 2009. **32**(3–4): p. 189–94.

[46] O'Connell, R.M., D.S. Rao, and D. Baltimore, *microRNA regulation of inflammatory responses.* Annu Rev Immunol, 2012. **30**: p. 295–312.

[47] Kawai, T. and S. Akira, *Toll-like receptors and their crosstalk with other innate receptors in infection and immunity.* Immunity, 2011. **34**(5): p. 637–50.

[48] Roach, J.C., et al., *The evolution of vertebrate Toll-like receptors.* Proc Natl Acad Sci U S A, 2005. **102**(27): p. 9577–82.

[49] Takeda, K. and S. Akira, *Toll-like receptors in innate immunity.* Int Immunol, 2005. **17**(1): p. 1–14.

[50] Chen, J.Q., P. Szodoray, and M. Zeher, *Toll-Like Receptor Pathways in Autoimmune Diseases.* Clin Rev Allergy Immunol, 2016. **50**(1): p. 1–17.

[51] Taganov, K.D., et al., *NF-kappaB-dependent induction of microRNA miR-146, an inhibitor targeted to signaling proteins of innate immune responses.* Proc Natl Acad Sci U S A, 2006. **103**(33): p. 12481–6.

[52] Hou, J., et al., *MicroRNA-146a feedback inhibits RIG-I-dependent Type I IFN production in macrophages by targeting TRAF6, IRAK1, and IRAK2.* J Immunol, 2009. **183**(3): p. 2150–8.

[53] Tili, E., et al., *Modulation of miR-155 and miR-125b levels following lipopolysaccharide/TNF-alpha stimulation and their possible roles in regulating the response to endotoxin shock.* J Immunol, 2007. **179**(8): p. 5082–9.

[54] Liu, G., et al., *miR-147, a microRNA that is induced upon Toll-like receptor stimulation, regulates murine macrophage inflammatory responses.* Proc Natl Acad Sci U S A, 2009. **106**(37): p. 15819–24.

[55] Au, K.Y., et al., *MiR-1303 regulates mycobacteria induced autophagy by targeting Atg2B.* PLoS One, 2016. **11**(1): p. e0146770.

[56] Husakova, M., *MicroRNAs in the key events of systemic lupus erythematosus pathogenesis.* Biomed Pap Med Fac Univ Palacky Olomouc Czech Repub, 2016. **160**(3): p. 327–42.

[57] de Yebenes, V.G., et al., *miR-181b negatively regulates activation-induced cytidine deaminase in B cells.* J Exp Med, 2008. **205**(10): p. 2199–206.

[58] Gonzalez-Martin, A., et al., *The microRNA miR-148a functions as a critical regulator of B cell tolerance and autoimmunity.* Nat Immunol, 2016. **17**(4): p. 433–40.

[59] Cobb, B.S., et al., *T cell lineage choice and differentiation in the absence of the RNase III enzyme Dicer*. J Exp Med, 2005. **201**(9): p. 1367–73.

[60] Koralov, S.B., et al., *Dicer ablation affects antibody diversity and cell survival in the B lymphocyte lineage*. Cell, 2008. **132**(5): p. 860–74.

[61] Honardoost, M.A., et al., *miR-326 and miR-26a, two potential markers for diagnosis of relapse and remission phases in patient with relapsing-remitting multiple sclerosis*. Gene, 2014. **544**(2): p. 128–33.

[62] Ceppi, M., et al., *MicroRNA-155 modulates the interleukin-1 signaling pathway in activated human monocyte-derived dendritic cells*. Proc Natl Acad Sci U S A, 2009. **106**(8): p. 2735–40.

[63] O'Connell, R.M., et al., *MicroRNA-155 promotes autoimmune inflammation by enhancing inflammatory T cell development*. Immunity, 2010. **33**(4): p. 607–19.

[64] Lu, L.F., et al., *Function of miR-146a in controlling Treg cell-mediated regulation of Th1 responses*. Cell, 2010. **142**(6): p. 914–29.

[65] Alamanos, Y. and A.A. Drosos, *Epidemiology of adult rheumatoid arthritis*. Autoimmun Rev, 2005. **4**(3): p. 130–6.

[66] Ahlmen, M., et al., *Influence of gender on assessments of disease activity and function in early rheumatoid arthritis in relation to radiographic joint damage*. Ann Rheum Dis, 2010. **69**(1): p. 230–3.

[67] Areskoug-Josefsson, K. and U. Oberg, *A literature review of the sexual health of women with rheumatoid arthritis*. Musculoskeletal Care, 2009. **7**(4): p. 219–26.

[68] Rossini, M., et al., *Prevalence and incidence of rheumatoid arthritis in Italy*. Rheumatol Int, 2014. **34**(5): p. 659–64.

[69] Smolen, J.S., et al., *Treating rheumatoid arthritis to target: 2014 update of the recommendations of an international task force*. Ann Rheum Dis, 2016. **75**(1): p. 3–15.

[70] Uhlig, T., R.H. Moe, and T.K. Kvien, *The burden of disease in rheumatoid arthritis*. Pharmacoeconomics, 2014. **32**(9): p. 841–51.

[71] Vojdani, A., *A potential link between environmental triggers and autoimmunity*. Autoimmune Dis, 2014. **2014**: p. 437231.

[72] Iborra, M., et al., *MicroRNAs in autoimmunity and inflammatory bowel disease: crucial regulators in immune response*. Autoimmun Rev, 2012. **11**(5): p. 305–14.

[73] Jimenez, S.A. and S. Piera-Velazquez, *Potential role of human-specific genes, human-specific microRNAs and human-specific non-coding regulatory RNAs in the pathogenesis of systemic sclerosis and Sjogren's syndrome*. Autoimmun Rev, 2013. **12**(11): p. 1046–51.

[74] Thamilarasan, M., et al., *MicroRNAs in multiple sclerosis and experimental autoimmune encephalomyelitis*. Autoimmun Rev, 2012. **11**(3): p. 174–9.

[75] Singh, R.P., et al., *The role of miRNA in inflammation and autoimmunity*. Autoimmun Rev, 2013. **12**(12): p. 1160–5.

[76] Chatzikyriakidou, A., et al., *miRNAs and related polymorphisms in rheumatoid arthritis susceptibility.* Autoimmun Rev, 2012. **11**(9): p. 636–41.

[77] Salehi, E., et al., *MicroRNAs in rheumatoid arthritis.* Clin Rheumatol, 2015. **34**(4): p. 615–28.

[78] Stanczyk, J., et al., *Altered expression of microRNA in synovial fibroblasts and synovial tissue in rheumatoid arthritis.* Arthritis Rheum, 2008. **58**(4): p. 1001–9.

[79] Wittmann, J. and H.M. Jack, *microRNAs in rheumatoid arthritis: midget RNAs with a giant impact.* Ann Rheum Dis, 2011. **70 Suppl 1**: p. i92–6.

[80] Shibuya, H., et al., *Overexpression of microRNA-223 in rheumatoid arthritis synovium controls osteoclast differentiation.* Mod Rheumatol, 2013. **23**(4): p. 674–85.

[81] Nakasa, T., et al., *Expression of microRNA-146 in rheumatoid arthritis synovial tissue.* Arthritis Rheum, 2008. **58**(5): p. 1284–92.

[82] Niimoto, T., et al., *MicroRNA-146a expresses in interleukin-17 producing T cells in rheumatoid arthritis patients.* BMC Musculoskelet Disord, 2010. **11**: p. 209.

[83] Zhu, S., et al., *The microRNA miR-23b suppresses IL-17-associated autoimmune inflammation by targeting TAB2, TAB3 and IKK-alpha.* Nat Med, 2012. **18**(7): p. 1077–86.

[84] Xu, K., et al., *Reduced apoptosis correlates with enhanced autophagy in synovial tissues of rheumatoid arthritis.* Inflamm Res, 2013. **62**(2): p. 229–37.

[85] Lin, J., et al., *A novel p53/microRNA-22/Cyr61 axis in synovial cells regulates inflammation in rheumatoid arthritis.* Arthritis Rheumatol, 2014. **66**(1): p. 49–59.

[86] Murata, K., et al., *Plasma and synovial fluid microRNAs as potential biomarkers of rheumatoid arthritis and osteoarthritis.* Arthritis Res Ther, 2010. **12**(3): p. R86.

[87] Churov, A.V., E.K. Oleinik, and M. Knip, *MicroRNAs in rheumatoid arthritis: altered expression and diagnostic potential.* Autoimmun Rev, 2015. **14**(11): p. 1029–37.

[88] Nakamachi, Y., et al., *MicroRNA-124a is a key regulator of proliferation and monocyte chemoattractant protein 1 secretion in fibroblast-like synoviocytes from patients with rheumatoid arthritis.* Arthritis Rheum, 2009. **60**(5): p. 1294–304.

[89] Niederer, F., et al., *Down-regulation of microRNA-34a* in rheumatoid arthritis synovial fibroblasts promotes apoptosis resistance.* Arthritis Rheum, 2012. **64**(6): p. 1771–9.

[90] Pandis, I., et al., *Identification of microRNA-221/222 and microRNA-323-3p association with rheumatoid arthritis via predictions using the human tumour necrosis factor transgenic mouse model.* Ann Rheum Dis, 2012. **71**(10): p. 1716–23.

[91] Stanczyk, J., et al., *Altered expression of microRNA-203 in rheumatoid arthritis synovial fibroblasts and its role in fibroblast activation.* Arthritis Rheum, 2011. **63**(2): p. 373–81.

[92] Miao, C.G., et al., *MicroRNA-152 modulates the canonical Wnt pathway activation by targeting DNA methyltransferase 1 in arthritic rat model.* Biochimie, 2014. **106**: p. 149–56.

[93] Miao, C.G., et al., *miR-375 regulates the canonical Wnt pathway through FZD8 silencing in arthritis synovial fibroblasts.* Immunol Lett, 2015. **164**(1): p. 1–10.

[94] Kurowska-Stolarska, M., et al., *MicroRNA-155 as a proinflammatory regulator in clinical and experimental arthritis.* Proc Natl Acad Sci U S A, 2011. **108**(27): p. 11193–8.

[95] Duroux-Richard, I., et al., *Circulating miRNA-125b is a potential biomarker predicting response to rituximab in rheumatoid arthritis.* Mediators Inflamm, 2014. **2014**: p. 342524.

[96] Mookherjee, N. and H.S. El-Gabalawy, *High degree of correlation between whole blood and PBMC expression levels of miR-155 and miR-146a in healthy controls and rheumatoid arthritis patients.* J Immunol Methods, 2013. **400-401**: p. 106–10.

[97] Pauley, K.M., et al., *Upregulated miR-146a expression in peripheral blood mononuclear cells from rheumatoid arthritis patients.* Arthritis Res Ther, 2008. **10**(4): p. R101.

[98] Filkova, M., et al., *Association of circulating miR-223 and miR-16 with disease activity in patients with early rheumatoid arthritis.* Ann Rheum Dis, 2014. **73**(10): p. 1898–904.

[99] Wang, H., et al., *Circulating microRNAs as candidate biomarkers in patients with systemic lupus erythematosus.* Transl Res, 2012. **160**(3): p. 198–206.

[100] Murata, K., et al., *Comprehensive microRNA analysis identifies miR-24 and miR-125a-5p as plasma biomarkers for rheumatoid arthritis.* PLoS One, 2013. **8**(7): p. e69118.

[101] Nagata, Y., et al., *Induction of apoptosis in the synovium of mice with autoantibody-mediated arthritis by the intraarticular injection of double-stranded MicroRNA-15a.* Arthritis Rheum, 2009. **60**(9): p. 2677–83.

[102] Philippe, L., et al., *The miR-17 approximately 92 cluster: A key player in the control of inflammation during rheumatoid arthritis.* Front Immunol, 2013. **4**: p. 70.

[103] Trenkmann, M., et al., *Tumor necrosis factor alpha-induced microRNA-18a activates rheumatoid arthritis synovial fibroblasts through a feedback loop in NF-kappaB signaling.* Arthritis Rheum, 2013. **65**(4): p. 916–27.

[104] Dong, L., et al., *Decreased expression of microRNA-21 correlates with the imbalance of Th17 and Treg cells in patients with rheumatoid arthritis.* J Cell Mol Med, 2014. **18**(11): p. 2213–24.

[105] Tardif, G., et al., *Regulation of the IGFBP-5 and MMP-13 genes by the microRNAs miR-140 and miR 27a in human osteoarthritic chondrocytes.* BMC Musculoskelet Disord, 2009. **10**: p. 148.

[106] Akhtar, N., et al., *MicroRNA-27b regulates the expression of matrix metalloproteinase 13 in human osteoarthritis chondrocytes.* Arthritis Rheum, 2010. **62**(5): p. 1361–71.

[107] Alsaleh, G., et al., *MiR-30a-3p negatively regulates BAFF synthesis in systemic sclerosis and rheumatoid arthritis fibroblasts.* PLoS One, 2014. **9**(10): p. e111266.

[108] Kim, S.W., et al., *MicroRNAs miR-125a and miR-125b constitutively activate the NF-kappaB pathway by targeting the tumor necrosis factor alpha-induced protein 3 (TNFAIP3, A20).* Proc Natl Acad Sci U S A, 2012. **109**(20): p. 7865–70.

[109] Hruskova, V., et al., *MicroRNA-125b: association with disease activity and the treatment response of patients with early rheumatoid arthritis.* Arthritis Res Ther, 2016. **18**(1): p. 124.

[110] Gao, J., et al., *microRNA-126 targeting PIK3R2 promotes rheumatoid arthritis synovial fibroblasts proliferation and resistance to apoptosis by regulating PI3K/AKT pathway.* Exp Mol Pathol, 2016. **100**(1): p. 192–8.

[111] O'Neill, L.A., *Boosting the brain's ability to block inflammation via microRNA-132.* Immunity, 2009. **31**(6): p. 854–5.

[112] Dong, S., et al., *MicroRNAs regulate osteogenesis and chondrogenesis.* Biochem Biophys Res Commun, 2012. **418**(4): p. 587–91.

[113] Yamasaki, K., et al., *Expression of microRNA-146a in osteoarthritis cartilage.* Arthritis Rheum, 2009. **60**(4): p. 1035–41.

[114] Li, J., et al., *Altered microRNA expression profile with miR-146a upregulation in CD4+ T cells from patients with rheumatoid arthritis.* Arthritis Res Ther, 2010. **12**(3): p. R81.

[115] Abou-Zeid, A., M. Saad, and E. Soliman, *MicroRNA 146a expression in rheumatoid arthritis: association with tumor necrosis factor-alpha and disease activity.* Genet Test Mol Biomarkers, 2011. **15**(11): p. 807–12.

[116] Zhou, Q., et al., *Decreased expression of miR-146a and miR-155 contributes to an abnormal Treg phenotype in patients with rheumatoid arthritis.* Ann Rheum Dis, 2015. **74**(6): p. 1265–74.

[117] Guo, M., et al., *miR-146a in PBMCs modulates Th1 function in patients with acute coronary syndrome.* Immunol Cell Biol, 2010. **88**(5): p. 555–64.

[118] Swingler, T.E., et al., *The expression and function of microRNAs in chondrogenesis and osteoarthritis.* Arthritis Rheum, 2012. **64**(6): p. 1909–19.

[119] Yang, S. and Y. Yang, *Downregulation of microRNA221 decreases migration and invasion in fibroblastlike synoviocytes in rheumatoid arthritis.* Mol Med Rep, 2015. **12**(2): p. 2395–401.

[120] Lu, M.C., et al., *Increased miR-223 expression in T cells from patients with rheumatoid arthritis leads to decreased insulin-like growth factor-1-mediated interleukin-10 production.* Clin Exp Immunol, 2014. **177**(3): p. 641–51.

[121] Fulci, V., et al., *miR-223 is overexpressed in T-lymphocytes of patients affected by rheumatoid arthritis.* Hum Immunol, 2010. **71**(2): p. 206–11.

[122] Murata, K., et al., *MicroRNA-451 down-regulates neutrophil chemotaxis via p38 MAPK.* Arthritis Rheumatol, 2014. **66**(3): p. 549–59.

[123] Krintel, S.B., et al., *Prediction of treatment response to adalimumab: a double-blind placebo-controlled study of circulating microRNA in patients with early rheumatoid arthritis.* Pharmacogenomics J, 2016. **16**(2): p. 141–6.

[124] Jiang, S., T.E. Hinchliffe, and T. Wu, *Biomarkers of an autoimmune skin disease—Psoriasis.* Genomics Proteomics Bioinformatics, 2015. **13**(4): p. 224–33.

[125] Ichihara, A., et al., *Increased serum levels of miR-1266 in patients with psoriasis vulgaris.* Eur J Dermatol, 2012. **22**(1): p. 68–71.

[126] Lovendorf, M.B., et al., *MicroRNA-223 and miR-143 are important systemic biomarkers for disease activity in psoriasis.* J Dermatol Sci, 2014. **75**(2): p. 133–9.

[127] Chandra, A., et al., *Genetic and epigenetic basis of psoriasis pathogenesis.* Mol Immunol, 2015. **64**(2): p. 313–23.

[128] Joyce, C.E., et al., *Deep sequencing of small RNAs from human skin reveals major alterations in the psoriasis miRNAome.* Hum Mol Genet, 2011. **20**(20): p. 4025–40.

[129] Dai, Y., et al., *Microarray analysis of microRNA expression in peripheral blood cells of systemic lupus erythematosus patients.* Lupus, 2007. **16**(12): p. 939–46.

[130] Dai, Y., et al., *Comprehensive analysis of microRNA expression patterns in renal biopsies of lupus nephritis patients.* Rheumatol Int, 2009. **29**(7): p. 749–54.

[131] Tang, Y., et al., *MicroRNA-146A contributes to abnormal activation of the type I interferon pathway in human lupus by targeting the key signaling proteins.* Arthritis Rheum, 2009. **60**(4): p. 1065–75.

[132] Otaegui, D., et al., *Differential micro RNA expression in PBMC from multiple sclerosis patients.* PLoS One, 2009. **4**(7): p. e6309.

[133] Brown, K.D., E. Claudio, and U. Siebenlist, *The roles of the classical and alternative nuclear factor-kappaB pathways: potential implications for autoimmunity and rheumatoid arthritis.* Arthritis Res Ther, 2008. **10**(4): p. 212.

14

Efficacy of SSEA-3 Positive Cells Derived from Synovial Tissue in Rheumatoid Arthritis

Rie Kurose and Takashi Sawai

Abstract

Rheumatoid arthritis (RA) is a refractory systemic autoimmune disease with chronic synovial inflammation. Sustained synovial inflammation leads to progressive destruction of bone and cartilage. Treatment to restore joints that have been destroyed irreversibly is not to be established yet even with the recent development of antirheumatic drugs and biological agents. Stage-specific embryonic antigen-3 (SSEA-3), a marker of human embryonic stem (ES) cell, acts as stem cells in the blood. SSEA-3 positive cells derived from RA synovial tissue have higher differentiating abilities than that of SSEA-3 negative cells and inhibitory effects on arthritis in collagen antibody-induced arthritis mice study. SSEA-3 positive cells derived from RA synovial tissue might have the inhibitory effect on arthritis and would be one of the cell sources for new RA treatment. The present manuscript is a brief review of mesenchymal stem cells in RA and described with the potential of RA cell therapy by SSEA-3 positive cells based on our research.

Keywords: rheumatoid arthritis, synovial tissue, SSEA-3

1. Introduction

Rheumatoid arthritis (RA) is a refractory systemic autoimmune disease with chronic synovial inflammation. Sustained synovial inflammation leads to progressive destruction of bone and cartilage. In the pathogenesis of RA, activated T cells and antigen-presenting cells such as monocytes and macrophages produce inflammatory cytokines such as tumor necrosis factor-α (TNF-α), interleukin (IL)-1β, IL-2, IL-6, and interferon-γ (INF-γ). They promote release of inflammatory mediators, infiltration of inflammatory cells, production of autoantibody, proliferation of the synovial cells, and activation of the osteoclasts, resulting in the bone and the cartilage destruction [1–3].

In the last few years, development of disease-modifying antirheumatic drugs (DMARDs) and biological agents targeting inflammatory cytokines has been major advances in the treatment of RA. Biological agents targeting inflammatory cytokines such as TNF-α, which has been shown to be a key factor in the pathology of RA, are effective for RA. These are known to improve disease activity and inhibit the progress of joint destruction. The best possible treatment goal for patients is clinical remission and consistently stopping continuing joint damage through erosions.

However, treatment to restore joints that have been destroyed irreversibly is not to be established yet. Also, DMARDs or biological agents can have serious side effects affecting the blood, liver, or kidneys rarely. Therefore, a novel RA treatment that enables restoration of destroyed joints is needed. Use of mesenchymal stem cells (MSCs) derived from bone marrow as a biological method for repairing articular cartilage defects have been investigated [4–8]. We think that the treatment by thus autologous cells can overcome these problems.

2. Mesenchymal stem cells in RA synovial tissue

2.1. Multipotency

MSCs are self-renewing, multipotent progenitor cells with multilineage potential to differentiate into various types of cells including chondrocytes, osteoblasts, and adipocytes [9–15]. While MSCs are most commonly isolated from bone marrow [13] and proliferate rapidly in vitro, they are also isolated from other tissues including adipose tissue [16], placenta [17], and umbilical cord blood [18]. Due to their accessibility and convenient expansion protocols, ethical dilemmas and risk of tumor formation, such as in ES cells and iPS cells, can also be avoided and therefore MSCs are easy to use in clinical application and have been recognized as promising candidates for cell therapy.

We investigated earlier the potential of chondrogenic differentiation of MSCs derived from bone marrow and synovial fluid in human osteoarthritis (OA) [19, 20]. Our study concluded that both bone marrow MSCs (BMMSCs) and synovial fluid MSCs (SFMSCs) had a potential of cell proliferation and chondrogenic differentiation. Both cells were fibroblast-like cells and had similar cell surface antigen in flow cytometry analysis, namely positive for CD13, CD44, and CD105 and negative for CD10, CD14, and CD45. However, aggrecan (AGC) mRNA expression in SFMSCs, which are traditionally associated with chondrogenic commitment, was a significant high compared to BMMSCs in vitro. According to other researches, SFMSCs are considered the same as synovial MSCs [21, 22]. Study of Sekiya et al. [23] reported that synovial MSCs are a candidate cell source for regenerative medicine of cartilage due to their high chondrogenic ability. They demonstrated that chondrogenic potentials of synovial MSCs between RA and OA patients were similar, as the weight of the pellet is a quantitative indicator of the ability of MSCs to produce chondrogenesis in vitro. Therefore, autologous synovial MSCs can be expected in cartilage regeneration for RA patients. According to previous reports [24], there was a negative relationship between chondrogenic potential of synovial MSCs and magnitude of synovitis in RA, and some properties of synovial MSCs vary dependent on the diseases patients have. Also, it was reported that chondrogenic potential in RA patients was inferior to that in OA patients. However, Jones et al. [24] reported that effective suppression of joint inflammation is necessary for the development of autologous MSC treatments aimed at cartilage regeneration in RA and synovial MSCs can be expected for RA patients with the inflammation well controlled as well as OA patients.

2.2. Immunosuppresive effect

Previous reports have suggested that synovial MSCs harvested from RA were capable of immunosuppression in vitro [24]. However, other reports have suggested that the immunomodulatory function of synovial MSCs seems to be disturbed and causes an inefficacy due to various factors within RA microenvironment and as a result of a direct contact with inflammatory cells and cytokines [25]. In RA synovial tissue, synovial MSCs appear to play an important role in controlling the inflammation and immune hemostasis.

3. Stage-specific embryonic antigen-3 (SSEA-3) positive cells in RA synovial tissue

3.1. SSEA-3

Multilineage differentiating stress enduring (Muse) cells are a novel type of pluripotent stem cells and recently reported as adult human MSCs without introducing exogenous genes. They are present in various organs such as pancreas, dermis, umbilical cord, fat, liver, trachea, bone marrow, spleen [26–31] and are contained at a proportion of several percent in cultured mesenchymal stem cells [26], 4–9% in human adipose tissue [27] and 1–2% in human skin fibroblasts [26]. Muse cells are able to differentiate into cells from all three embryonic germ layers both spontaneously and under media-specific induction. Also, Muse cells have a low tumor-forming ability compared with embryonic stem (ES) cells and a high efficiency of change to iPS cells by Yamanaka gene introduction [32]. They can migrate to damaged tissues by intravenous injection in vivo, spontaneously differentiate into cells compatible with the targeted tissue, and contribute to tissue repair. Thus, Muse cells will be expected to play an important role in regenerative therapy by further studies. SSEA-3 is a marker of human embryonic stem cell. Muse cells are able to be isolated as SSEA-3 positive cells from cultured mesenchymal cells.

SSEA-3 positive cells are autologous cells and act as stem cells in the blood and also possess immunosuppression effects [28–31]. Therefore, they could be one of novel cell sources as cell therapy in RA. We studied the possibility of SSEA-3 positive cells derived from RA synovial tissue.

3.2. SSEA-3 as cell therapy in RA

3.2.1. SSEA-3 positive cells in RA synovial tissue

We used synovial tissue harvested from 13 RA patients at the time of joint surgery in our hospital (**Table 1**) [33]. Diagnosis of RA for all patients was based on the American College of Rheumatology (ACR) criteria in 1987 [34] or the ACR/European League Against Rheumatism

Pts.	Age	M/F	Stage	Class	R/L	Surgery
1	73	M	IV	III	R	total knee arthroplasty
2	45	F	I	II	L	arthroscopic synovectomy
3	78	M	III	I	R	total knee arthroplasty
4	82	F	IV	II	R	total knee arthroplasty
5	77	M	IV	II	L	total knee arthroplasty
6	84	F	IV	II	R	total knee arthroplasty
7	69	F	III	II	R	total elbow arthroplasty
8	77	F	III	II	L	total elbow arthroplasty
9	66	F	IV	II	R	2nd, 4th PIP arthrodesis
10	69	F	IV	III	L	1st IP arthrodesis
11	61	F	IV	II	R	wrist arthroplasty
12	62	F	IV	II	R	1st IP arthrodesis
13	66	F	III	I	L	total hip arthroplasty

Pts, patients; M/F, male or female; R/L, right or left; PIP, proximal interphalangeal joint; IP, interphalangeal joint.

Table 1. Clinical data of patients with RA (n = 13) for this study.

(EULAR) classification criteria in 2010 [35]. Approval for this study was obtained from the Ethics of Human Experiments Committee at Hirosaki University Graduate School of Medicine, Hirosaki, Japan. Informed consent was obtained from all patients.

Immunohistochemical staining was performed to investigate the localization of SSEA-3 positive cells in RA synovial tissue. Harvested synovial tissue was immediately fixed in 4% paraformaldehyde/PBS and embedded in paraffin in a usual manner. Rat monoclonal antibody specific for human SSEA-3 (Merck Millipore, Darmstadt, Germany) was used as a primary antibody. Immunoreactivity was detected by incubation with a biotinylated anti-rat IgG antibody (Vectastain ABC kit; Vector Laboratories, Burlingame, CA, USA), followed by streptavidin-biotin reaction (Vectastain ABC kit). Immunohistochemical staining for SSEA-3 showed a few positive cells in RA synovial tissue (**Figure 1a–c**).

Harvested synovial tissue was minced, digested with 3 mg/mL collagenase Type V (Wako Pure Chemical Industries: Osaka, Japan) for 3 hours at 37°C, and cultured in the αMEM (Sigma-Aldrich: Tokyo, Japan) containing 10% fetal bovine serum (FBS) (Thermo Fisher Scientific: Waltham, MA, USA) and antibiotics (100 units/mL penicillin G and 100 μg/mL streptomycin) (Thermo Fisher Scientific) at 37°C in a 5% CO_2 incubator. SSEA-3 positive cells were sorted by suspending 1×10^6 synovial cells at passage 2 in 100 ml FACS buffer containing 1 ml of EDTA, 5 ml of BSA, and 44 ml of FluoroBrite DMEM (Thermo Fisher Scientific, Waltham, MA, USA). Cells were collected by using antibody specific for SSEA-3, approximately 1% in cultured cells (**Figure 1d**).

SSEA-3 positive cells strongly expressed CD44, CD90, and CD105 and lacked CD34 (**Figure 2**) in flow cytometry assay. SSEA-3 negative cells were similar to positive cells in immunophenotype, but they weakly expressed CD105.

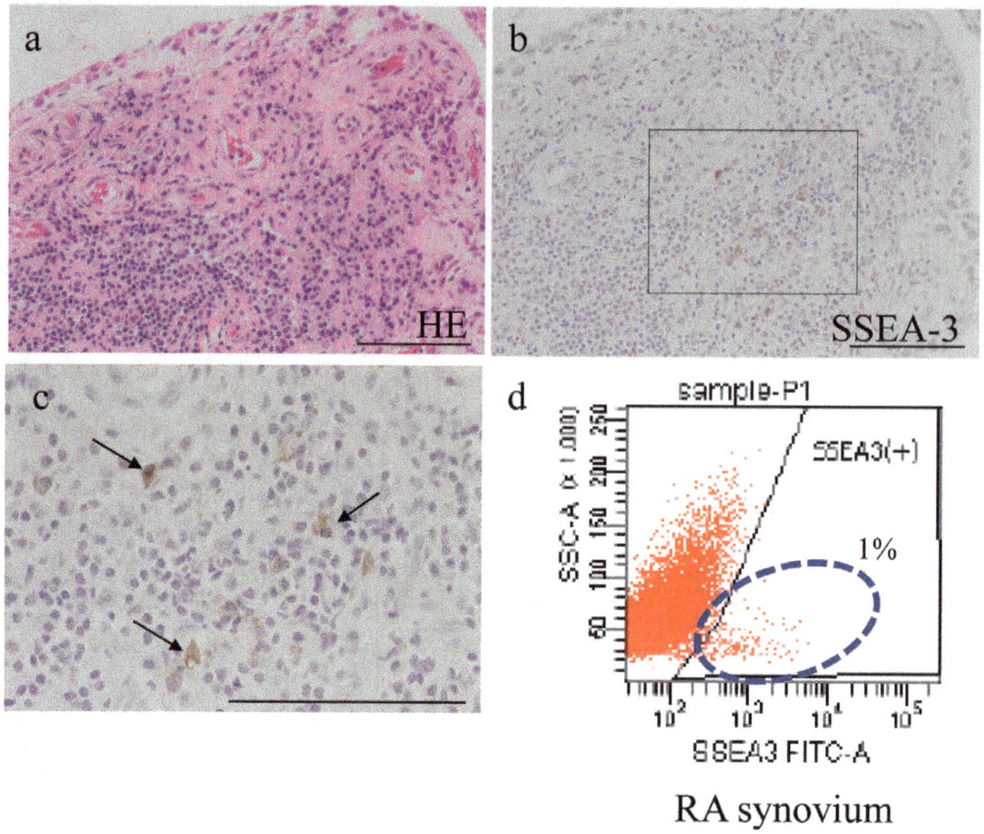

Figure 1. (a) RA synovial tissue. Hematoxylin and eosin (HE) staining. (b) Immunohistochemical staining specific for SSEA-3 in RA synovial tissue. (c) Magnified feature of (b). Bar = 100 **mm**. (d) Ratio of SSEA-3 positive cells in cultured cells derived from RA synovial tissue.

Histological staining after differentiation induction culture showed differentiation into osteoblasts, adipocytes, and chondrocytes from the cultured SSEA-3 positive cells (**Figure 3**). In all mRNA expression of alkaline phosphatase (ALP) and bone morphogenetic protein 2 (BMP2) for osteogenic differentiation, peroxisome proliferator-activated receptor gamma (PPARγ) for adipogenic differentiation and type II collagen (COL2A1), sex determining region Y (SRY)-Box 9 (SOX9) and aggrecan (AGG) for chondrogenic differentiation, SSEA-3 positive cells showed higher gene expression level than SSEA-3 negative cells although there were individual differences (**Figure 4**). These results indicate possibility of higher differentiation ability of SSEA-3 positive cells.

3.2.2. *Inhibitory effect on arthritis*

Collagen antibody-induced arthritis (CAIA) mice were established as the animal model for RA [36]. Induction of CAIA mice was performed on *scid/scid* mice, 7 weeks old (CLEA Japan), in which they were injected with 1.5 mg of 5-clone cocktail (arthrogen-CIA arthrogenic monoclonal antibody (mAb), Chondrex, Redmond, WA) by intraperitoneal (IP) injection at Day 0. Fifty micrograms of lipopolysaccharide (LPS) (Chondrex) was injected by IP injection at Day 3. 3×10^4. SSEA-3 positive cells labeled with cell tracker green (CTG) (Thermo Fisher Scientific) were suspended in PBS, filtered, then intravenously injected via the tail vein after the injection of LPS at Day 3. SSEA-3 negative cells labeled with CTG were used in the same procedure as control. Mice were scored for clinical arthritis; paws were assessed for signs of redness and swelling.

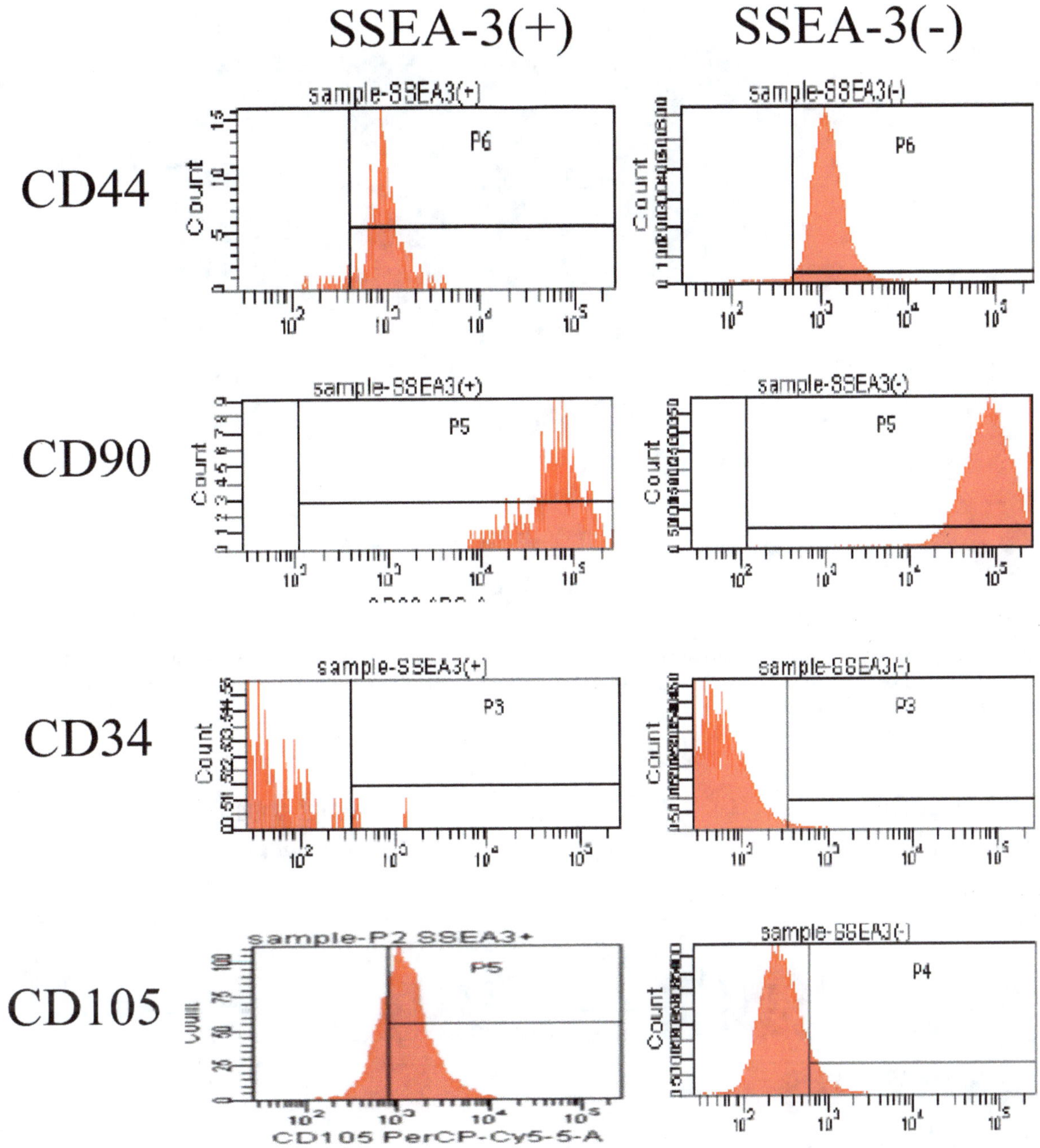

Figure 2. Representative flow cytometry analysis data.

Each paw was given a score of 0–4, giving a total maximum score of 16. (0, normal paw; 1, mild but definite redness and swelling in each joint of the digit or wrist/ankle; 2, moderate redness and swelling in two joints of the wrist/ankle with digit involvement; 3, severe redness and swelling in whole paw; 4, maximum inflammation within the wrist/ankle with many digits involved) [37]. **Figure 5a** displays the arthritis score of CAIA mice in the both transplanted groups after mAb injection. The group transplanted with SSEA-3 positive cells (n = 3) consisted of mice with intravenously transplanted SSEA-3 positive cells labeled with cell tracker green (CTG) seen in **Figure 5b**, while the group transplanted with SSEA-3 negative cells (n = 3) consisted mice with the transplanted SSEA-3 negative cells in the same procedure. Arthritis in the SSEA-3 negative cells group remained for 28 days, while arthritis score in the SSEA-3 positive cells group improved faster after peak inflammation (**Figure 5a**). There was a significant

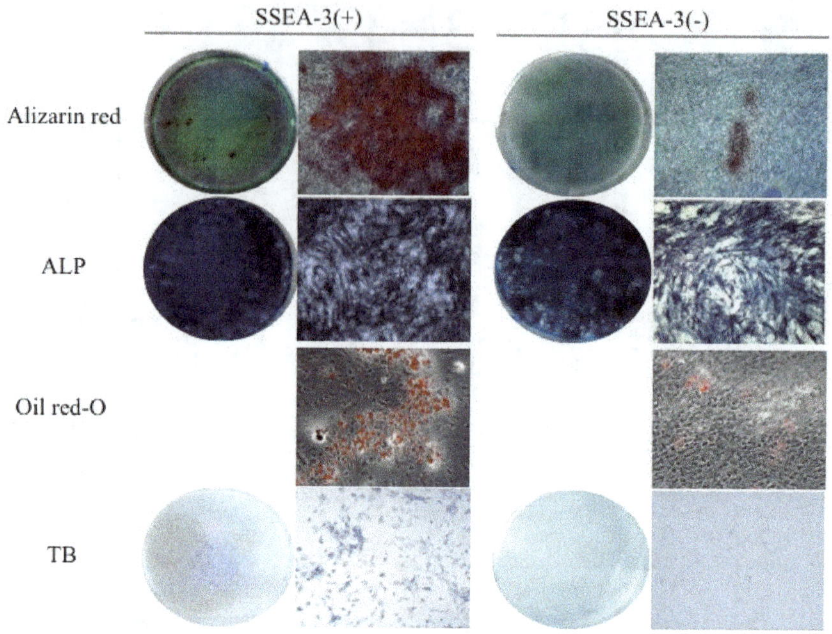

Figure 3

Figure 3. Multipotency of SSEA-3 positive cells derived from RA synovial cells. Osteogenesis was shown by alizarin red and alkaline phosphatase (ALP) staining. Adipogenesis was shown by oil red-O staining and chondrogenesis was shown by toluidine blue (TB) staining.

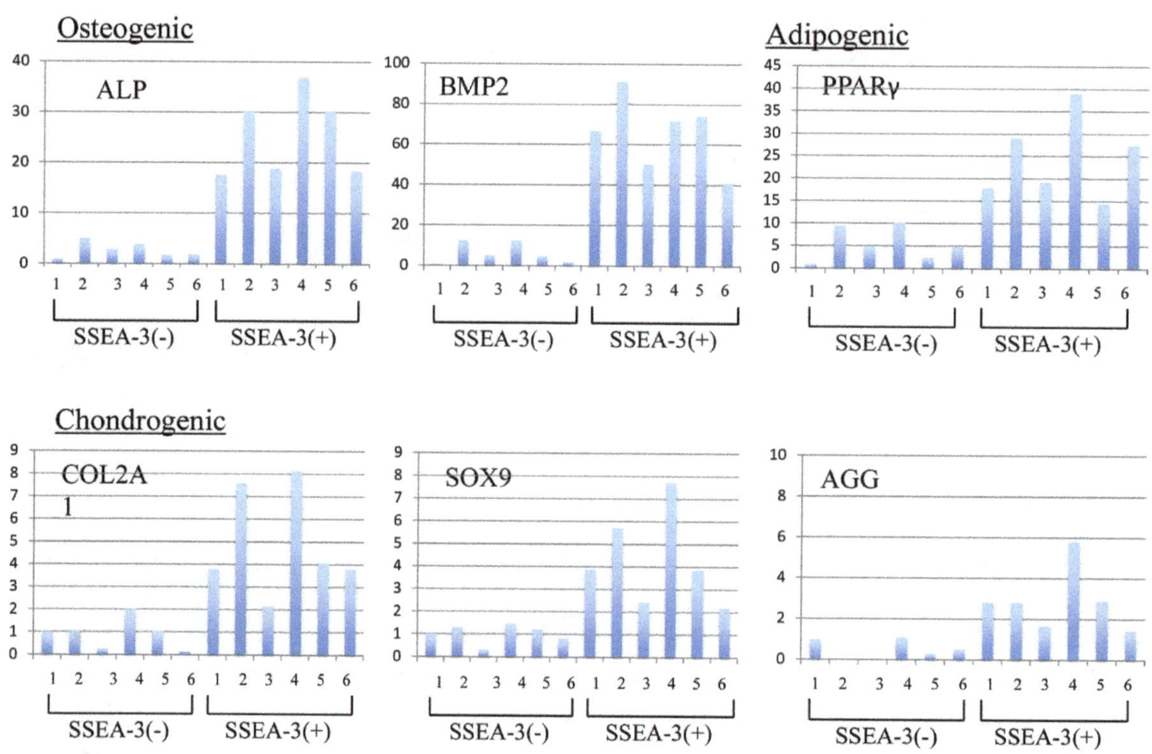

Figure 4. Real-time polymerase chain reaction (PCR) analysis. Results are reported as the mean of three independent experiments and the messenger RNA (mRNA) value of glyceraldehydes-3-phosphate-dehydrogenase (GAPDH) was set as an internal control. Osteogenesis was shown by the expression of ALP mRNA and BMP-2 mRNA, adipogenesis was shown by the expression of PPARγ mRNA and chondrogenesis was shown by the expression of COL2A1 mRNA, SOX9 and AGG. Each data represents an average of three times. Note that the x-axis numbers represent patients in **Table 1**. The mRNA values of y-axis were arbitrary set.

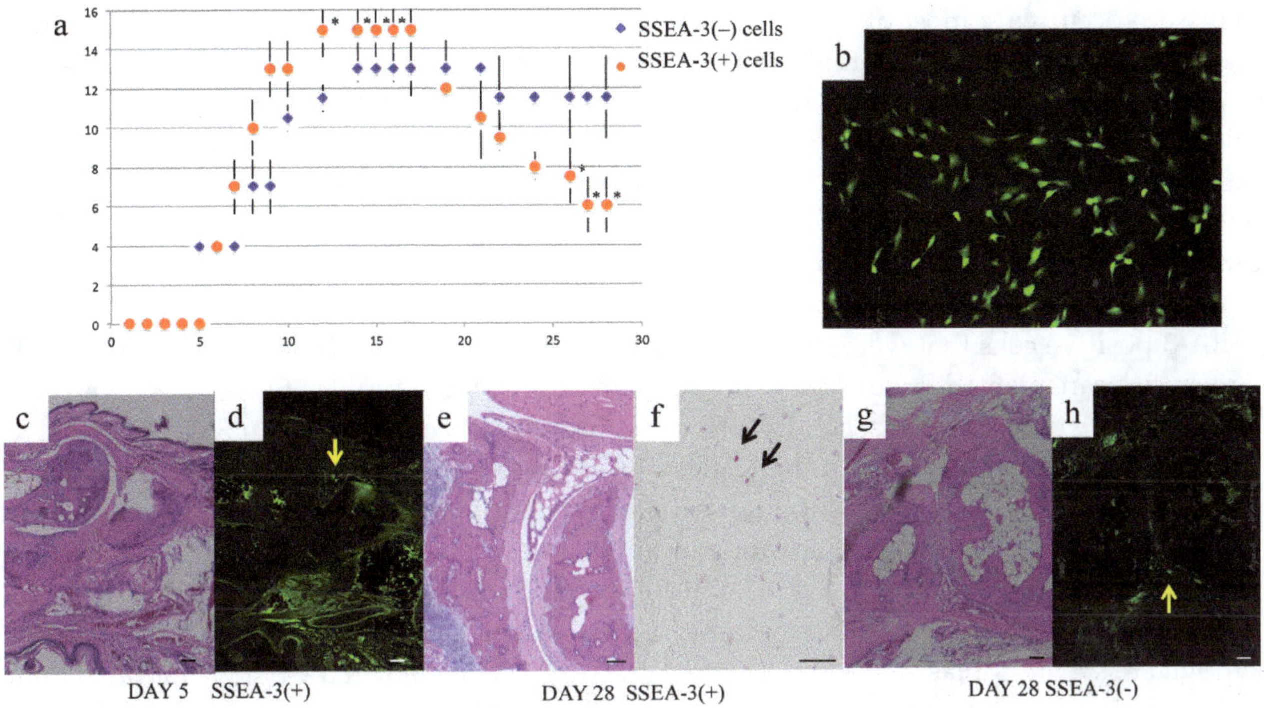

Figure 5. (a) Arthritis score of CAIA mice after mAb injection. SSEA-3 (–) cells group consisted of mice transplanted with SSEA-3 negative cells. SSEA-3 (+) cells group consisted of mice transplanted with SSEA-3 positive cells. Both groups contained three mice. Each score shows average values of three mice and * means $p < 0.05$. The X-axis means the day from day 0 when the monoclonal antibody cocktail was administered. (b) Cell tracker green (CTG)-labeled SSEA-3 positive cells (10X). (c, d and e, f) histology of joint of CAIA mouse after CTG-labeled SSEA-3 positive cells injections on day 5 and 28, respectively. Arrows shows CTG-labeled cells and positive cells for SSEA-3 in immunohistochemical staining. Bar = 100 **mm.** (g and h) representative histology of joint of CAIA mouse after CTG-labeled SSEA-3 negative cells injections on day 28. Bar = 100 **mm**.

improvement in arthritis in the SSEA-3 positive cells group. On Day 5, CTG-labeled cells were detected in the synovial tissue (**Figure 5c** and **d**) and were still present on Day 28 (**Figure 5e** and **f**) in the group transplanted with SSEA-3 positive cells. **Figure 5e** shows representative joint in the group transplanted with SSEA-3 positive cells on Day 28 and **Figure 5f** shows SSEA-3 positive cells in synovial tissue in the immunohistochemical staining of **Figure 5e**. **Figure 5g** and **h** show the progression of joint destruction in the group transplanted with SSEA-3 negative cells on Day 28. CTG-labeled cells were not detected in other healthy organs on Day 28 by fluorescent microscopy (data not shown). These results indicate that SSEA-3 positive cells have the inhibitory effect on arthritis and systemic administration of them is safety.

4. Conclusions

In our study, SSEA-3 positive cells were detected in RA synovial tissue even under pathological conditions such as RA. Although the synovial tissue we used was collected from various RA disease stages and surgical sites, SSEA-3 positive cells were detected with values of approximately 0.5–1% in all cultured SFMSCs. Collected SSEA-3 positive cells had higher gene expression level and differentiation ability in vitro compared with SSEA-3 negative cells that were occupying most of mesenchymal stem cells. Wakao S., et al., reported that Muse and non-Muse cells had differentiation ability of osteocytes, chondrocytes, and adipocytes, while differentiation ability in non-Muse cells was lower [31]. We think that SSEA-3 positive cells in this study had a similar nature as Muse cells, considering also the results that SSEA-3 positive cells strongly expressed CD105 in FACS analysis. SSEA-3 positive cells can be systemically administered by intravenous administration like Muse cells and have possibility of differentiation into osteoblasts, adipocytes, and chondrocyte. These suggest the possibility of repairing degenerative cartilage and destroyed joints in RA. In the CAIA mice experiment, SSEA-3 positive cells that were systemically administered had an inhibitory effect on arthritis. In the transplanted group consisting of mice transplanted with SSEA-3 positive cells, arthritis score quickly decreased after the onset of arthritis compared with SSEA-3 negative cells group. There were some previous studies on immunosuppressive effect of BMMSCs [38–40] and SFMSCs [24] as mentioned earlier. Especially, SFMSCs extracted from healthy subjects are able to inhibit T-cell proliferation [25]. However, immunomodulatory function of SFMSCs and SSEA-3 positive cells may be disturbed and cause an inefficacy of SFMSCs and SSEA-3 positive cells in inflammatory environment like uncontrolled RA [41]. In RA synovial tissue, fibroblast-like synoviocytes (FLS) are key players in the perpetuation of joint inflammation and destruction. The link between FLS and SFMSCs plays an important role in controlling the inflammation and immune hemostasis in RA. In our mice study, autologous SSEA-3 positive cells proliferated in vitro might have altered the balance of immune regulation with FLS.

Our study suggests the possibility of inhibiting arthritis and joint destruction by SSEA-3 positive cells derived from synovial tissue in RA. Further study of SSEA-3 positive cells for clinical application in humans will lead to future development as a new treatment in RA.

Author details

Rie Kurose[1]* and Takashi Sawai[2]

*Address all correspondence to: riekuro@hirosaki-u.ac.jp

1 Department of Orthopaedic Surgery, Hirosaki University Graduate School of Medicine, Hirosaki, Japan

2 Department of Histopathology, Tohoku University, Sendai, Japan

References

[1] Lefevre S, Knedla A, Tennie C, Kampmann A, Wunrau C, Dinser R, Korb A, Schnäker EM, Tarner IH, Robbins PD, Evans CH, Stürz H, Steinmeyer J, Gay S, Schölmerich J, Pap T, Müller-Ladner U, Neumann E. Synovial fibroblasts spread rheumatoid arthritis to unaffected joints. Nature Medicine. 2009;**15**(12):1414-1420

[2] Karouzakis E, Neidhart M, Gay RE, Gay S. Molecular and cellular basis of rheumatoid joint destruction. Immunology Letters. 2006;**106**:8-13

[3] Muller-Ladner U, Pap T, Gay RE, Neidhart M, Gay S. Mechanisms of disease: The molecular and cellular basis of joint destruction in rheumatoid arthritis. Nature Clinical Practice. Rheumatology. 2005;**1**:102-110

[4] Wakitani S, Goto T, Pineda SJ, Young RG, Mansour JM, Caplan AI, Goldberg VM. Mesenchymal cell-based repair of large, full-thickness defects of articular cartilage. The Journal of Bone and Joint Surgery. American Volume. 1994;**76**:579-592

[5] Ponticiello MS, Schinagl RM, Kadiyala S, Barry FP. Gelatin-based resorbable sponge as a carrier matrix for human mesenchymal stem cells in cartilage regeneration therapy. Journal of Biomedical Materials Research. 2000;**52**:246-255

[6] Im GI, Kim DY, Shin JH, Hyun CW, Cho WH. Repair of cartilage defect in the rabbit with cultured mesenchymal stem cells from bone marrow. Journal of Bone and Joint Surgery. British Volume (London). 2001;**83**:289-294

[7] Wakitani S, Imoto K, Yamamoto T, Saito M, Murata N, Yoneda M. Human autologous culture expanded bone marrow mesenchymal cell transplantation for repair of cartilage defects in osteoarthritic knees. Osteoarthritis and Cartilage. 2002;**10**:199-206

[8] Katayama R, Wakitani S, Tsumaki N, Morita Y, Matsushita I, Gejo R, Kimura T. Repair of articular cartilage defects in rabbits using CDMP1 gene-transfected autologous mesenchymal cells derived from bone marrow. Rheumatology. 2004;**43**(8):980-985

[9] Wakitani S, Saito T, Caplan AI. Myogenic cells derived from rat bone marrow mesenchymal stem cells exposed to 5-azacytidine. Muscle & Nerve. 1995;**18**:1417-1426

[10] Jaiswal N, Haynesworth SE, Caplan AI, Bruder SP. Osteogenic differentiation of purified, culture-expanded human mesenchymal stem cells in vitro. Journal of Cellular Biochemistry. 1997;**64**:295-312

[11] Johnstone B, Hering TM, Caplan AI, Goldberg VM, Yoo JU. In vitro chondrogenesis of bone marrow-derived mesenchymal progenitor cells. Experimental Cell Research. 1998;**238**:265-272

[12] Yoo JU, Barthel TS, Nishimura K, Solchaga L, Caplan AI, Goldberg VM, Johnstone B. The chondrogenic potential of human bone-marrow-derived mesenchymal progenitor cells. The Journal of Bone and Joint Surgery. American Volume. 1998;**80**:1745-1757

[13] Pittenger MF, Mackay AM, Beck SC, Jaiswal RK, Douglas R, Mosca JD, Moorman MA, Simonetti DW, Craig S, Marshak DR. Multilineage potential of adult human mesenchymal stem cells. Science. 1999;**284**:143-146

[14] Tsutsumi S, Shimazu A, Miyazaki K, Pan H, Koike C, Yoshida E, Takagishi K, Kato Y. Retention of multilineage differentiation potential of mesenchymal cells during proliferation in response to FGF. Biochemical and Biophysical Research Communications. 2001;**288**:413-419

[15] Jiang Y, Jahagirdar BN, Reinhardt RL, Schwartz RE, Keene CD, Ortiz-Gonzalez XR, Reyes M, Lenvik T, Lund T, Blackstad M, Du J, Aldrich S, Lisberg A, Low WC, Largaespada DA, Verfaillie CM. Pluripotency of mesenchymal stem cells derived from adult marrow. Nature. 2002;**418**:41-49

[16] Zuk PA, Zhu M, Mizuno H, Huang J, Futrell JW, Katz AJ, Benhaim P, Lorenz HP, Hedrick MH. Multilineage cells from human adipose tissue: implications for cell-based therapies. Tissue Engineering. 2001;**7**:211-228

[17] Zhang Y, Li C, Jiang X, Zhang S, Wu Y, Liu B, Tang P, Mao N. Human placenta-derived mesenchymal progenitor cells support culture expansion of long-term culture-initiating cells from cord blood CD34+ cells. Experimental Hematology. 2004;**32**:657-664

[18] Bieback K, Kern S, Kluter H, Eichler H. Critical parameters for the isolation of mesenchymal stem cells from umbilical cord blood. Stem Cells. 2004;**22**:625-634

[19] Kurose R, Ichinohe S, Tajima G, Horiuchi S, Kurose A, Sawai T, Shimamura T. Characterization of human synovial fluid cells of 26 patients with osteoarthritis knee for cartilage repair therapy. International Journal of Rheumatic Diseases. 2010;**13**:68-74

[20] Kurose R, Sawai T. Cell-Based Therapy for Human OA. In: Osteoarthritis - Progress in Basic Research and Treatment. InTech Open Access Books; 2015

[21] Jones EA, English A, Henshaw K, Kinsey SE, Markham AF, Emery P, McGonagle D. Enumeration and phenotypic characterization of synovial fluid multipotential mesenchymal progenitor cells in inflammatory and degenerative arthritis. Arthritis and Rheumatism. 2004;**50**:817-827

[22] Jones EA, Crawford A, English A, Henshaw K, Mundy J, Corscadden D, Chapman T, Emery P, Hatton P, McGonagle D. Synovial fluid mesenchymal stem cells in health and early osteoarthritis: detection and functional evalution at the singlecell level. Arthritis and Rheumatism. 2008;**58**:1731-1740

[23] Kohno Y, Mizuno M, Ozeki N, Katano H, Komori K, Fujii S, Otabe K, Horie M, Koga H, Tsuji K, Matsumoto M, Kaneko H, Takazawa Y, Muneta T, Sekiya I. Yields and chondrogenic potential of primary synovial mesenchymal stem cells are comparable between rheumatoid arthritis and osteoarthritis patients. Stem Cell Research & Therapy. 2017;**8**(1):115

[24] Jones E, Churchman SM, English A, Buch MH, Horner EA, Burgoyne CH, Reece R, Kinsey S, Emery P, McGonagle D, Ponchel F. Mesenchymal stem cells in rheumatoid synovium: enumeration and functional assessment in relation to synovial inflammation level. Annals of the Rheumatic Diseases. 2010;**69**(2):450-457

[25] Djouad F, Bony C, Haupl T, Uze G, Lahlou N, Louis-Plence P, Apparailly F, Canovas F, Rème T, Sany J, Jorgensen C, Noël D. Transcriptional profiles discriminate bone marrow-derived and synovium-derived mesenchymal stem cells. Arthritis Research & Therapy. 2005;**7**:1304-1315

[26] Kuroda Y, Kitada M, Wakao S, Nishikawa K, Tanimura Y, Makinoshima H, Goda M, Akashi H, Inutsuka A, Niwa A, Shigemoto T, Nabeshima Y, Nakahata T, Nabeshima Y, Fujiyoshi Y, Dezawa M. Unique multipotent cells in adult human mesenchymal cell populations. Proceedings of the National Academy of Sciences of the United States of America. 2010;**107**:8639-8643

[27] Ogura F, Wakao S, Kuroda Y, Tsuchiyama K, Bagheri M, Heneidi S, Chazenbalk G, Aiba S, Dezawa M. Human adipose tissue possesses a unique population of pluripotent stem cells with nontumorigenic and low telomerase activities: potential implications in regenerative medicine. Stem Cells and Development. 2014;**23**(7):717-728

[28] Wakao S, Akashi H, Kushida Y, Dezawa M. Muse cells, a novel type of non-tumorigenic pluripotent stem cells, reside in human mesenchymal tissues. Pathology International. 2014;**64**(1):1-9

[29] Kuroda Y, Wakao S, Kitada M, Murakami T, Nojima M, Dezawa M. Isolation, culture and evaluation of multilineage-differentiating stress enduring (muse) cells. Nature Protocols. 2013;**8**(7):1391-1415

[30] Wakao S, Kuroda Y, Ogura F, Shigemoto T, Dezawa M. Regenerative effects of mesenchymal stem cells: Contribution of muse cells, a novel pluripotent stem cell type that resides in mesenchymal cells. Cell. 2012;**1**:1045-1060

[31] Wakao S, Kitada M, Kuroda Y, Shigemoto T, Matsuse D, Akashi H, Tanimura Y, Tsuchiyama K, Kikuchi T, Goda M, Nakahata T, Fujiyoshi Y, Dezawa M. Multilineage-differentiating stress-enduring (muse) cells are a primary source of induced pluripotent stem cells in human fibroblasts. Proceedings of the National Academy of Sciences of the United States of America. 2011;**108**(24):9875-9880

[32] Takahashi K, Tanabe K, Ohnuki M, Narita M, Ichisaka T, Tomoda K, Yamanaka S. Induction of pluripotent stem cells from adult human fibroblasts by defined factors. Cell. 2007;**131**:861-872

[33] Kurose R, Sawai T, Oishi K, Liu X, Sasaki A, Kurose A, Kumagai N, Fujishima Y, Ishibashi Y. Possibility of inhibiting arthritis and joint destruction by SSEA-3 positive cells derived from synovial tissue in rheumatoid arthritis. Regenerative Therapy. 2017;**7**:82-88

[34] Arnett FC, Edworthy SM, Bloch DA, McShane DJ, Fries JF, Cooper NS, Healey LA, Kaplan SR, Liang MH, Luthra HS, Medsger TA, Mitchell DM, Neustadt DH, Pinals RS, Schaller JG, Wilder JTRL, Hunder GG. The American Rheumatism Association 1987 revised criteria for the classification of rheumatoid arthritis. Arthritis and Rheumatism. 1988;**31**(3):315-324

[35] Aletaha D, Neogi T, Silman AJ, Funovits J, Felson DT, Bingham CO 3rd, Birnbaum NS, Burmester GR, Bykerk VP, Cohen MD, Combe B, Costenbader KH, Dougados M, Emery P, Ferraccioli G, Hazes JM, Hobbs K, Huizinga TW, Kavanaugh A, Kay J, Kvien TK, Laing T, Mease P, Ménard HA, Moreland LW, Naden RL, Pincus T, Smolen JS, Stanislawska-Biernat E, Symmons D, Tak PP, Upchurch KS, Vencovsky J, Wolfe F, Hawker G. Rheumatoid

arthritis classification criteria: an American College of Rheumatology/European League Against Rheumatism collaborative initiative. Annals of the Rheumatic Diseases. 2010, 2010;**69**(9):1580-1588

[36] Nandakumar KS, Bäcklund J, Vestberg M, Holmdahl R. Collagen type II (CII)-specific antibodies induce arthritis in the absence of T or B cells but the arthritis progression is enhanced by CII-reactive T cells. Arthritis Research & Therapy. 2004;**6**(6):R544-R550

[37] P1 H, Saito T, Yamaki K, Mizutani N, Brand DD, Waritani T, Terato K, Yoshino S. Collagen antibody-induced arthritis in mice: development of a new arthritogenic 5-clone cocktail of monoclonal anti-type II collagen antibodies. Journal of Immunological Methods. 2009;**343**(1):49-55

[38] Ozawa K, Sato K, Oh I, Ozaki K, Uchibori R, Obara Y, Kikuchi Y, Ito T, Okada T, Urabe M, Mizukami H, Kume A. Cell and gene therapy using mesenchymal stem cells (MSCs). Journal of Autoimmunity. 2008;**30**:121-127

[39] Liu Y, Mu R, Wang S, Long L, Liu X, Li R, Sun J, Guo J, Zhang X, Guo J, Yu P, Li C, Liu X, Huang Z, Wang D, Li H, Gu Z, Liu B, Li Z. Therapeutic potential of human umbilical cord mesenchymal stem cells in the treatment of rheumatoid arthritis. Arthritis Research & Therapy. 2010;**12**(6):R210

[40] Sarah P. Rheumatoid arthritis: Umbilical cord stem cells—The birth of a new treatment for RA? Nature Reviews Rheumatology. 2011;**7**:69

[41] El-Jawhari JJ, El-Sherbiny YM, Jones EA, McGonagle D. Mesenchymal stem cells, autoimmunity and rheumatoid arthritis. The Quarterly Journal of Medicine. 2014;**107**(7):505-514

Permissions

All chapters in this book were first published in NDPRA, by InTech Open; hereby published with permission under the Creative Commons Attribution License or equivalent. Every chapter published in this book has been scrutinized by our experts. Their significance has been extensively debated. The topics covered herein carry significant findings which will fuel the growth of the discipline. They may even be implemented as practical applications or may be referred to as a beginning point for another development.

The contributors of this book come from diverse backgrounds, making this book a truly international effort. This book will bring forth new frontiers with its revolutionizing research information and detailed analysis of the nascent developments around the world.

We would like to thank all the contributing authors for lending their expertise to make the book truly unique. They have played a crucial role in the development of this book. Without their invaluable contributions this book wouldn't have been possible. They have made vital efforts to compile up to date information on the varied aspects of this subject to make this book a valuable addition to the collection of many professionals and students.

This book was conceptualized with the vision of imparting up-to-date information and advanced data in this field. To ensure the same, a matchless editorial board was set up. Every individual on the board went through rigorous rounds of assessment to prove their worth. After which they invested a large part of their time researching and compiling the most relevant data for our readers.

The editorial board has been involved in producing this book since its inception. They have spent rigorous hours researching and exploring the diverse topics which have resulted in the successful publishing of this book. They have passed on their knowledge of decades through this book. To expedite this challenging task, the publisher supported the team at every step. A small team of assistant editors was also appointed to further simplify the editing procedure and attain best results for the readers.

Apart from the editorial board, the designing team has also invested a significant amount of their time in understanding the subject and creating the most relevant covers. They scrutinized every image to scout for the most suitable representation of the subject and create an appropriate cover for the book.

The publishing team has been an ardent support to the editorial, designing and production team. Their endless efforts to recruit the best for this project, has resulted in the accomplishment of this book. They are a veteran in the field of academics and their pool of knowledge is as vast as their experience in printing. Their expertise and guidance has proved useful at every step. Their uncompromising quality standards have made this book an exceptional effort. Their encouragement from time to time has been an inspiration for everyone.

The publisher and the editorial board hope that this book will prove to be a valuable piece of knowledge for researchers, students, practitioners and scholars across the globe.

List of Contributors

Naoko Yagishita and Yoshihisa Yamano
Department of Rare Diseases Research, Institute of Medical Science, St. Marianna University School of Medicine, Kawasaki, Kanagawa, Japan

Satoko Aratani
Institute of Medical Science, Tokyo Medical University, Shinjuku-ku, Tokyo, Japan
Department of Future Medical Science, Institute of Medical Science, Tokyo Medical University, Shinjuku-ku, Tokyo, Japan
Physician, Student and Researcher Support Center, Tokyo Medical University, Shinjukuku, Tokyo, Japan

Hidetoshi Fujita
Institute of Medical Science, Tokyo Medical University, Shinjuku-ku, Tokyo, Japan
Department of Future Medical Science, Institute of Medical Science, Tokyo Medical University, Shinjuku-ku, Tokyo, Japan

Kusuki Nishioka
Institute of Medical Science, Tokyo Medical University, Shinjuku-ku, Tokyo, Japan

Toshihiro Nakajima
Department of Rare Diseases Research, Institute of Medical Science, St. Marianna University School of Medicine, Kawasaki, Kanagawa, Japan
Institute of Medical Science, Tokyo Medical University, Shinjuku-ku, Tokyo, Japan
Department of Future Medical Science, Institute of Medical Science, Tokyo Medical University, Shinjuku-ku, Tokyo, Japan
Physician, Student and Researcher Support Center, Tokyo Medical University, Shinjukuku, Tokyo, Japan
Integrated Genome Editing Section (iGES), Tokyo Medical University, Shinjuku-ku, Tokyo, Japan
Bayside Misato Medical Center, Niida, Kochi, Japan

Leszek Królicki
Nuclear Medicine Department, Medical University of Warsaw, Warsaw, Poland

Adrian Michno
Department of Diagnostic Imaging, Bródno Hospital, Warsaw, Poland

Maria H. Kazakova and Victoria S. Sarafian
Department of Medical Biology, Faculty of Medicine, Medical University-Plovdiv, Bulgaria

Agnieszka Paradowska-Gorycka and Barbara Stypińska
Department of Biochemistry and Molecular Biology, National Institute of Geriatrics, Rheumatology and Rehabilitation, Warsaw, Poland

Hulya Bukulmez
Department of Pediatrics, Division of Pediatric Rheumatology, MetroHealth Medical Center, Case Western Reserve University, Cleveland, Ohio, United States

Vladimira Schwartzova, Branislav Borza and Peter Kizek
Dental Clinic, Kosice, Slovakia

Marcel Riznic
Department of Stomatology and Maxillofacial Surgery, Kosice, Slovakia

Reem Hamdy A. Mohammed
Department of Rheumatology/Clinical Immunology and Rehabilitation, School of Medicine, Cairo University-FRCP, Egypt

Hesham Ibrahim I. Elmakhzangy
Department of Gastroenterology/Hepatology and Tropical Medicine, School of Medicine,Cairo University, Egypt

Codrina Ancuta and Cristina Pomirleanu
Rheumatology Department, Clinical Rehabilitation Hospital, Rheumatology 2 Department, 'Grigore T. Popa' University of Medicine and Pharmacy, Iasi, Romania

Claudia Mihailov
Clinical Port Hospital of Constanta, Faculty of Medicine, 'Ovidius' University of Constanta, Constanta, Romania

Eugen Ancuta
'Elena Doamna' Cinical Hospital, Research Department, Iasi, Romania

Daniela Opris
Internal Medicine and Rheumatology Department, 'Sfanta Maria' University Hospital, 'Carol Davila' University of Medicine and Pharmacy, Bucuresti, Romania

Sevdalina Nikolova Lambova
Department of Propaedeutics of Internal Diseases, Faculty of Medicine, Medical University, Plovdiv, Bulgaria

Codrina Ancuta
2nd Rheumatology Department, Clinical Rehabilitation Hospital, University of Medicine and Pharmacy "Grigore T Popa", Iasi, Romania

Claudia Mihailov
2nd Medical Department, Clinical CF Hospital of Constanta, Faculty of Medicine, "Ovidius" University of Constanta, Romania

Eugen Ancuta
"Elena Doamna" Clinical Hospital, Iasi, Romania

Selim Nalbant
Department of Internal Medicine, Medical Faculty of Maltepe University, Istanbul, Turkey

Ahmet Merih Birlik
Department of Immunology and Rheumatology of Medical School of Dokuz Eylul Universty, Izmir, Turkey

Codrina Ancuta
2nd Rheumatology Department, Clinical Rehabilitation Hospital, "Grigore T. Popa" University of Medicine and Pharmacy, Iasi, Romania

Cristina Iordache
Ergonomics Department, School of Dentistry, "Grigore T. Popa" University of Medicine and Pharmacy, Iasi, Romania

Eugen Ancuta
Research Department, "Elena Doamna" Clinical Hospital, Iasi, Romania

Claudia Mihailov
2nd Medical Department, Clinical Port Hospital of Constanta, Faculty of Medicine, 'Ovidius' University of Constanta, Romania

Merih Birlik
Department of Internal Medicine, Division of Rheumatology, Faculty of Medicine, Dokuz Eylül University, Izmir, Turkey

Ayşe Koçak and Duygu Harmancı
Department of Molecular Medicine, Graduate School of Health Sciences, Dokuz Eylül University, Izmir, Turkey

Rie Kurose
Department of Orthopaedic Surgery, Hirosaki University Graduate School of Medicine, Hirosaki, Japan

Takashi Sawai
Department of Histopathology, Tohoku University, Sendai, Japan

Index

www.ingramcontent.com/pod-product-compliance
Lightning Source LLC
LaVergne TN
LVHW080956210926
848485LV00004B/838

* 9 7 8 1 6 3 9 8 9 1 4 0 5 *